Cardiology

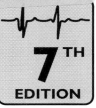

7TH EDITION

Desmond G. Julian MA MD FRCP FACC
Emeritus Professor of Cardiology
University of Newcastle-upon-Tyne, UK

J. Campbell Cowan MA DPhil FRCP
Consultant Cardiologist
Yorkshire Heart Centre
The General Infirmary at Leeds
Leeds, UK

James M. McLenachan MD FRCP
Consultant Cardiologist
Yorkshire Heart Centre
The General Infirmary at Leeds
Leeds, UK

WB Saunders Company Ltd
Edinburgh London New York Philadelphia Sydney Toronto

WB Saunders Company Ltd   24–28 Oval Road
London NW1 7DX

The Curtis Center
Independence Square West
Philadelphia, PA 19106-3399, USA

Harcourt Brace & Company
55 Horner Avenue
Toronto, Ontario M8Z 4X6, Canada

Harcourt Brace & Company, Australia
30–52 Smidmore Street
Marrickville, NSW 2204, Australia

Harcourt Brace & Company, Japan
Ichibancho Central Building, 22-1 Ichibancho
Chiyoda-ku, Tokyo 102, Japan

A catalogue record for this book is available from the British Library

ISBN 0-7020-2211-X

Typeset by J&L Composition Ltd, Filey, North Yorkshire
Printed and bound by WBC, Bridgend, Mid Glamorgan.

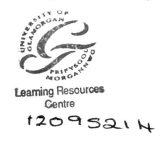

Contents

Preface   ix

1   **Normal Myocardial Function**   1

2   **The Electrical Activity of the Heart: the Electrocardiogram**   9
    The cardiac action potential   9
    The electrocardiogram   11

3   **The Symptoms of Heart Disease**   32
    Dyspnoea   32
    Cardiac pain   34
    Palpitation   36
    Oedema   36
    Ascites   37
    Cyanosis   37
    Haemoptysis   38
    Syncope   38
    Functional capacity   40

4   **The Physical Signs of Heart Disease**   41
    The arterial pulse   41
    The venous pulse and pressure   44
    Inspection of the chest   47
    Palpation of the chest   47
    Percussion of the heart   49
    Auscultation: heart sounds and murmurs   49
    General examination of patients with cardiac disease   60

5   **Non-invasive Investigation of the Heart**   61

6   **Invasive Investigations**   82

7   **Diseases of the Coronary Arteries – Causes, Pathology and
    Prevention**   92
    The coronary circulation   92
    Coronary artery Disease   93

8 Coronary Heart Disease – Angina and Unstable Angina 106

9 Coronary Heart Disease – Myocardial Infarction 123
Treatment of acute infarction 133
Complications of acute myocardial infarction and their
management 138
Late complications of infarction 145
Risk stratification at hospital discharge 148
Drug treatment at discharge 149
Rehabilitation 151

10 Heart Failure 153
The pathophysiology of heart failure 154
Clinical syndromes of heart failure 159
The management of cardiac failure 162
Acute circulatory failure (shock) 170
Cardiac transplantation 173

11 Disorders of Rate, Rhythm and Conduction 177
Mechanisms of arrhythmias 177
Disturbances of rate and rhythm 179
Disorders of conduction 202
Investigation of arrythmias 208
Management of arrythmias 208

12 Diseases of the Pericardium and Myocardium 223
The pericardium 223
Cardiomyopathy and myocarditis 233

13 Rheumatic Fever and its Sequelae 245

14 Disorders of the Cardiac Valves 252
Mitral valve disease 252
Aortic valve disease 274
Tricuspid valve disease 286
Pulmonary valve disease 288
Infective endocarditis 289

15 Congenital Heart Disease 297
The varieties of congenital heart disease 299

16 Hypertension and Heart Disease 321
Aetiology of hypertension 323
Pathophysiology of hypertension 328
The decision to treat 332

17 Diseases of the Aorta 338

18 Disorders of the Lungs and Pulmonary Circulation **345**
Pulmonary embolism 345
Pulmonary hypertension 349
Pulmonary heart disease 353

19 Systemic Disorders and the Heart **357**
Infections and the heart 357
Endocrine and metabolic diseases 360
Miscellaneous disorders 366
Anaemia and the heart 371
Pregnancy and the heart 372

20 Psychological Aspects of Heart Disease **376**
Psychological factors in the genesis of hypertension and
coronary disease 376
Anxiety state and the heart 377

21 Surgery and the Heart **379**
Anaesthesia and general surgery in patients with heart
disease 379
Surgery for heart disease 382

**22 Practical Guidelines for the Management of Cardiac
Emergencies** **391**
Acute myocardial infarction 391
Cardiac arrest 392
Management of tachyarrythmias 397
Management of pulmonary oedema 402
Management of pulmonary embolism 402
Management of cardiac tamponade 403
Temporary cardiac pacing 405
Hypertensive crisis 406

23 Clinical Trials and their Influence on Clinical Practice **407**

Index **417**

Preface

The first edition of this book was written in 1970. The succeeding quarter of a century has witnessed major advances in cardiology. This has been particularly true of the five years since the last edition and is reflected in the extensive changes which we have undertaken in preparing this edition.

The text has been thoroughly revised and a number of chapters rewritten or extended. The clinical manifestations of coronary disease, previously described in a single chapter, are now described in two chapters, one dealing with angina and the second dealing with myocardial infarction. We believe that this greater depth of coverage reflects both the importance of these subjects in UK practice and also the rapid developments which have occurred in recent years. Cardiac investigations, previously described in a single chapter, have also been subdivided into two chapters, reflecting the natural division into invasive and non-invasive investigations. Many figures have been replaced when newer imaging methods have afforded greater clarity. Finally we have incorporated a chapter dealing specifically with clinical trials as it is these which have formed the basis of the rapid developments in the specialty.

Despite these extensive revisions, we recognize that certain aspects in the introductory text are relatively unchanging. The chapters dealing with the fundamentals of history taking and examination, which have proved such a strength of previous editions, are retained in their previous format.

In its original conception, this book was intended as an introductory text for medical students. It has subsequently achieved a much wider readership, including nurses, junior hospital doctors preparing for membership and general practitioners. The book has in addition achieved an international readership, reaching countries with differing disease profiles and a range of healthcare provision. We have endeavoured to retain the characteristics necessary to interest this diverse readership. We hope, moreover, that we have been able to convey to all our readers the ethos of a dynamic, rapidly evolving specialty.

As in previous editions, we would like to thank many colleagues. We are indebted to Dr J. I. Hall and Dr D. P. Hammersley for providing illustrations retained from early editions and to many colleagues for providing clinical recordings, particularly Drs S. Hunter, A. Zezulka and Professor R. J. C. Hall. We are also indebted to Mrs S. Rutter for assistance in typing the manuscript.

Newcastle-upon-Tyne, 1998   D. G. Julian
Leeds, 1998   J. Campbell Cowan
Leeds, 1998   J. M. McLenachan

Normal Myocardial Function

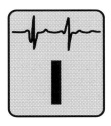

The primary function of the heart is to provide the tissues and organs of the body with a flow of oxygenated blood sufficient for their metabolic needs. In order to do this, it must pump a cardiac output of about 5 litres/min at rest (in the adult), and be able to increase this to 15 litres/min or more on exercise. It must also adjust to great variations in peripheral resistance and venous return without substantially altering arterial, venous or intracardiac pressures.

The ways in which the ventricles as a whole respond to changing demands can be, to a considerable extent, explained by the structure and function of the sarcomere, the fundamental unit of cardiac contraction.

The structure and function of the sarcomere

Each muscle cell contains, amongst other structures, a nucleus, numerous mitochondria, and a number of parallel fibrils. Each fibril is made up of functional sub-units or sarcomeres. The sarcomere is composed of parallel actin and myosin filaments, arranged with the thin actin filaments attached to its limiting membrane (or Z line) and interdigitating with the thicker myosin filaments which are placed centrally (Fig. 1.1).

The myosin filaments are lined with a series of 'heads', which can flex, thus bringing them into contact with the actin filaments. The filaments are propelled past each other by the repeated making and breaking of cross-bridges between the actin and myosin filaments. In addition to actin the thin filaments contain two regulatory proteins, troponin and tropomyosin (Fig. 1.1). The thread-like tropomyosin molecules lie in the trough between the two twisting strands of actin molecules. Troponin molecules are attached to the tropomyosin molecules at regular intervals. In the resting state, when the calcium level is low, the myosin-binding sites on the actin filament are blocked by tropomyosin, preventing cross-bridge formation. When activation

1

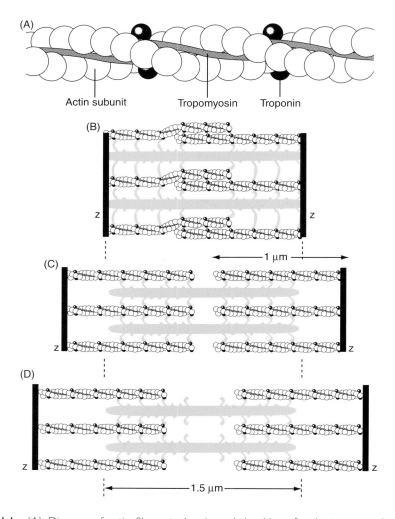

Fig. 1.1 (A) Diagram of actin filament, showing relationships of actin, tropomyosin and troponin. (B, C, D) Relationships of actin (thin horizontal lines) and myosin (thick horizontal bars) in the sarcomere. In (B) the actin filaments are overriding one another. In (C) all bridges (vertical lines) are available for binding. In (D) the sarcomere is overextended; some sites are not engaged. Contraction is maximal when the greatest number of sites is available for interaction as in (C).

causes a rise in calcium level, calcium ions bind with troponin, altering the position of the adjacent tropomyosin molecule and exposing the myosin-binding sites on the actin filament. Following cross-bridge formation there is a change in the angle of the cross-bridge, following which the cross-bridge disengages. The repeated making and breaking of many cross-bridges causes the thick filament to row itself into the space between the thin filaments. The energy for cross-bridge recycling is provided by adenosine triphosphate (ATP).

The number of cross-bridges that develop is dependent upon the number of calcium molecules available; the more bridges there are for interaction, the more forceful will be the resulting contraction.

Starling's law

The law of the heart, as enunciated by Starling, states that the more myocardial fibres are stretched (or the greater the diastolic volume of the heart) within physiological limits, the greater the energy of the ensuing contraction. Beyond these limits, the energy of contraction falls off. Two aspects of sarcomere function contribute to Starling's law:

- as the sarcomere is progressively stretched to its optimal length, and the diastolic fibre lengthens proportionately, the force of contraction progressively increases. This is partly due to the fact that over the normal operating range the opposing actin filaments overlap, interfering with actin–myosin cross-bridge formation (Fig. 1.1). With stretch the degree of overlap decreases and hence force generation increases;
- recent evidence suggests that calcium sensitivity of the contractile proteins increases with increase in length, providing a greater degree of activation for a given calcium concentration.

Excitation–contraction coupling

During systole there is a 50-fold increase in intracellular calcium concentration. The cardiac action potential is responsible for the increase in intracellular calcium in two ways:

- calcium ions enter the cell from the extracellular space during the plateau phase of the action potential (see Chapter 2);
- the spike of the action potential triggers the release of calcium from intracellular stores within the sarcoplasmic reticulum.

The energy supply of the myocardial cell

Energy is produced in the heart by the process of oxidative phosphorylation. This results from the conversion of the energy produced by the oxidation of substrates such as glucose, lactate and fatty acids into the energy of adenosine triphosphate (ATP) and creatine phosphate (CP). These substances provide the energy source for muscular contraction. Normally, free fatty acids are the main substrate, but in ischaemia the glycolytic pathway is stimulated. This, however, cannot substitute for oxidative phosphorylation and inevitably ischaemia leads to a fall in ATP levels and a consequent impairment of myocardial function.

The mechanics of the myocardium

Two important characteristics of heart muscle are the force with which it contracts, and the velocity with which it shortens, for these determine the volume of blood expelled during systole. Three major factors are responsible for the force and velocity of cardiac contraction:

- 'preload' – the extent to which the muscle is stretched prior to contraction;
- 'afterload' – the load that the ventricle faces during contraction;
- the contractile state of the myocardium.

Preload

If other factors are held constant, the force with which the heart contracts depends on the extent to which it has been stretched prior to contraction (Fig. 1.2). This is a restatement of Starling's law. In effect, the preload is the volume of the ventricle at the end of diastole, i.e. the *end-diastolic volume*. The end-diastolic volume is largely determined by the venous return, which is, in turn, dependent upon a number of influences including the blood volume and venous tone. Another important factor affecting venous return is the distensibility (compliance) of the ventricle. Atrial contraction contributes appreciably to ventricular end-diastolic volume as it occurs immediately before ventricular systole. This atrial component of ventricular filling assumes particular importance when the ventricle is hypertrophied because passive filling is then impeded by the indistensibility (lack of compliance) of the ventricle.

Afterload

The ventricle has to develop sufficient tension during systole to expel blood into the aorta in the face of the resistance (or, more correctly, impedance) imposed by the aortic valve, aorta and peripheral arterial vessels.

The contractile state of the myocardium

If the end-diastolic volume and the aortic impedance are held constant, the force and velocity of contraction of the myocardium depend upon its contractile state. For a given end-diastolic volume, therefore, changes in contractility can alter the performance of the ventricle (see

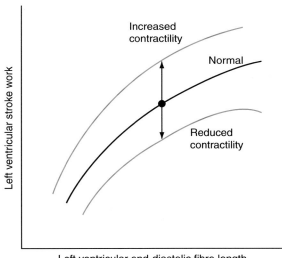

Fig. 1.2 The relationship between end-diastolic fibre length and left ventricular stroke work. For any given end-diastolic fibre length, increased contractility, such as is produced by sympathetic action, produces more stroke work. Reduced contractility, as occurs in cardiac failure, produces less work. Similarly, if the arrows were drawn horizontally instead of vertically, it would be seen that, for any given amount of work, increased contractility enables this to be performed at a smaller end-diastolic fibre length. In cardiac failure, a given amount of stroke work can be achieved only with a greater end-diastolic fibre length.

Fig. 1.2). Myocardial contractility is largely dependent upon the activity of the cardiac sympathetic nerves, but it can also be increased by circulating catecholamines, tachycardia, and inotropic drugs such as dopamine and dobutamine. Myocardial contractility is depressed by ischaemia and by a number of drugs, particularly antiarrhythmic agents.

Mechanisms which lead to an increased ventricular performance, such as an enlarged end-diastolic volume or sympathetic stimulation, also cause an increase in myocardial oxygen consumption. The greater ventricular performance does not necessarily, therefore, mean an increase in cardiac efficiency. Indeed, the increase in myocardial oxygen consumption is disproportionately great in relation to the increase in work performed.

The effect of exercise

Cardiovascular changes take place as soon as exercise is anticipated — as a result of vagal inhibition and a generalized sympathetic discharge. Both heart rate and myocardial contractility increase. The resistance vessels in the muscles dilate whilst those supplying the kidneys, abdominal viscera and skin constrict. The overall effect is to increase cardiac output and, specifically, the blood supply to the muscles.

With the onset of exercise, further dilatation of muscular arterioles and capillaries occurs and venous return is augmented by the pumping action of the muscles. The systolic blood pressure rises, the increase roughly corresponding to the severity of the exercise. Diastolic pressure changes little.

The pressure and volume changes in the heart and great vessels during the cardiac cycle (Fig. 1.3)

The pressure and volume changes of the cardiac cycle fall into a number of phases:

Isovolumetric contraction. With the onset of left ventricular systole, the mitral valve closes and the pressure in the ventricle rises rapidly. Until the aortic valve opens, the volume of the ventricle remains unchanged.

Ejection. As soon as the aortic valve opens, blood is rapidly ejected from the ventricle into the aorta. This phase is followed by one of relatively slow ejection.

Isovolumetric relaxation. Shortly after ejection ceases, the aortic valve closes. As the ventricle relaxes, the pressure within it falls rapidly, but until it has fallen to the level present in the left atrium, the volume in the ventricle remains unchanged.

Ventricular filling. When the pressure in the ventricle falls below that in the atrium, the mitral valve opens and a period of rapid ventricular filling ensues. This is followed by a slow phase, or diastasis, during which the pressure rises slowly. This continues until atrial contraction propels more blood through the mitral valve and causes a small increase in left ventricular volume and pressure prior to the onset of the next ventricular systole.

Atrial pressure waveform

In the left atrium, there are three waves in the cardiac cycle, the crests being designated 'a', 'c' and 'v', and the troughs 'x', 'y' and 'z' (Fig. 1.3):

- the 'a' wave is due to atrial contraction, which is followed by a 'z' trough associated with atrial relaxation;

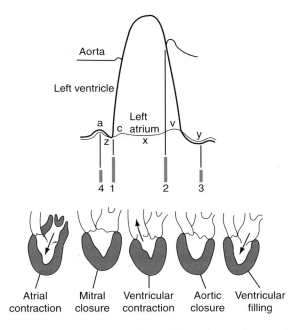

Fig. 1.3 Pressure pulses in the left atrium, left ventricle and aorta (see text).

- the 'c' wave is a result of upward movement of the mitral valve cusps, with a subsequent 'x' descent as the mitral valve ring descends as the ventricle contracts;
- the 'v' wave is due to a build up of pressure in the atrium with increasing pulmonary venous return during the latter portion of ventricular systole, with the mitral valve closed. This rising pressure is terminated when the mitral valve opens. At this point, the peak of the 'v' wave is produced. The 'y' descent follows as blood flows into the ventricle during ventricular diastole.

From the opening of the mitral valve to its closure at the onset of ventricular systole, the pressures in the atrium and the ventricle are almost identical.

Right heart pressures

Events on the right side of the heart mirror those on the left but they take place slightly later so that tricuspid valve closure occurs shortly after mitral valve closure, and closure of the pulmonary valve follows that of the aortic valve. The timing of pulmonary valve closure varies with respiration. The increased negative pressure in the thorax during inspiration results in an augmented venous return to the right side of the heart. As a consequence of this transient increase in blood flow, ejection of blood in the right side of the heart is delayed and pulmonary valve closure occurs relatively later during inspiration than it does during expiration.

Further reading

Levick, J. R. (1991) *An Introduction to Cardiovascular Physiology*. London: Butterworths.

The Electrical Activity of the Heart: the Electrocardiogram

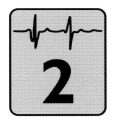

Electrical activity is a basic characteristic of the heart and is the stimulus for cardiac contraction. Disturbances of electrical function are common in heart disease. Their registration on an electrocardiogram (ECG) plays an essential role in the diagnosis and management of myocardial infarction, and of rhythm and conduction abnormalities. The ECG also provides important information about the presence of atrial and ventricular enlargement and can contribute to the detection of electrolyte disorders and drug intoxication.

THE CARDIAC ACTION POTENTIAL

The ECG is best understood by first considering some electrical and chemical features of the myocardial cell. Resting cells have a potassium concentration (about 140 mmol/litre) which is high in comparison with that in the extracellular tissues (about 4 mmol/litre), whereas extracellular sodium concentration is much greater than intracellular. This ionic disequilibrium between the cell and its environment is maintained by a sodium–potassium exchange pump which simultaneously transports potassium ions into the cell and sodium ions out of the cell.

During diastole there is a relative negative potential within the cell of the order of 90 mV – the *transmembrane resting potential*. This is primarily due to two factors, the high concentration of potassium ions intracellularly and the high permeability of the cell membrane to potassium ions. As a result, potassium ions tend to diffuse out of the cell down their concentration gradient, creating a negative charge in the interior of the cell, which offsets and almost balances the concentration gradient for potassium.

The cardiac action potential (Fig. 2.1A) arises due to a sequence of changes in permeability to sodium, calcium and potassium ions (Fig. 2.1A and Table 2.1). At rest, the cell membrane is relatively

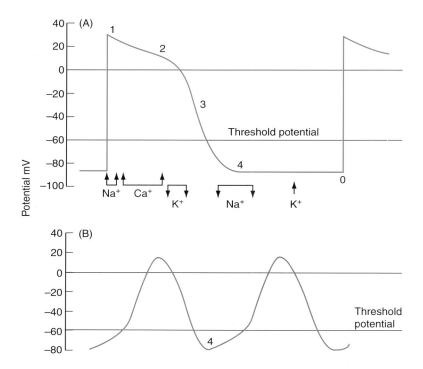

Fig. 2.1 (A) Transmembrane potential. Phase 0 corresponds with depolarization, and phases 1, 2 and 3 with repolarization. Phase 4 is the period of diastolic rest. When the cell is electrically stimulated, the transmembrane potential is reduced to the threshold potential, after which the process of depolarization is self-perpetuating. (B) Transmembrane potential in a pacemaking cell. In these cells, phase 4 is a period of slow depolarization. When the threshold potential is reached the cell rapidly becomes depolarized.

impermeable to sodium ions. The rapid upstroke of the action potential is due to a sudden increase in sodium permeability, causing a rapid influx of sodium ions. This sodium current is short-lived, because the ion channels which open to cause the increase in sodium permeability rapidly close once again. The first inward sodium current is succeeded by a slower inward current, comprised predominantly of calcium ions and to a lesser extent sodium ions. This slow inward current is responsible for the plateau phase of the cardiac action potential, preventing the cell from repolarizing rapidly like a nerve.

During the plateau of the action potential permeability to potassium ions is reduced. Repolarization to the resting potential is achieved by a gradual increase in potassium permeability once again, accompanied by a gradual decrease in the slow inward current.

Table 2.I   Ionic currents in a myocardial cell

Current	Ion	Function
Fast inward current	Na^+	Rapid depolarization
Slow inward current	Ca^{2+} (mainly)	Plateau maintenance Excitation–contraction coupling
Outward curves	K+	Repolarization Resting membrane potential

Pacemaker activity

In a pacemaking or automatic cell (Fig. 2.1B) diastole is not stable. A gradual fall in potassium permeability causes a gradual decline in the resting potential to less negative values. When the transmembrane potential reaches its threshold, the cell automatically becomes depolarized. This characteristic forms the basis of automaticity.

The groups of automatic cells, which are present in the sinus node, the junctional tissue in the neighbourhood of the atrioventricular (AV) node, the bundle of His, the bundle branches and the Purkinje cells of the ventricles vary from each other in their rate of spontaneous depolarization. In the normal heart, the cells of the sinus node have the shortest spontaneous depolarization time (phase 4) and so have the fastest firing rate. The sinus node dominates the heart because impulses spreading from it discharge the other potential pacemakers before they are ready for a spontaneous depolarization. If one of the other areas develops a faster rate, a new and 'ectopic' focus assumes the role of pacemaker. Conversely, if the rate of sinus node discharge is reduced for any reason, a pacemaker from lower in the conduction system may provide an 'escape' focus. In general terms, the more distal the location in the conduction system, the slower and less reliable is the escape pacemaker.

THE ELECTROCARDIOGRAM

The genesis of the ECG

Relation to the cardiac action potential

The ECG is the summation on the body surface of the individual action potentials from throughout the heart. To explain how the ECG arises, a single resting cell may be represented by a square with a positive charge on the outside and a negative one within. A muscle strip can be represented diagrammatically as a series of such squares (Fig. 2.2). If a cell at one end is stimulated, it becomes depolarized and its surface is negatively charged in relation to its fellows. As the electrical impulse spreads from one cell to the next, there is a progressively advancing negative charge. Immediately in front of it is a positive charge of equal magnitude. This combination of negative and positive charges in close proximity is termed a *dipole* with, in this case, the positive charge preceding the negative. The advancing dipole sets up an electrical field which can be detected by an exploring electrode paired with an indifferent electrode. By convention, relative positivity in the exploring electrode is represented by an upright deflection and negativity by a downward one. Therefore, as the positive front of the dipole approaches the electrode, an upright deflection is recorded; as it retreats, the deflection is negative.

The whole heart can be regarded as a large number of muscle strips arranged in a complex fashion. At any one time in the cardiac cycle there are numerous dipoles moving in different directions; as viewed from a single electrode many of these cancel each other out. The total electrical activity at any one moment in time can be summed and represented by a single electrical force of a certain magnitude and in a certain direction which is termed the *instantaneous vector*. All the

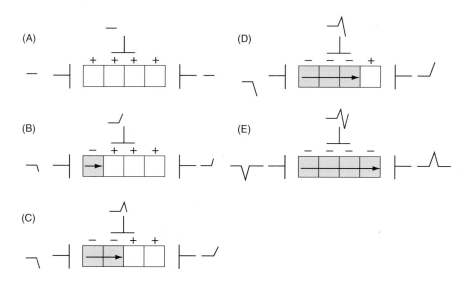

Fig. 2.2 The recording produced from electrodes during depolarization of a muscle strip. By convention, an upstroke (a positive deflection) is recorded as depolarization proceeds towards that electrode, and a negative deflection is obtained from an electrode facing the opposite direction.

instantaneous vectors occurring throughout the cardiac cycle form the *cardiac vector*.

The pathways of conduction and the ECG

The sinus node is situated in the right atrium close to the entrance of the superior vena cava. The AV node lies in the right atrial wall immediately above the tricuspid valve. The fibres of the AV bundle (of His) arise from the AV node and run along the posterior border of the septum between the ventricles (Fig. 2.3). On reaching the muscular part of the septum, they split into right and left bundle branches and then spread out in the subendocardium of the ventricles as the Purkinje system. The right bundle is a slender, compact structure. The left bundle soon splits into two or more divisions or fascicles, one of which proceeds anteriorly, sharing the same blood supply as the right bundle, and another is directed posteriorly.

In the usual sequence of events, the electrical impulse arises in the sinus node and spreads across the atria to reach the AV node. It can then only reach the ventricles by passing into the rapidly conducting AV bundle and its branches.

The first part of the ventricles to be activated is the septum, followed by the endocardium. Finally, the impulse spreads outwards to the epicardium.

The spread of the cardiac impulse gives rise to the main deflections of the ECG: P, QRS and T waves (Fig. 2.4):

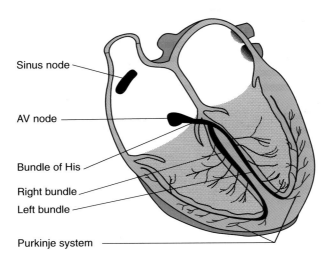

Sinus node

AV node

Bundle of His

Right bundle

Left bundle

Purkinje system

Fig. 2.3   The pathways of conduction.

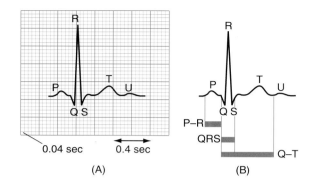

Fig. 2.4   (A) Normal ECG complexes. (B) PR, QRS and QT segments.

- *the P wave* is the first deflection of the cardiac cycle and represents atrial depolarization;
- *the PR interval* represents the time taken for the cardiac impulse to spread over the atrium and through the AV node and His–Purkinje system;
- *the QRS complex* represents the spread of depolarization through the ventricles;
- *the T wave* represents ventricular repolarization.

Electrodes and leads

A conventional electrocardiogram (ECG) consists of tracings from 12 or more leads. The term 'lead' refers to the ECG obtained as a result of recording the difference in potential between a pair of electrodes.

The bipolar (standard) leads. In these leads, the electrodes are attached to the limbs. In lead I the positive electrode is attached to the left arm and the negative to the right arm. In lead II the positive electrode is attached to the left leg and the negative to the right arm. In lead III the positive is attached to the left leg and the negative to the left arm. They may thus be depicted as:

- lead I = left arm minus right arm (LA−RA);
- lead II = left leg minus right arm (LL−RA);
- lead III = left leg minus left arm (LL−LA).

It can be deduced from these equations that lead II should be equal to the sum of leads I and III.

The position from which the heart is viewed by each of these leads is shown in Fig. 2.5.

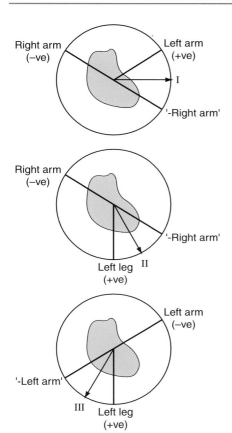

Fig. 2.5   Diagram of the effective position of the bipolar (standard) leads. In lead I, the positive electrode is attached to the left arm and the negative to the right arm. In effect, lead I is the sum of the potentials from the left arm with those that would be obtained from an electrode diametrically opposite the right arm. The resultant force is directed midway between these two points. Similar principles can be applied to derive the effective direction of the leads II and III.

Einthoven regarded each limb used in the recording of the bipolar ECG as an apex of an equilateral triangle, equidistant electrically from the heart at the centre. Although useful, this hypothesis is only approximately true, as it assumes that the body is a homogeneous sphere, which it clearly is not.

Unipolar leads. These have an exploring electrode placed on a chosen site linked with an indifferent electrode with a very small potential. In an attempt to obtain a central terminal with 'zero potential', Wilson connected all three limb electrodes through 5000 Ω resistances to form the indifferent electrode.

Unipolar chest leads.   When unipolar leads are recorded from the chest wall, the exploring electrode is connected to the positive pole of the ECG and the negative to the central terminal of Wilson (Fig. 2.6A). By convention, the following sites are normally selected (Fig. 2.6B):

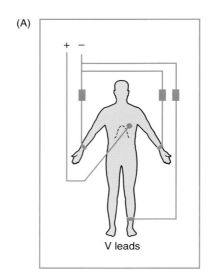

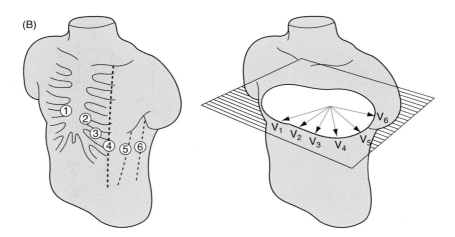

Fig. 2.6 (A) Each lead is recorded with respect to an 'indifferent' terminal, created by linking together the three limb electrodes. (B) The sites of electrode placement on the precordium.

- V1, the fourth intercostal space just to the right of the sternum;
- V2, the fourth intercostal space just to the left of the sternum;
- V3, midway betwen V2 and V4;
- V4, the fifth intercostal space in the mid-clavicular line;

- V5, the left anterior axillary line at the same horizontal level as V4;
- V6, the left mid-axillary line at the same horizontal level as V4.

Additional leads can be taken from V3R and V4R, sites on the right side of the chest equivalent to V3 and V4. Occasionally, leads may be placed at higher levels, for example the second, third or fourth inter-costal spaces or further laterally (V7 and V8).

Unipolar limb leads. In these leads, the exploring electrode is placed on one limb, and the negative pole is connected to Wilson's central terminal, modified by the omission of the connection from the limb under study to the central terminal (Fig. 2.7). This modification augments the voltage of the ECG, and the leads so derived are referred to as 'a' leads. They are designated as follows:

- aVR, right arm lead;
- aVL, left arm lead;
- aVF, left foot lead.

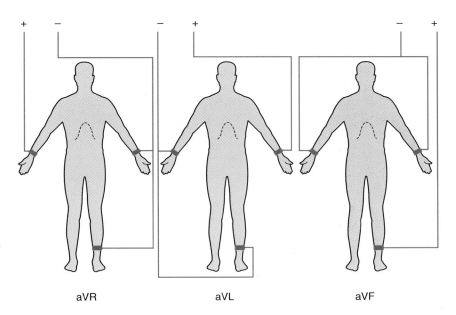

aVR   aVL   aVF

Fig. 2.7 The attachment of unipolar limb leads. Note that the limb under study is not attached to the central (negative) terminal.

The normal electrocardiogram

Normally, ECGs are recorded at a rate of 25 mm/s and the ECG paper is printed with thin vertical lines 1 mm apart and thick vertical lines 5 mm apart (Fig. 2.8). The interval between the thin lines represents 0.04 s and that between two thick lines 0.20 s. If the heart rhythm is regular, the rate can be counted by dividing the number of small squares between two consecutive R waves into 1500 or large squares into 300. If the rhythm is irregular, one can multiply the number of complexes in 6 s (i.e. 15 cm) by 10. Special rulers simplify the calculation of rate.

There are also thin horizontal lines at 1-mm intervals and thick horizontal lines at 5-mm intervals. An ECG recording is standardized so that 1 mV gives a deflection of 10 mm on the paper. The height of a deflection therefore indicates its voltage.

The P wave

The normal P wave (Fig. 2.9A) results from the spread of electrical activity across the atria (the activity of the sinus node itself cannot be detected in the ECG). Because the impulse spreads from right to left, the P wave is upright in leads I, II and aVF, is inverted in aVR and may be upright, biphasic or inverted in lead III, aVL and V1. It should not be higher than 3 mm in the bipolar leads or 2.5 mm in the unipolar leads, or greater than 0.10 s in duration.

When abnormal, the P wave may become:

- *inverted* (i.e. negative in the leads in which it is usually positive). This indicates depolarization of the atria in an unusual direction, and that the pacemaker is not in the sinus node, but is situated

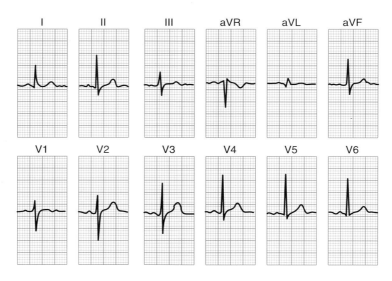

Fig. 2.8   Normal 12-lead electrocardiogram. Note the progression in the upright deflection from 'r' over the right ventricle (V1) to an 'R' over the left ventricle (V6).

either elsewhere in the atrium, in the AV node or below this; or there is dextrocardia;

- *broadened and notched*, due to delayed depolarization of the left atrium when this chamber is enlarged (P mitrale) (Fig. 2.9B). In V1, the P wave is then usually biphasic with a small positive wave preceding a deep and broad negative one;
- *tall and peaked*, exceeding 3 mm, as a result of right atrial enlargement (P pulmonale) (Fig. 2.9C);
- *absent* or invisible due to the presence of junctional rhythm or sino-atrial block;
- replaced by flutter or fibrillation waves.

PR interval

This is measured from the beginning of the P wave to the beginning of the QRS complex (i.e. to the onset of the Q wave if there is one, and to the onset of the R wave if there is not). This interval corresponds to the time taken for the impulse to travel from the sinus node to the ventricular muscle. There is an iso-electric segment between the end of the P wave and the beginning of the QRS, whilst the impulse is passing through the AV node and the specialized conducting tissue, as an insufficient amount of tissue is being electrically stimulated to produce a deflection detectable on the body surface.

The PR interval varies with age and with heart rate. The upper limit in children is 0.16, in adolescents 0.18 and in adults 0.20 s, although it may be even longer in a few normal individuals. The faster the heart rate the shorter is the PR interval. It is regarded as abnormally short if it is less than 0.10 s. A shortened PR interval is seen when the impulse originates in the junctional tissue and in the Wolff–Parkinson–White syndrome (see p. 187). The PR interval is prolonged in some forms of heart block (see p. 202).

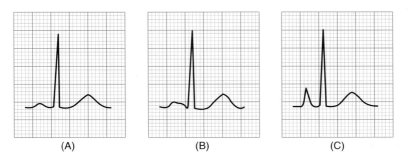

(A)   (B)   (C)

Fig. 2.9   P wave appearances in lead II. (A) Normal. (B) Broadened and notched (P mitrale). (C) Tall and peaked (P pulmonale).

The QRS complex

The QRS complex represents depolarization of the ventricular muscle. The components of the QRS complex are defined as follows (Fig. 2.10):

- the R wave is any positive (upward) deflection of the QRS. If there is more than one R wave, the second is denoted R'; an R wave of small voltage may be denoted r;
- a negative (downward) deflection preceding an R wave is termed Q;
- a negative deflection following an R wave is termed S;
- if the ventricular complex is entirely negative (i.e. there is no R wave), the complex is termed QS.

The whole complex is often referred to as the QRS complex irrespective of whether one or two of its components are absent.

Ventricular depolarization starts in the middle of the left side of the septum and spreads across to the right (phase 1 of ventricular depolarization) (Fig. 2.11). Subsequently, the main free walls of the ventricles are activated, the impulse spreading from within outwards and from below upwards. Because of the dominating bulk of the left ventricle, the direction of the vector of phase 2 is to the left and posteriorly. Finally, the base of both ventricular walls and the interventricular septum are depolarized. The appearances of the QRS in different leads can be largely explained by the major vectors of these phases as is seen in Fig. 2.11. In leads facing the left ventricular surface, there is a small Q wave due to septal depolarization and a large R wave due to left ventricular depolarization. On the right side of the heart, as seen from V1, there is usually an r wave due to septal depolarization and a large S wave due to left ventricular forces directed away from the electrode.

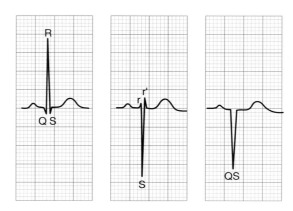

Fig. 2.10   Variations in the QRS complex (see text).

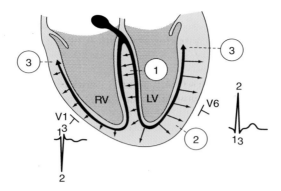

Fig. 2.11   Genesis of the QRS complex. Note that the first phase, directed from left to right across the septum, produces a Q wave in V6 and an R wave in V1. The second phase, due mainly to depolarization of the left ventricle from endocardium to epicardium, results in a tall R wave in V6 and a deep S wave in V1. Finally, depolarization of the basal parts of the ventricles may produce a terminal S wave in V6 and a terminal R wave in V1.

Pathological Q waves.   As mentioned, small, narrow Q waves are normally to be found in leads facing the left ventricle (e.g. lead I, aVL, aVF, V5 and V6). These Q waves do not normally exceed 2 mm in depth, or 0.03 s in width. It should be noted that QS waves are normal in aVR, and are common in V1. Abnormally broad and deep Q waves are often a feature of myocardial infarction (see p. 125). Q waves in lead III are difficult to evaluate but can be ignored if there are no Q waves either in lead II or in aVF, or if they do not exceed 0.03 s. Usually, a 'normal' Q wave in lead III diminishes or disappears on deep inspiration because of an alteration in the position of the heart, whilst the 'pathological' Q wave of infarction persists.

The QRS complex should not exceed 0.10 s in duration, and usually is in the range 0.06–0.08 s. Broad QRS complexes occur in bundle branch block (p. 25), in ventricular hypertrophy and in ventricular ectopic beats.

The T wave

The T wave is due to repolarization of the ventricles. If repolarization (the T wave) occurred in the same direction as depolarization (the QRS complex) the T wave would be directed in an opposite way to that of the QRS. In fact, depolarization takes place from endocardium to epicardium, whereas repolarization takes place from epicardium to endocardium. Because of this, the T wave usually points in the same direction as the major component of the QRS complex. Thus, the T wave is normally upright in leads I and II as well as in V3 to V6, is inverted in aVR, and may be upright or inverted in lead III, aVL, aVF and V1 and V2.

The T waves are usually not taller than 5 mm in standard leads and 10 mm in precordial leads. Unusually tall and peaked T waves may be seen in hyperkalaemia and in early myocardial infarction. Flattened T waves are seen when the voltage of all complexes is low, as in myxoedema, as well as in hypokalaemia and in a large number of other conditions in which it may be regarded as a non-specific abnormality. Slight T wave inversion is also often non-specific, and may be due to such influences as hyperventilation, posture and smoking. The most important causes of T wave inversion are:

- myocardial ischaemia and infarction;
- ventricular hypertrophy;
- bundle branch block.

Detailed descriptions of T wave changes will be found in the subsequent section on abnormalities of the ST segment, and also under the subheadings dealing with ventricular hypertrophy, bundle branch block and myocardial infarction.

The QT interval

The QT interval represents the total time from the onset of ventricular depolarization to the completion of repolarization. It is measured from the beginning of the Q wave (or the R wave if there is no Q wave) to the end of the T wave. Its duration varies with heart rate, becoming shorter as the heart rate increases. In general, the QT interval at heart rates between 60 and 90 per minute does not exceed in duration half the preceding RR interval. The measurement of the QT interval is often difficult as the end of the T wave cannot always be clearly identified, and the relationship between heart rate and duration of the QT is a complex one. Tables are available in textbooks of electrocardiography giving normal QT intervals. In practice, the main importance of a prolonged QT interval is that it is associated with a risk of ventricular tachycardias (particularly torsades de pointes, p.198), and sudden death. A long QT is sometimes an inherited abnormality but may result from such drugs as quinidine, procainamide, disopyramide, amiodarone and tricyclic antidepressants.

The ST segment

The ST segment is that part of the electrocardiogram between the end of the QRS complex and the beginning of the T wave (Fig. 2.12). The point of junction between the S wave and the ST segment is known as the J point. The ST segment occurs during a period of unchanging polarity in the ventricles, corresponding with phase 2 of the action

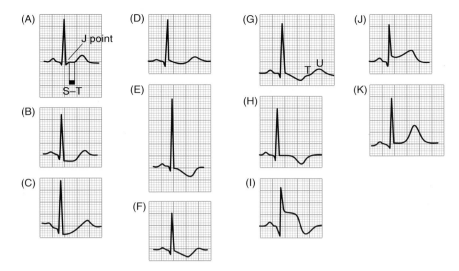

Fig. 2.12 Normal and abnormal ST segments and T waves. (A) Normal ST segment with J point. (B) Horizontal ST depression in myocardial ischaemia. (C) ST segment sloping upwards in sinus tachycardia. (D) ST sagging in digitalis therapy. (E) Asymmetrical T wave inversion associated with ventricular hypertrophy. (F) Similar pattern sometimes seen without voltage changes in hypertrophy – 'strain'. (G) ST sagging and prominent U waves of hypokalaemia. (H) Symmetrically inverted T wave of myocardial ischaemia or infarction. (I) ST elevation in acute myocardial infarction. (J) ST elevation in acute pericarditis. (K) Peaked T wave in hyperkalaemia.

potential (see Fig. 2.1). The normal ST segment is situated on the iso-electric line but curves upwards.

Displacements of the ST segment and variations in its shape are of great importance in electrocardiographic diagnosis. The characteristic abnormalities of the ST segment are illustrated in Fig. 2.12. In some normal individuals, particularly young people of African descent, slight ST elevation is seen. This may be up to 1 mm in standard leads and 2 mm in the right precordial leads. Depression of more than 0.5 mm is abnormal. When ST elevation occurs in normal individuals, it is often preceded by a slight notch on the downstroke of the R wave:

- *acute myocardial infarction.* The ST segment is elevated with a curve which is convex upwards in the leads facing the infarct. At a later stage ST segment elevation becomes less pronounced as T wave inversion develops. These changes are considered in more detail on p. 125;
- *pericarditis.* This also causes ST elevation, but the ST segments are concave upwards and the changes are widespread rather than localized as in myocardial infarction;

- *digitalis therapy* depresses the ST segment, particularly in leads II and III, so that there is a gentle sagging, but the T wave remains upright or flattened;
- *ventricular hypertrophy.* ST segment depression may occur in leads facing the relevant ventricle and be accompanied by asymmetrical T wave inversion. This contrasts with the symmetrical T wave inversion seen in myocardial infarction and ischaemia;
- *acute myocardial ischaemia.* The ST segment is horizontally depressed or slightly downward sloping from the J point onwards;
- *sinus tachycardia.* There may be ST depression which slopes upwards from the J point;
- *hypothermia.* There is a prominent J wave (the junction of the S wave and the ST segment) (Fig. 2.13).

The U wave

The U wave is a broad, low-voltage wave present in most normal ECGs. Its cause is unknown; it may become unusually prominent in hypokalaemia and with digitalis therapy.

Abnormal ECG patterns

Left ventricular hypertrophy (Fig. 2.14)

Hypertrophy of the left ventricle increases the amplitude of R waves in left chest leads and S waves in right chest leads. Where there is septal hypertrophy, deep but narrow Q waves are seen in left chest leads. When left ventricular hypertrophy becomes advanced, the T wave may become flattened in the leads in which the R wave is tall; eventually ST depression and T wave inversion may occur.

Many efforts have been made to lay down criteria for the diagnosis of left ventricular hypertrophy. None is satisfactory as many factors contribute to the amplitude of ECG waves, including the thickness of the chest wall and the age of the patient. The following criteria have gained wide acceptance:

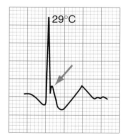

Fig. 2.13 ECG in hypothermia. The arrow indicates the characteristic prominent J wave.

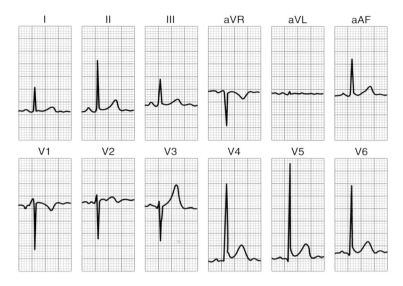

Fig. 2.14   Left ventricular hypertrophy. Note the deep S wave in lead VI and the tall R waves in leads V5 and V6.

- R in V5 or V6 plus S in V1 greater than 35 mm. This criterion applies only in individuals over 25 years of age. In younger persons, R in V5 or V6 plus S in V1 should exceed 40 mm before the diagnosis of left ventricular hypertrophy can be made;
- R in V5 or V6 greater than 25 mm;
- R in aVL greater than 13 mm;
- R in aVF greater than 20 mm.

Right ventricular hypertrophy (Fig. 2.15)

When the right ventricle becomes hypertrophied, the leads facing the right ventricle (particularly in V1, V3R and V4R) show dominant R waves instead of the usually dominant S wave. The diagnostic criterion for right ventricular hypertrophy is:

- R wave in V1 equal to or greater than the S wave and at least 5 mm tall.

As with left ventricular hypertrophy, ST depression and T wave inversion may develop in the leads with tall R waves.

Left bundle branch block (Fig. 2.16)

When the left branch of the bundle is blocked, the interventricular septum is activated from the right instead of from the left side and the

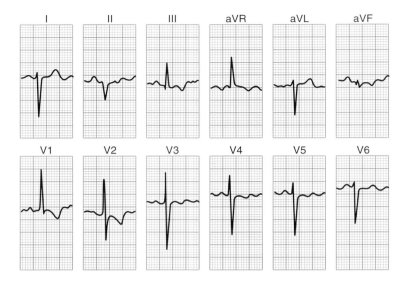

Fig. 2.15 Right ventricular hypertrophy. Note the tall R waves in leads V1 and V2, and associated T wave inversion extending across the chest leads to V5. There is right axis deviation.

initial vector (phase 1) is directed to the left. Because of this, the normal initial q wave in the left ventricular leads is lost, being replaced by a small r wave. Right ventricular depolarization, which follows, produces an r in V1 and an s in V6. The left ventricle is finally depolarized resulting in an R' in V6 and a broad S in V1. The QRS duration is increased to 0.12 s or more.

The abnormal left ventricular depolarization sequence in left bundle branch block causes secondary repolarization changes. Consequently, the ST segment and T wave are abnormal. This prevents interpretation of other factors causing ST and T wave changes, such as ischaemia and infarction.

Right bundle branch block (Fig. 2.17)

In this disorder, the right branch of the bundle is blocked, but the septum is activated from left to right, as in the normal heart. The left ventricular q wave is preserved, as is the initial r wave over right chest leads. The left ventricle is then depolarized, producing an S wave in right chest leads and an R wave in left chest leads. Finally, depolarization reaches the right ventricle, and so produces an R' in the right chest leads and a deep broad S wave in the left chest leads. An M pattern is

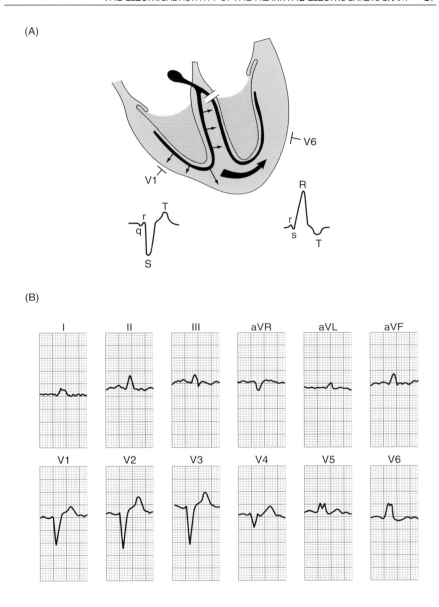

Fig. 2.16   Left bundle branch block. (A) The initial vector is abnormal in being from right to left across the septum, thus producing an initial r wave in V6 and a q wave in V1. (B) 12-lead ECG demonstrating features of left bundle branch block.

(A)

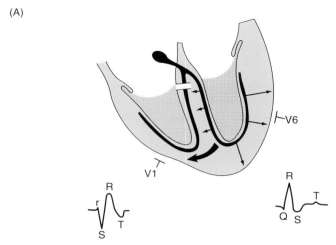

(B)

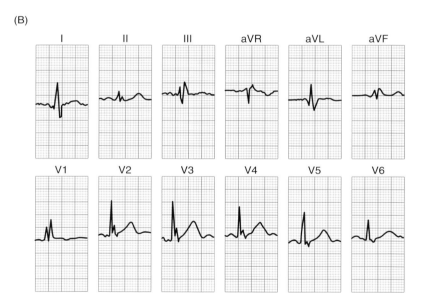

Fig. 2.17 Right bundle branch block. (A) The septum is depolarized normally from left to right and hence a small q is preserved in left ventricular leads and a small r in right ventricular leads. Left ventricular depolarization produces an s wave in V1 and an R wave in V6. Late depolarization of the right ventricle results in a prominent R' wave in V1 and broad S wave in V6. (B) 12-lead ECG showing features of right bundle branch block.

thus seen in the right chest leads, such as V1. It is also common to see T wave abnormalities in leads V2 and V3.

The mean frontal QRS axis

As pointed out on p. 13, the total electrical activity at any one moment of time can be summated and represented by a single electrical force of a certain magnitude and in a certain direction, termed the instantaneous vector. All the instantaneous vectors occurring during the inscription of the QRS complex can be averaged, the direction of the vector so derived being called the mean QRS axis. It is customary to measure this only in the frontal plane, based on the orientation of the limb leads (Fig. 2.18). The limb lead with the tallest R wave will be closest to the QRS axis.

An alternative method of deriving the mean frontal QRS axis is to find in which of the leads I, II, III, aVR, aVL and aVF, the deflections of the QRS above and below the line are most nearly equal. The mean frontal QRS axis is at right angles to this lead.

Left axis deviation is present when the axis is less than −30° and right axis deviation when the axis is greater than +110°.

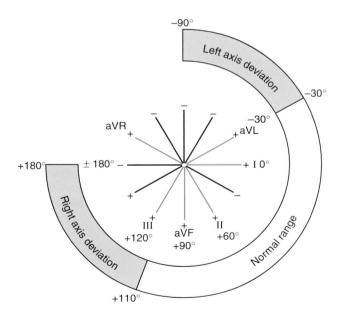

Fig. 2.18   Hexaxial reference system. The orientation of the limb leads in the frontal plane is shown, together with the normal range for the mean frontal QRS axis.

Calculation of the mean frontal QRS axis is of limited value except in a few conditions such as the differentiation of ostium primum from ostium secundum atrial septal defects (see p. 303).

Left axis deviation is often due to block in the anterior division (fascicle) of the left bundle branch, and when associated with right bundle branch block is a frequent precursor of complete heart block.

Right axis deviation commonly accompanies right ventricular hypertrophy, but may be due to block of the posterior fascicle of the left bundle.

ECG interpretation

ECG interpretation is largely a matter of experience and pattern interpretation. However, while building experience, it is useful to develop a method of 'systematic' ECG analysis. This is most easily performed by asking oneself a number of questions in a logical sequence about P, QRS and T waves in turn. A simple system is presented in Table 2.2.

Table 2.2   A system of ECG interpretation

Rate and rhythm
   What is the rate (see p. 18)?
   Is it regular or irregular?

P wave
   Are P waves present?
   Is the P wave axis normal (p. 18)?
   Is there evidence of left or right atrial enlargement (p. 19)?

PR interval (normal range 0.12–0.20 s)
   Is the PR interval normal?
   Is each QRS complex preceded by a P wave?
   Is there evidence of a slurred QRS upstroke (delta wave) (pp. 19, 187)?

QRS complex
   Is the QRS duration within normal limits (0.08–0.11 s)?
   Is there evidence of bundle branch block (pp. 25, 26)?
   Is the QRS axis normal (p. 29)?
   Are pathological Q waves present (p. 21)?
   Is there a normal R wave progression across the chest leads (p. 18)?

ST segment and T wave
   Is there abnormal ST elevation or depression (p. 22)?
   Are the T waves upright (except aVR and V1)?

QT interval
   Is the QT interval normal (in general less than 0.44 s)?

Further reading

Goldman, M. J. (1986) *Principles of Clinical Electrocardiography*, 12th edn. Los Altos, California: Lange.
Hampton, J. R. (1997) *The ECG in practice*, 3rd edn. Edinburgh: Churchill Livingstone.
Noble, D. (1979) *The Initiation of the Heartbeat*, 2nd edn. Oxford: Clarendon.
Schamroth, L. (1982) *An Introduction to Electrocardiography*, 6th edn. Oxford: Blackwell.

The Symptoms of Heart Disease

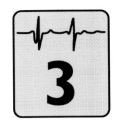

DYSPNOEA

Dyspnoea – difficulty with breathing – is the commonest symptom of heart failure. The term implies discomfort in the act of respiration, a consciousness of laboured breathing. It is, of course, also a symptom of respiratory disease and occurs in normal individuals on exercise.

No single explanation so far advanced accounts for all cases of dyspnoea. Furthermore, because it is subjective the degree of distress depends, in part, upon individual perceptions. Thus, some patients do not complain of breathlessness in spite of obviously laboured respiration, whereas others claim to be short of breath although their capacity for exercise is normal.

Mechanisms

The dyspnoea of cardiac disease may be due to the following factors:

Increased work of breathing. It is probable that in most cases of cardiac failure the discomfort arises in overworked respiratory muscles. In left-sided cardiac failure, engorgement of the pulmonary veins and capillaries occurs; if the pulmonary capillary pressure exceeds 25 mmHg, fluid may exude from the alveolar walls or even into the alveoli. These changes make the lung more rigid (less compliant) and require more respiratory work for a given volume of air inspired.

Reduced vital capacity. This is due to pulmonary venous congestion and, occasionally, to hydrothorax or ascites.

Reflex hyperventilation. The pulmonary stretch receptors may be abnormally stretched by congestion of the lungs.

Bronchial narrowing. Bronchial narrowing by spasm or fluid may occur in cardiac failure and adds to the work of breathing.

Hypoxaemia and carbon dioxide retention. These may both contribute to dyspnoea. They are seldom important factors in patients with left-sided heart failure, in whom the carbon dioxide tension is normal or low as a result of hyperventilation, and there is little hypoxaemia except when there is pulmonary oedema. In cyanotic congenital heart disease, hypoxaemia is severe.

Clinical features

The patient with cardiac dyspnoea breathes rapidly and shallowly. This pattern contrasts with that of the anxious individual who has deep and sighing respiration, and 'is unable to take a deep breath' or 'fill his lungs with air'. It also differs from the deep breathing of patients with diabetic keto-acidosis or renal failure.

Dyspnoea in patients with cardiac disease is usually slowly progressive, although it may be suddenly exacerbated by the onset of atrial fibrillation or the occurrence of pulmonary infarction or infection. At first it occurs only on effort, but as the disease process advances, less and less exercise is required to provoke breathlessness until it may eventually be present at rest.

Orthopnoea. Orthopnoea is dyspnoea when lying flat. There are several possible explanations for its occurrence in left heart failure:

- when an individual lies flat there is increased venous return, which in the patient on the verge of failure may increase pulmonary venous congestion, and thereby decrease pulmonary compliance and vital capacity;
- the vital capacity is reduced in the recumbent posture by the relatively high position of the diaphragm, which may be further displaced upwards by ascites or an enlarged liver.

Orthopnoea usually occurs when there is already a considerable limitation of exercise tolerance, but is occasionally an early symptom. Many patients learn for themselves that they are more comfortable propped up by three or four pillows.

Paroxysmal dyspnoea. In patients with left-sided cardiac failure, attacks of dyspnoea may develop without an obvious precipitating cause. They are most apt to occur during sleep (paroxysmal nocturnal dyspnoea). The mechanism is probably the same as that of orthopnoea, but the sensory unawareness of the sleeping state prevents the patient from correcting the situation by sitting up. The victim wakes up intensely short of breath and frightened. He sits on the side of the bed or struggles to the window. The attack may pass off spontaneously within a few minutes, or progress to acute pulmonary oedema.

Acute pulmonary oedema. In this condition, fluid accumulates in the alveoli as a result of a high pulmonary capillary pressure. Such attacks occur in patients with mitral stenosis, acute myocardial infarction and other left-sided cardiac lesions. There is often a provoking factor such as an arrhythmia or respiratory infection.

The patient is intensely dyspnoeic with noisy breathing, cough and frothy sputum which is often blood-tinged. The skin is usually moist, cold and cyanosed. The pulse is fast and may be irregular. Crepitations may be heard throughout the chest in a severe attack. In some patients, rhonchi, due to fluid in the bronchi, predominate and the clinical picture may resemble bronchial asthma. Pulmonary oedema is usually visible on a chest radiograph (see p. 68).

Cheyne–Stokes respiration. In Cheyne–Stokes respiration, there is a periodic waxing and waning in the depth of respiration, over a period of about 1 min. As William Stokes wrote in 1854:

> It consists in the occurrence of a series of inspirations, increasing to maximum, and then declining in force and length, until a state of apparent apnoea is established. In this condition the patient may remain for such a length of time as to make his attendants believe that he is dead, when a low inspiration, followed by one more decided marks the commencement of a new ascending and then descending series of inspirations.

This pattern of breathing is seen during sleep in some normal individuals, but its occurrence in the conscious patient suggests advanced left ventricular failure. It also occurs in patients with cerebral vascular disease, particularly if they have received morphine.

The cause of Cheyne–Stokes breathing is not yet established but it seems likely that the prolonged lung-to-brain circulation time disturbs the normal feedback mechanisms for respiratory control.

CARDIAC PAIN

There are two major causes of cardiac pain: myocardial ischaemia and pericarditis.

Myocardial ischaemia and infarction (see also Chapters 8 and 9)

A transient and reversible inadequacy of the coronary circulation gives rise to that type of chest pain known as angina pectoris. If the reduction in coronary blood flow is such as to cause death of an area of myocardium (myocardial infarction), the pain is usually more severe and prolonged.

The term angina pectoris was adopted by William Heberden, who described the characteristics of the syndrome in 1768. He wrote:

> There is a disorder of the breast marked with strong and peculiar symptoms, considerable for the kind of danger belonging to it, and not extremely rare which deserves to be mentioned more at length. The seat of it, and the sense of strangling, and anxiety with which it is attended, may make it not improperly called angina pectoris.
>
> They who are afflicted with it, are seized while they are walking (more especially if it be uphill, and soon after eating) with a painful and most disagreeable sensation in the breast, which seems as if it were to extinguish life, if it were to increase or continue; but the moment they stand still, all this uneasiness vanishes.
>
> In all other respects the patients are, at the beginning of this disorder, perfectly well, and in particular have no shortness of breath, from which it is totally different. The pain is sometimes situated in the upper part, sometimes in the middle, sometimes at the bottom of the os sterni, and often more inclined to the left than to the right side. It likewise very frequently extends from the breast to the middle of the left arm.

Heberden clearly described the four cardinal features of angina - pectoris:

- the location – in the retrosternal region and its radiation particularly to the left arm;
- the character – often a strangling feeling;
- the relationship to exertion;
- the duration (usually 1–10 min).

For a more detailed description of angina pectoris, see p. 106.

Angina pectoris most commonly occurs in response to exercise in patients with coronary artery disease. The same symptom can be provoked by paroxysmal tachycardia, when there is insufficient time during diastole for the coronary arteries to fill and meet the increased oxygen demands of the tachycardia. Angina is a frequent symptom in aortic stenosis because of the inability of the coronary circulation to match the oxygen requirements of extreme left ventricular hypertrophy. Other conditions which may cause or exacerbate angina pectoris are coronary arterial spasm, aortic regurgitation, syphilitic aortitis, anaemia, hyperthyroidism and mitral stenosis.

There seems little doubt that the cause of angina pectoris is myocardial hypoxia secondary to inadequate coronary blood flow. The site of angina appears to be the myocardium; the stimulus to the pain has not been determined but may be due to a chemical substance related to oxygen lack or to a phenomenon analogous to cramp. The impulses arising in the myocardium pass through afferent sympathetic fibres to reach the upper thoracic sympathetic ganglia and are then directed to the upper four or five thoracic spinal nerves. In this way, the same segments of the spinal cord receive sensations from the heart as receive sensory impulses from the anterior chest wall and the inner aspect of the arm, forearm and hand. The pain is perceived as arising in the territory supplied by the corresponding spinal somatic nerves, rather than in the organ itself.

The pain of myocardial infarction is similar to that of angina pectoris in its location and character, but its duration is longer (usually more than 30 min), it is usually more severe, and it has no relationship to exertion.

Pericarditis (see also Chapter 12)

Pain is a characteristic feature of pericarditis, and appears to arise in the parietal pericardium, the visceral pericardium being insensitive. It is usually sharp, but may be of an aching nature. It is situated in the retrosternal region, and radiates to the neck, back or upper abdomen, but rarely the arms. It may be exacerbated by inspiration, swallowing and movement, and by body posture such as lying flat.

PALPITATION

Palpitation may be defined as an awareness of the heart beat. It takes several different forms including a thumping sensation in the chest, a throbbing in the neck, a consciousness of missed or extra beats, or a racing of the heart. Anxious individuals are often distressed by the sinus tachycardia associated with emotion. Even normal individuals may be disagreeably conscious of their heart action when lying on the left side. Palpitation is, therefore, a common symptom in those without heart disease.

A careful history can sometimes help in distinguishing the cause of palpitation. Ectopic beats frequently give rise to the sensation of jumping of the heart, missed beats or extra beats. Patients with paroxysmal arrhythmias are frequently aware of both the sudden onset and sudden termination of the arrhythmia. Patients with atrial fibrillation may be able to describe the chaotic irregularity of the heart beat.

In assessing the significance of palpitation it is important to enquire about associated symptoms such as dizziness, dyspnoea or chest discomfort as these may be features of a rapid arrhythmia causing haemodynamic compromise.

OEDEMA

Oedema – the accumulation of fluid in the interstitial tissues – is an important but relatively late manifestation of cardiac failure. It does not usually occur except in the presence of a raised venous pressure, and salt and water retention. Oedema is preceded by a gain in body weight of some 3–5 kg due to an increase in the extracellular fluid.

Normally, fluid exudes into the tissues at the arterial ends of capillaries because the hydrostatic pressure of approximately 30 mmHg exceeds the colloid osmotic pressure of 25 mmHg. Fluid is reabsorbed at the venous ends because the hydrostatic pressure at this point is approximately 12 mmHg. Oedema occurs when there is inadequate reabsorption of fluid from the tissues. A high venous pressure alone can, by increasing the hydrostatic force at the venous ends of the capillaries, cause oedema, as it does, for example, in vena caval obstruction. Raised venous pressure is nearly always a factor in cardiac oedema, but is seldom the sole explanation, for the retention of salt and water almost invariably antedates the appearance of the oedema.

The location of oedema in cardiac failure is determined by local factors, particularly gravity. In the ambulant patient, it occurs bilaterally in the lower legs and feet; in those kept in bed, it accumulates in the sacral area. When the oedema is very great, it may affect the whole of the lower limbs, the genitalia, the abdominal and chest walls and even the face (anasarca).

In the oedema of cardiac failure, the tissues dimple ('pit') when pressure is applied to them by the thumb.

ASCITES

The intraperitoneal accumulation of fluid is a manifestation of advanced heart disease, usually occurring later than peripheral oedema but for similar reasons. In some conditions, however, such as tricuspid valve disease and constrictive pericarditis, ascites may be even more evident than oedema and is probably then, in part, a consequence of portal hypertension secondary to cardiac cirrhosis of the liver.

CYANOSIS

Cyanosis, a blue discoloration of the skin or mucous membranes, is more a sign than a symptom of heart disease and is often first noticed by relatives when the affected individual exercises or is exposed to cold temperatures. It is usually due to a large proportion of reduced haemoglobin in the superficial capillaries and venules. It has been observed that cyanosis appears when the amount of reduced haemoglobin in the blood of these vessels exceeds 5 g/100 ml. Cyanosis results either from oxygen desaturation of the arterial blood or from an unusually large extraction of oxygen in the peripheral tissues. When the cyanosis is due to arterial oxygen desaturation, it is considered to be 'central' in origin because it is caused by a disorder in the heart or lungs. When the cause of the cyanosis is high oxygen extraction in the tissues, it is said to be 'peripheral'.

Central cyanosis is due either to blood bypassing the lungs as it is shunted from the venous side of the circulation to the arterial, as a result of congenital heart disease, or to inadequate oxygenation of the blood in the lungs, as in some varieties of lung disease. Clubbing of the digits is a common accompaniment of cyanotic congenital heart disease.

Peripheral cyanosis, a consequence of diminished blood flow through the skin and mucous membranes, occurs in normal people when they are cold, and in patients with a low cardiac output due to such conditions as mitral stenosis and acute circulatory failure.

The differentiation of central from peripheral cyanosis is usually not difficult. In peripheral cyanosis the skin is cold, and the cyanosis does not affect the warm mucous membranes such as those of the tongue. Furthermore, peripheral cyanosis can be abolished by warming the skin. The central origin of the cyanosis can be confirmed by measuring the arterial oxygen saturation which is usually less than 85%.

Rarely, central cyanosis may be due not to arterial oxygen desaturation but to methaemoglobinaemia or sulphaemoglobinaemia as a result of taking certain drugs.

HAEMOPTYSIS

The expectoration of blood is not uncommon in patients with heart disease. Several mechanisms are involved; examination of the sputum may help to determine which of them is responsible.

Frank haemoptysis – the coughing up of pure blood – occurs in mitral stenosis, due to the rupture of pulmonary or bronchial veins, or to pulmonary infarction. When there is pulmonary infection, the sputum may be purulent or rusty in appearance. In pulmonary oedema, the frothy sputum may be pink or streaked with blood.

Of course, patients with heart disease may also have haemoptysis due to other types of lung disease such as tuberculosis, bronchiectasis and bronchial neoplasm.

SYNCOPE

Syncope is a transient loss of consciousness due to inadequate cerebral blood flow or perfusion pressure. Cerebral blood flow and perfusion pressure depend upon the cardiac output, the arterial blood pressure and the resistance of the cerebral circulation. Cerebral arteries are relatively uninfluenced by the autonomic system but are dilated by carbon dioxide.

The commonest type of syncope is that of the simple faint (*vaso-motor or vasodepressor syncope*). It is often a response to emotion, but various physical factors such as blood loss, debility after infection and pain may contribute to its occurrence. It is believed to result mainly from dilatation of the arterial resistance vessels in the muscles. The fall in blood pressure causes a diminished perfusion pressure in the brain and loss of consciousness. Fainting of this kind usually develops when standing, rarely when sitting and virtually never when lying or walking. The first symptom is usually a sense of weakness, accompanied by yawning or sighing, sweating, nausea and 'a sinking feeling' in the stomach. After seconds or minutes, unconsciousness ensues; this is transient because the subject usually falls flat on the ground and this posture leads to an improvement in cerebral blood flow. In a severe attack, the face is pale, the pupils are dilated and respiration is slow. The heart rate is usually diminished and the radial pulse difficult to feel, although carotid artery pulsation can be detected without difficulty.

Micturition syncope occurs in adult men with nocturia. Consciousness is lost immediately after passing urine. It is particularly likely after considerable alcohol consumption. It may be due to reflex vasodilatation secondary to sudden relief of distension of the bladder combined with the vasodilator effects of alcohol and a warm bed.

Cardiac rhythm disturbance may be responsible for syncope. A catastrophic fall in cardiac output may result if the heart rate is either extremely slow or very fast. In supraventricular and ventricular tachycardias the ventricular rate sometimes exceeds 180/min, leaving insufficient time for adequate filling of the heart. An important and dangerous form of syncope is the *Adams–Stokes attack*, which is a brief episode of cardiac arrest due to either asystole or ventricular fibrillation. This characteristically occurs in patients with heart block in whom either the ventricular pacemaker suddenly fails, or in whom ventricular arrhythmias are superimposed on the heart block. In most cases, effective cardiac action returns in 10–15 s, but if the attack is more prolonged convulsions may occur. The return of consciousness is accompanied by flushing as blood flows once more through vessels dilated by hypoxia.

Syncope on exertion.   This is a characteristic feature of severe aortic stenosis (see p. 274), and may be due to an inability of the heart to supply an adequate blood flow in the face of the increased demands of the muscles. Patients with aortic stenosis are also susceptible to syncope due to heart block or ventricular arrhythmias.

Carotid sinus syncope.   This is a condition occurring in elderly individuals in whom light pressure on the carotid sinus produces extreme cardiac slowing or reflex hypotension.

Postural syncope.   When a normal individual stands up, pooling of blood in the legs is prevented by arteriolar and venous constriction, and there is an acceleration of the heart rate together with an increase in plasma catecholamine levels. Postural syncope, due to orthostatic hypotension, occurs in patients with autonomic disorders, including diabetic neuropathy and tabes dorsalis, as well as in some otherwise normal elderly individuals in whom these compensatory mechanisms do not function. Some hypotensive agents, particularly antiadrenergic drugs such as guanethidine, lead to orthostatic hypotension.

Syncope of cardiac origin also occurs in other conditions in which there may be a sudden fall in cardiac output such as massive pulmonary embolism, acute myocardial infarction and mitral valve obstruction due to left atrial myxoma or ball-valve thrombus.

FUNCTIONAL CAPACITY

On the basis of recommendations of the New York Heart Association, patients may be divided into four classes depending on the severity of their symptoms:

Class 1   the patients, although they have heart disease, can with-
            stand normal physical activity without symptoms
Class 2   the patient develops symptoms on moderate or severe
            exertion but not at rest or with mild exertion
Class 3   symptoms are present even on mild exertion
Class 4   symptoms are present at rest.

Such a classification is of value provided its limitations are borne in mind. Thus, many patients with severe heart disease have few or no complaints, whereas those who have an anxiety neurosis, or are anaemic or pregnant, may have dyspnoea in the absence of heart disease.

Further reading

Criteria Committee of the New York Heart Association (1964) *Diseases of the Heart and Blood Vessels (Nomenclature and Criteria for Diagnosis)*. Boston: Little, Brown.

The Physical Signs of Heart Disease

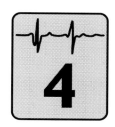

Signs are small measurable things but interpretations are illimitable.

George Eliot *Middlemarch*

THE ARTERIAL PULSE

The elastic structure of the aorta and its major branches enables them to act as both reservoirs and conduits. As a consequence, they are able to convert the highly pulsatile discontinuous blood flow from the ventricles into a more continuous flow in the peripheral vessels. The pressure pulse recorded a short distance above the aortic valve shows a sharp upstroke, produced by the rapid ejection of blood from the left ventricle, followed by a slower downstroke, as the rate of flow into peripheral arteries exceeds that from the left ventricle into the aorta (Fig. 4.1). This descending limb of the pulse wave is interrupted by the *dicrotic notch*, as the column of blood, briefly retreating towards the ventricle at the onset of diastole, is halted by aortic valve closure. As the main wave of the pulse travels peripherally, secondary waves are produced at the points of branching of the arteries. These are reflected backwards and summate with the main wave. Consequently, the peak systolic pressure in a peripheral artery may be higher than that in the central aorta.

When the arterial pulse is examined, the following characteristics should be noted:

- the rate;
- the rhythm;
- the amplitude;
- the character or wave form.

It is customary to feel the right radial artery to determine the rate and rhythm of the heart, but the amplitude and quality of the pulse is better appreciated in the brachial or carotid arteries. One should also

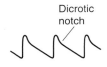

Dicrotic
notch

Fig. 4.1   The normal arterial pulse wave.

search for pulsation in the radial, brachial, carotid, femoral, dorsalis pedis and posterior tibial arteries on both sides.

The heart and pulse rate.   The rate of the pulse, if regular, can be calculated by multiplying the number of beats in 15 s by 4. If it is irregular, the number of beats in 30 s should be doubled. The pulse rate in normal resting adults ranges from 60 to 100/min. A rate of less than 60/min is most commonly due to sinus bradycardia (see p. 180), but may also be due to junctional rhythm or heart block. Rates in excess of 100/min (tachycardia) are most often due to sinus tachycardia associated with emotion or exercise; the heart rate may exceed 200 beats per minute on vigorous exercise. If the rate exceeds 120/min at rest in adults, some form of arrhythmia is likely (see Chapter 11).

Pulse rhythm.   The normal pulse is regular or exhibits sinus arrhythmia. An occasional irregularity in an otherwise regular pulse suggests ectopic beats, and a coupling of beats (pulsus bigeminus or bigeminy) is due to the alternation of normal and ectopic beats. A totally irregular pulse suggests atrial fibrillation.

The amplitude and character of the pulse.   The amplitude of the pulse depends on the pulse pressure, i.e. the difference between the systolic and diastolic pressures. The pulse is of small volume when the pulse pressure is small. This is the case when there is a low stroke volume and peripheral vasoconstriction as occurs in acute myocardial infarction, the shock syndrome, mitral stenosis and pericardial constriction or tamponade. In aortic stenosis, the pulse is small and prolonged and has a slow upstroke. This is called an *anacrotic* pulse if the wave has a notch on its upstroke (Fig. 4.2). *Pulsus bisferiens* is a pulse of moderate or large volume in which a double beat can be felt. This sign suggests a combination of aortic stenosis and regurgitation but is not diagnostic.

A large pulse, associated with a large stroke volume occurs in aortic regurgitation, anaemia, pregnancy and thyrotoxicosis. When a large volume pulse rises rapidly and collapses suddenly (Fig. 4.2) it is described as a *collapsing* pulse; this is also called a *waterhammer* pulse after a Victorian toy of this name. This type of pulse is encountered when there is a rapid runoff of blood during diastole as in aortic regurgitation, persistent ductus arteriosus and arteriovenous fistulae. It is best felt by placing the palm of the hand on the patient's vertically elevated forearm, thereby increasing the retrograde flow of blood during diastole.

A reduction in systolic pressure of up to 10 mmHg may occur on inspiration in normal people, probably because the capacity of the

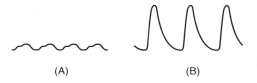

Fig. 4.2 (A) The pulse of severe aortic stenosis. (B) The rapidly rising and collapsing pulse of aortic regurgitation.

(A)   (B)

pulmonary vascular bed enlarges and reduces the return of blood to the left ventricle. This is partly compensated for by a simultaneous increase in right ventricular output. A more substantial inspiratory fall, which occurs in obstructive airways disease, especially asthma, and pericardial constriction, produces *pulsus paradoxus*. In obstructive lung disease the reduction in arterial pressure is the consequence of the increased negativity of the intrathoracic pressure. In pericardial constriction and tamponade, this may be due to the right ventricle being unable to compensate for the augmented pulmonary vascular capacity by increasing its output. Another and probably more important explanation is that an inspiratory increase in the right ventricle occurs at the expense of left ventricle, as they are both confined within an indistensible pericardium.

In *pulsus alternans*, the beats are evenly spaced in time but are alternately large and small in volume. This is most readily detected when the blood pressure is being measured, for as the cuff is being deflated only alternate beats are heard at first. After a fall of a further 5 or 10 mmHg, every beat is audible. The mechanism of pulsus alternans is not well understood, but is usually associated with left ventricular failure.

The *absence* of a peripheral pulse indicates an anatomical aberration, or narrowing or occlusion of the artery proximal to it. In coarctation of the aorta, pulsation of the femoral arteries is delayed compared with that of the radial arteries.

Blood pressure recording

Precise measurement of the blood pressure can be obtained only by intra-arterial catheterization but a sphygmomanometer is sufficiently accurate for clinical purposes. This instrument consists of a manometer linked to an inflatable bag, surrounded by an inelastic cuff. The size of bag and cuff is of importance in ensuring accuracy, large cuffs being required for the obese and small for children. The cuff must fit around the arm snugly, being neither loose nor touching any article of clothing. It should be applied about 2 cm above the antecubital space with the rubber bag over the medial aspect of the arm.

Manometers are of two types: mercury and aneroid. The mercury type requires care in ensuring that there is no loss or oxidation of mercury and that the air vent at the top of the tube is open. Aneroid manometers are as accurate as mercury instruments, provided they are calibrated regularly.

It is best for the patient to be reclining comfortably, but the blood pressure can be taken satisfactorily with the patient sitting or standing provided the limb is supported and at the same level as the heart. Using a mercury manometer, one's eye should be in line with the top of the meniscus.

The patient should be warm, comfortable and in a quiet environment, and should have stayed in the same position for 5 min before the blood pressure recording; if in doubt, several recordings should be made.

The cuff should be inflated until the pulsations of the brachial artery can no longer be felt. The pressure is then raised by a further 20 mmHg and released at a rate of about 2 mmHg a second. As the pressure falls, sounds (Korotkoff sounds) are heard as blood begins to pass through the artery which has been occluded. At first these are faint and tapping; then a swishing quality is noted. The sounds become crisper and more intense and, as the pressure falls further, there is an abrupt muffling (fourth phase) and, finally, the sounds disappear altogether (fifth phase). Sometimes there is a period of silence after the first appearance of the sounds before they reappear, known as the auscultatory gap, which is particularly common in the presence of hypertension.

The systolic pressure is that at which the sounds are first heard. Intra-arterial pressure recordings suggest that the fifth phase usually represents the diastolic pressure better than the fourth but in some individuals, particularly if they are vasodilated, the sounds may never disappear; this may also be due to overextension of the elbow. To avoid inconsistency between different observers and repeated observations, the pressures both at muffling and disappearance should be noted.

When blood pressure measurements are taken in the leg, the patient should be lying on his abdomen, with a large cuff covering the mid-thigh region, and the stethoscope placed in the popliteal fossa.

Certain circumstances make blood pressure estimations difficult. In the shock syndrome, blood pressure readings from a sphygmomanometer may be grossly inaccurate. In atrial fibrillation and other arrhythmias, the blood pressure may vary from beat to beat; the average of a number of beats should be taken for both the systolic and diastolic pressures.

THE VENOUS PULSE AND PRESSURE (Fig. 4.3)

Inspection of the veins in the neck is an essential but often neglected part of cardiac diagnosis. The external jugular vein is easily seen, but is so often obstructed as it passes through the fascial plane that it cannot be relied upon as a guide to the true venous pressure. The internal jugular vein cannot be directly visualized, but it imparts a broad pulsation to the tissues of the neck overlying it. Its undulations can be

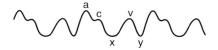

Fig. 4.3   The venous pulse. Note the 'a' wave due to atrial systole and the 'c' wave occurring at the time of tricuspid valve closure. The upstroke of the 'v' wave occurs as the atrium is filling passively during ventricular systole; the descent from the peak of 'v' to 'y' occurs as blood flows from the atrium to the ventricle after tricuspid valve opening.

seen in virtually all individuals, if the correct technique of examination is used; occasionally, especially in the obese or bullnecked, it cannot be identified.

There are normally three peaks:

- 'a' corresponding to atrial systole;
- 'c' occurring at the time of tricuspid valve closure;
- 'v' at the time of tricuspid valve opening.

There are two troughs:

- 'x' corresponding to the descent of the tricuspid valve ring as the right ventricle contracts;
- 'y' trough representing the fall in pressure as blood flows into the right ventricle.

As it is usually not possible to see the 'c' wave in the jugular pulse, the normal venous pulse in the neck is composed of two positive and two negative waves (Fig. 4.3).

It is essential to observe both the *waveform* and the *pressure level* of the jugular venous pulse. The pressure should not be determined until the characteristics of the wave form have been identified. The patient should be reclining with the chest, head and neck at 45°, and with the muscles of the neck relaxed. If venous pulsation cannot be seen with the patient at 45°, he should be placed more horizontally until it can.

The venous waveform.   In differentiating venous from arterial pulsation the following points are important: the venous pulse normally shows two positive pulsations in each cardiac cycle compared with the single pulsation in the arteries; the venous pulse cannot usually be felt, although it can be readily seen, whereas the arterial pulsation is more easily felt than seen; the venous pulse waves can be obliterated by light pressure at the root of the neck. Pressure on the abdomen, by increasing venous return to the thorax, increases the venous pressure in the neck transiently and permits it to be visualized more easily.

The venous pressure. With the patient in the semi-recumbent position, the vertical height of the top of the venous column above the sternal angle is observed. In normal individuals, this does not exceed 2 cm; it is increased by factors which augment venous return including pregnancy, anxiety, exercise and anaemia. If these causes cannot be invoked, raised venous pressure is usually due to right-sided cardiac failure; it is important to exclude non-pulsating engorgement due to obstruction of the superior vena cava.

Hepato-jugular reflux. If pressure is exerted on the relaxed abdomen, venous return to the right atrium is increased, and the jugular venous pressure rises accordingly. In normals this rise is very transient; in patients with heart failure, it may remain high as long as pressure is exerted on the abdomen.

The timing of venous waves may be difficult; it is essential either to feel the carotid artery pulsation on the other side of the neck or to listen for the first heart sound in order to allow identification of the 'a' wave which precedes these two events.

Giant 'a' wave (Fig. 4.4).   This develops when the right atrium contracts forcefully against the increased resistance provided by a stenotic tricuspid valve, or hypertrophied right ventricle.

Cannon waves.   These are large venous pulsations due to atrial contraction against a closed tricuspid valve. They occur intermittently in complete heart block and in ventricular tachycardia when atrial and

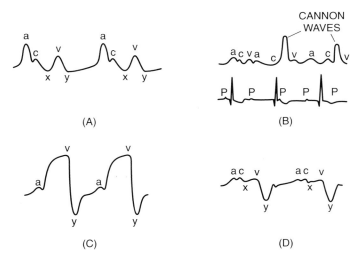

Fig. 4.4   (A) The giant 'a' wave. (B) Intermittent cannon waves in complete heart block, occurring at the time of synchronous atrial and ventricular contraction. (C) The systolic venous pulsation of tricuspid regurgitation. (D) The venous pulse in pericardial constriction, showing the rapid 'y' descent, followed by a plateau.

ventricular systoles coincide (Fig. 4.4). In junctional rhythms, atrial and ventricular contractions are synchronous and cannon waves occur with every heart beat.

Systolic venous pulsation ('cv' wave).   This is due to blood regurgitating into the venous system during ventricular systole and is characteristic of tricuspid regurgitation (Fig. 4.4).

In pericardial constriction, the venous pressure is greatly raised, and there is a sharp 'y' descent as blood rushes into the right ventricle in the early part of diastole (Fig. 4.4). Another feature of this condition is elevation of venous pressure during inspiration because the increase in venous return at this time cannot be accommodated by the constricted right ventricle.

INSPECTION OF THE CHEST

Abnormalities of the thorax and lungs may cause changes in the position of the heart; they may also result from or cause heart disease. Funnel chest (pectus excavatum) and kyphoscoliosis may lead to displacement of the heart. Cardiac enlargement associated with advanced congenital heart disease in childhood may cause deformity of the sternum and ribs.

The rate and pattern of breathing should be noted. The respiratory rate is often increased in left ventricular failure. Prolonged expiration suggests obstructive airway disease.

The cardiac impulse is frequently visible, particularly when there is heart disease. It is often possible to see the exaggerated apical impulse of left ventricular hypertrophy, the displaced apex of left ventricular dilatation, the left parasternal pulsation of right ventricular hypertrophy or the abnormal pulmonary arterial pulsation in the second and third left interspaces in pulmonary hypertension.

PALPATION OF THE CHEST

The apex beat

In the normal individual, the maximal thrust of the left ventricle – the apex beat – can be felt at or just internal to the mid-clavicular line in the fifth intercostal space. If it is displaced, one should determine whether this is due to abnormalities of the thoracic cage or lungs. After the apex beat has been located and assessed, the whole precordium should be explored with the palm of the hand in the search for abnormal pulsation.

The ventricular impulse may be abnormal in a number of different ways:

- left ventricular hypertrophy produces a sustained heaving or thrusting apex beat;
- left ventricular dilatation displaces the apex downwards and outwards. If there is a large left ventricular stroke volume, as in aortic regurgitation, the impulse is vigorous, but when myocardial contractility is impaired as by ischaemic heart disease, it may be diffuse and feeble;
- in mitral stenosis, the apex beat often has a characteristic abrupt tapping quality due to the vibrations associated with the loud first sound;
- in patients with a left ventricular aneurysm the outward movement of the aneurysmal segment during systole gives rise to an abnormal sustained apical impulse;
- in patients with hypertrophic obstructive cardiomyopathy a characteristic double impulse can sometimes be palpated, the first phase representing the onset of systole and the second contraction against an obstructed outflow.

Right ventricular impulse

The right ventricular impulse in the left parasternal region is not usually palpable in health, except in children and thin adults. In right ventricular hypertrophy, as occurs in pulmonary stenosis and pulmonary hypertension (particularly secondary to mitral stenosis) there is a sustained lifting impulse along the left sternal edge. When there is right ventricular dilatation associated with a high right ventricular output (as in atrial septal defect), the impulse is vigorous but less sustained. In severe mitral regurgitation, systolic pulsation of the enlarged left atrium may also cause a left parasternal heave.

Pulmonary arterial pulsation can quite often be felt in the second left intercostal space when there is pulmonary hypertension or high pulmonary blood flow. Occasionally, the pulsation of an aneurysm can be detected in the aortic area.

Vibrations may be felt over the precordium corresponding to audible sounds and murmurs. When they are associated with heart sounds, they may be described as 'shocks'. Shocks may accompany any loud heart sound.

Thrills

Thrills are the tactile equivalent of murmurs. They do not occur in the absence of loud murmurs and have no significance beyond that possessed by the murmur. Thrills are usually best felt by the palm of the hand when the patient is sitting upright and holding his breath in full expiration. The commonest thrills are the following:

- an apical systolic thrill corresponding with the loud systolic murmur of mitral regurgitation;
- a systolic thrill between the apex and the left sternal edge in ventricular septal defect;
- a systolic thrill in the second right intercostal space, occasionally over the sternum and the third or fourth left intercostal space, in aortic stenosis. This is often associated with a systolic thrill over the carotid arteries;
- a systolic thrill in the second or third left intercostal spaces in pulmonary stenosis;
- diastolic and presystolic thrills at the apex in mitral stenosis (best felt with the patient rotated to the left);
- a continuous systolic and diastolic thrill below the left clavicle in persistent ductus arteriosus.

It is rare for the murmurs of aortic or pulmonary regurgitation to be accompanied by a thrill.

After the chest has been palpated, the opportunity should be taken to palpate the abdomen. Particular attention should be paid to the liver. Enlargement, often tender, is a characteristic feature of rightsided heart failure. Systolic pulsation may be felt in tricuspid regurgitation, and presystolic pulsation in tricuspid stenosis.

PERCUSSION OF THE HEART

A crude estimate of the size of the heart may be made by percussion, but this is much less accurate than radiology and it has little place in diagnosis. It is sometimes of value in the diagnosis of pericardial effusion, as in this condition the area of cardiac dullness may be extended to the right of the sternum and to the second left intercostal space. In emphysema, the area of cardiac dullness may be reduced.

AUSCULTATION: HEART SOUNDS AND MURMURS

Vibrations within the heart give rise to sounds which are loud enough to be audible through a stethoscope and to be registered graphically by a phonocardiogram. If the noise is brief and transient, it is termed a heart sound; if more prolonged, it is a murmur. Careful auscultation, combined with the other methods of physical examination, provides information about the heart which even the most sophisticated modern techniques of investigation can scarcely match.

The physician should always use a stethoscope with which he is familiar. The earpieces should fit comfortably; the tubing should be short (not greater than 30 cm) and thick-walled. Both types of endpiece (diaphragm and bell) are necessary. The rigid diaphragm is best for hearing high-frequency sounds and murmurs such as the second heart sound and the diastolic murmur of aortic regurgitation. The bell pressed *lightly* on the chest is superior to the diaphragm for the low-pitched third and fourth heart sounds and the mid-diastolic and presystolic murmurs of mitral stenosis.

Traditionally, there are four areas of auscultation:

- aortic (right second intercostal space);
- pulmonary (left second intercostal space);
- tricuspid (lower sternal);
- mitral (apex beat).

These designations are somewhat misleading, especially with regard to the aortic valve, because aortic murmurs (especially if diastolic) are often maximal at the left sternal edge at the level of the fourth inter-costal space. The opening snap of mitral stenosis is also best heard in this area. Auscultation should never be restricted to the traditional areas; one should start on one side of the precordium and gradually move the stethoscope towards the other areas. One may begin in the pulmonary area in order to identify the first and second heart sounds, while palpating the carotid artery whose pulsation occurs just after the first heart sound. The aortic area may be listened to next, before moving obliquely across the sternum to the lower left sternal edge, thence to the tricuspid area, to the mitral area and into the axilla. One should then listen particularly in the aortic, pulmonary and lower left sternal edge areas with the patient sitting up and holding the breath in full expiration. The apical area should be listened to with the patient rotated into the left lateral position. If mitral stenosis is suspected, the patient should exercise by sitting forward and backwards several times, and then lie down again in the left lateral position.

Success in auscultation depends upon listening selectively for indi-vidual sounds and murmurs. Initially, the first heart sound should be identified and assessed before turning one's attention to the second heart sound and to any additional sounds. Having noted any normal or abnormal sounds, one should then listen for systolic and, later, for diastolic murmurs.

The heart sounds

The first sound

The first sound occurs at the time of closure of the atrioventricular valves. Although some have attributed the sound to the impact of closure, it seems more likely that it is due to the tensing of the cusps as they are projected into the atrium at the beginning of ventricular systole. Both tricuspid and mitral valves contribute to the sound. As these valves close slightly asynchronously, the first heart sound, in health, may be narrowly split. As the mitral component is louder, the first heart sound is usually best heard at the apex.

The intensity of the first heart sound is related to the extent of upward movement of the cusps when the ventricles contract. In the normal resting heart the valve cusps come into light contact with each other before the onset of ventricular systole which, therefore, projects them only a short distance. If the cusps are well down in the ventricular chamber, ventricular systole forces them rapidly upwards and causes a loud sound. This situation arises when the atrium contracts immediately before the ventricle (short PR interval) and when the left atrial pressure is abnormally high, as in mitral stenosis. In complete heart block, the relationship between atrial and ventricular systole changes from cycle to cycle, and the first sound varies in intensity accordingly. When the cusps are rigid, as in calcific mitral valve disease, the first sound is soft or inaudible.

The second sound

The second heart sound is related to the closure of the semilunar valves. Normally, it is single on expiration but splits into its aortic and pulmonary components during inspiration (Fig. 4.5). This phenomenon is accounted for by the prolongation of right ventricular systole associated with the increased flow into the right side of the heart occurring with inspiration. Splitting is best heard in the second left intercostal space. Abnormally wide splitting of the second sound, due to delay in pulmonary valve closure, occurs when the right ventricle is over-burdened by either a volume load (as in atrial septal defect) or a pressure load (as in pulmonary stenosis), or when there is a delay in electrical activation of the right ventricle (as in right bundle branch block). In atrial septal defect, there is usually 'fixed' splitting of the second heart sound because the increase in venous return on inspiration affects the filling of both ventricles.

When there is left bundle branch block and when the left ventricle is overburdened, as by systemic hypertension or aortic stenosis, the aortic component of the sound may be delayed. This produces 'reversed' splitting; the sound being single on inspiration and split on expiration (Fig. 4.6).

The intensity of the second heart sound may be increased by systemic or pulmonary hypertension, but this is not a reliable sign. The

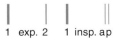

Fig. 4.5 Normal splitting of the second heart sound during inspiration, with the aortic component preceding the pulmonary.

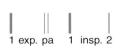

Fig. 4.6 'Reversed' splitting of the second sound. Due to delay in left ventricular emptying, the aortic component follows the pulmonary component of the second sound on expiration. On inspiration, the pulmonary component is, as usual, delayed and is superimposed on the aortic component.

aortic component of the second sound may be reduced or inaudible in aortic stenosis, particularly if the aortic valve is calcified, and the pulmonary component may be soft or absent in pulmonary stension. Both first and second sounds may be soft when the heart is separated from the chest wall by fat, pericardial effusion or emphysematous lung, or when the cardiac output is low as in shock.

The third sound (Fig. 4.7A)

The third sound occurs at the end of the period of rapid filling of the ventricles. It is probably due to sudden tensing of the valve structures and ventricular walls at this time. It is usually generated in the left ventricle and is best heard at or internal to the apex. The sound is low-pitched and distant, and is often heard only with the lightly applied stethoscope bell. Although normal in the young, it is a pathological finding in the middle-aged and elderly. Its presence implies either left ventricular failure or abnormally rapid filling of the ventricle, as in mitral regurgitation, pregnancy or anaemia. Occasionally, a third heart sound can be heard over the right ventricle in right ventricular failure. In pericardial constriction, there is a very early third heart sound of higher frequency associated with the sudden limitation to ventricular filling.

The fourth or atrial sound (Fig. 4.7B)

This sound resembles the third heart sound in being low-pitched and best heard at the apex, and probably has a similar mechanism. In this instance, the ventricular distension results from atrial contraction; the

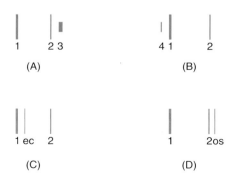

Fig. 4.7 (A) The third heart sound. (B) The fourth or atrial sound. (C) The ejection click (ec). (D) The opening snap.

fourth sound immediately precedes the first heart sound. It is rarely heard in health, and is usually a sign of either ventricular failure or hypertrophy. Thus, a fourth heart sound is heard over the left ventricle in some cases or aortic stenosis, hypertension and ischaemic heart disease. A right ventricular fourth heart sound may be heard at the left sternal edge in pulmonary stenosis and pulmonary hypertension.

Gallop rhythm

This term is applied to a cadence of three heart sounds which may be heard in the presence of tachycardia. It may be due to a third heart sound, to a fourth heart sound or to the superimposition of the two ('summation gallop').

Additional sounds in systole

Early systolic sounds (ejection sounds or clicks) occur at the time of aortic and pulmonary valve opening (Fig. 4.7C). The clicks may arise from sudden tensing of the opening cusps or from distension of the great vessels. Aortic clicks are almost invariable in valvar aortic stenosis provided the cusps are not calcified, and may be present in systemic hypertension. Pulmonary systolic clicks occur under conditions in which the pulmonary artery is dilated, as it is in valvar pulmonary stenosis and in pulmonary hypertension. They are usually heard best in held expiration.

   Clicks occurring later in systole are usually due to ballooning of a mitral valve cusp (mitral valve prolapse). A systolic clicking or crunching may occur in pneumothorax.

The opening snap (Fig. 4.7D)

This is one of the most important signs in auscultation and is virtually diagnostic of mitral stenosis. It occurs at the time of mitral valve opening and is presumed to be due to sudden tension of stenosed but pliant cusps. It is soft or absent if the mitral valve is rigid from fibrosis or calcification. It is heard best at the left sternal edge in the fourth intercostal space or between this point and the apex beat and has a snapping quality. Unlike splitting of the second sound and the third heart sound with which it may be confused, it can often be heard widely over the precordium (see Table 4.1).

Heart murmurs

Murmurs appear to result from vibrations set up by turbulent blood flow. Turbulence is encouraged by high velocity of flow, by abrupt change in the calibre of a vessel or chamber and by reduced blood

Table 4.1 The differentiation of splitting of the second heart sound, the opening snap, and the third heart sound (of the left ventricle)

	Splitting of second sound (normal)	Splitting of second sound (fixed)	Splitting of second sound (reversed)	Opening snap	Third heart sound
Interval between first component of second sound and 'extra' sound	0–0.05 s (maximal on inspiration)	0.03–0.08 s (at all phases)	0.01–0.03 s (maximal on expiration)	0.03–0.12 s	0.10–0.16 s
Effect of inspiration	Widens	Unaffected	Narrows	None	None
Character		Abrupt – heard best with diaphragm		'Snap' – heard best with diaphragm	Low-pitched – heard best with bell
Site of maximal intensity		Second left intercostal space		Lower left sternal edge	At apex
Radiation		Left sternal edge		All cardiac areas	Localized (usually)

viscosity. Murmurs therefore develop when there is rapid flow through a valve, valvar narrowing, or anaemia.

The following features of a murmur should be noted: its timing in the cardiac cycle, its location and radiation, its intensity and its quality.

Murmurs may occur either in systole or in diastole; they may continue from one into the other.

Murmurs are usually best heard at the place on the chest wall closest to their site of origin or in the direction of blood flow. Thus, the murmur of aortic stenosis is loudest over the aortic valve (the third left intercostal space), or in the second right intercostal space, or in the neck. On the other hand, the diastolic murmur of aortic regurgitation is usually maximal at the fourth left intercostal space and is less well heard in the 'aortic area'.

The intensity of murmurs can be classified in six grades:

Grade 1   Only just audible, even under good auscultatory conditions
Grade 2   Soft
Grade 3   Moderately loud
Grade 4   Loud and accompanied by a palpable thrill
Grade 5   Very loud but not audible with the stethoscope away from the chest
Grade 6   So loud as to be audible with the stethoscope lifted from the chest wall.

The quality of a murmur may be 'blowing', 'rumbling', 'harsh' or 'musical'. These are poor descriptions of what is heard; only with experience can one appreciate what is meant by such terms. Murmurs may also be described as low, medium or high pitched.

Systolic murmurs

These are usually midsystolic or pansystolic (holosystolic) in timing.

Midsystolic murmurs start after the opening of the aortic and pulmonary valves, increase in intensity to a maximum in midsystole and decrease and disappear before the second heart sound (Fig. 4.8A). Because of their configuration, they are sometimes called 'diamond-shaped', and are also termed 'ejection' because they arise during ejection of blood from the ventricles into great arteries. Murmurs arising at the aortic and pulmonary valves are characteristically midsystolic.

The murmur of aortic stenosis, which is often harsh, is usually best heard in the second right intercostal space, although sometimes it is maximal at the lower left sternal edge or even at the apex. It frequently radiates to the neck. The murmur of subaortic stenosis is loudest at the lower left sternal edge. The murmur of pulmonary valve stenosis is maximal at the second left intercostal space, that of infundibular

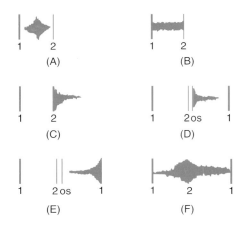

Fig. 4.8   (A) A midsystolic murmur. (B) A pansystolic murmur. (C) An early diastolic murmur. (D) A mid-diastolic murmur, following an opening snap in mitral stenosis. (E) The presystolic murmur of mitral stenosis. (F) The continuous murmur of a persistent ductus arteriosus.

pulmonary stenosis most intense at the third or fourth left intercostal space. The murmurs of aortic and pulmonary stenosis are often loud and accompanied by thrills.

A systolic murmur due to high flow in the pulmonary artery is characteristic of atrial septal defect but also occurs in conditions associated with a high cardiac output such as pregnancy, thyrotoxicosis and anaemia. These murmurs are usually of no more than grade 3 intensity and are not associated with thrills.

Quite frequently, particularly in children, midsystolic murmurs may be heard in the pulmonary area for which no organic cause can be found. These may be termed 'functional' or 'benign'. Such murmurs are neither intense nor accompanied by a thrill. They usually vary with position and respiration.

Pansystolic (holosystolic) murmurs persist from the first to the second heart sound and only occur as a result of mitral regurgitation, tricuspid regurgitation or ventricular septal defect, for it is only in these conditions that a pressure difference exists across the defective valve or septum throughout systole (Fig. 4.8B). In mitral regurgitation, the murmur is maximal at or just internal to the apex beat, and radiates into the axilla. It may be maximal in late systole.

The murmur of tricuspid regurgitation is usually loudest in the xiphisternal region, or at the lower left sternal edge. It frequently radiates to the apex and may therefore be readily confused with that of mitral regurgitation, but differs in becoming louder on inspiration, due to the increase in venous return at this time.

The murmur of ventricular septal defect is usually loud and is maximal at the lower left sternal edge.

Murmurs may be confined to early or late systole; those associated with a prolapsed mitral cusp characteristically follow a midsystolic click.

Assessing the significance of a systolic murmur

One can usually determine the cause of a systolic murmur by taking into account its location and radiation, its intensity, its character and its association with other abnormal findings. The duration of the murmur is also of value if one can be certain whether it is midsystolic or pansystolic, but even experts may be unsure on this point.

In aortic stenosis, there is usually a loud murmur at the lower left sternal edge and aortic area which is associated with a thrill, a small flat pulse and left ventricular hypertrophy. If the valve cusps are not calcified, there is an early systolic ('ejection') click; if the stenosis is severe, there may be reversed splitting of the second sound.

In aortic valve sclerosis, a common finding in the elderly, there is an aortic systolic murmur in the absence of any of the other features of aortic stenosis.

In pulmonary stenosis, the loud murmur in the pulmonary or lower left sternal area is accompanied by right ventricular hypertrophy, a soft and late pulmonary component of the second sound and a systolic thrill.

In severe mitral regurgitation, the apical systolic murmur, which is well heard from cardiac apex to axilla, is usually accompanied by left ventricular enlargement, a third heart sound and a mid-diastolic flow murmur. In tricuspid regurgitation, the murmur in the tricuspid area is usually increased by inspiration, and is associated with systolic pulsation in the jugular veins.

It is of particular importance to determine whether a systolic murmur is of the 'benign' variety, for the misinterpretation of such a murmur as organic may lead to unwarranted cardiac invalidism. Benign systolic murmurs are seldom of more than grade 2 intensity, are never pansystolic, are usually best heard in the pulmonary area and are not associated with cardiac enlargement or with abnormal heart sounds. Similar murmurs are encountered in pregnancy, thyrotoxicosis and anaemia, and these conditions should be excluded before a murmur is accepted as being of no significance. The pulmonary systolic murmur of atrial septal defect resembles a benign systolic murmur but is accompanied by wide splitting of the second heart sound, and often by a mid-diastolic murmur due to high flow across the tricuspid valve. One can usually be confident of the benign nature of a murmur on physical examination alone. Only if there are other features such as cardiomegaly or abnormal sounds is further investigation with ECG, radiography and echocardiography necessary.

Diastolic murmurs

Diastolic murmurs are of three main varieties: early diastolic, mid-diastolic and presystolic.

Early (immediate) diastolic murmurs

These murmurs occur shortly after closure of the aortic or pulmonary valves at the beginning of diastole (Fig. 4.8C). They are due to regurgitation through one or other of these valves when pressure in the aorta or pulmonary artery exceeds that of the related ventricle. The murmur decreases in intensity as diastole continues. The murmur is usually soft, high-pitched and blowing, and is best heard by using the diaphragm chest piece with the patient sitting forward, in full expiration. The murmur of aortic regurgitation is usually loudest at the third or fourth left intercostal space close to the sternum, but is occasionally maximal in the second right intercostal space.

The uncommon early diastolic murmur of pulmonary regurgitation (the Graham Steell murmur) is best heard in the left second, third and fourth intercostal spaces. It is similar in character to that of aortic regurgitation but is increased by inspiration and is accompanied by signs of pulmonary hypertension.

Mid-diastolic murmurs

Mid-diastolic murmurs are associated with flow through the atrioventricular valves and necessarily start an appreciable time after the second heart sound. The most important cause is mitral stenosis, in which there is a low-pitched murmur maximal in a localized area at or internal to the apex beat. The murmur is most easily heard with the bell of the stethoscope and with the patient lying in the left lateral position, preferably after exercise (Fig. 4.8D). It is frequently associated with an opening snap, a presystolic murmur and a loud first heart sound.

In tricuspid stenosis, a murmur due to a similar mechanism occurs, but in this condition it is maximal in the xiphisternal or lower left sternal region. This murmur is often of a rather scratchy character and is accentuated by inspiration. Mid-diastolic murmurs may also occur when there is a large flow through atrioventricular valves. Such flow murmurs in the mitral area occur in association with mitral regurgitation, ventricular septal defect and persistent ductus arteriosus. A high-flow tricuspid murmur occurs in atrial septal defect. Another mid-diastolic murmur is that due to rheumatic valvulitis (the Carey Coombs murmur). A mid-diastolic murmur may also be heard, in the absence of mitral valve disease, in patients with severe aortic regurgitation (the Austin Flint murmur). This may be due to the aortic regurgitant flow pushing the aortic cusp of the mitral valve across the mitral valve orifice, thereby causing turbulence as blood is also flowing simultaneously from the left atrium to the left ventricle.

Presystolic murmurs

Presystolic murmurs are produced when atrial systole propels blood through narrowed mitral or tricuspid valves. The presystolic murmur of mitral stenosis leads up to the loud first sound of that condition (Fig. 4.8E); it is most easily heard with the patient lying in the left lateral position with the bell of the stethoscope placed at or internal to the apex beat. The presystolic murmur of tricuspid stenosis is maximal in the xiphisternal region or at the lower left sternal edge and is accentuated by inspiration.

Continuous murmurs

The term 'continuous' is applied to a murmur which starts during systole and continues into diastole; it is not necessarily continuous throughout the cardiac cycle. The commonest types are the venous hum and the murmur of persistent ductus arteriosus.

The venous hum is common in childhood, but may be heard in anaemic or pregnant adults. It is due to high blood flow in the jugular veins and can be diminished or abolished by lying the patient flat, or by constricting the veins by pressure. It is usually loudest in the neck, but may be audible over the upper chest.

The murmur in persistent ductus arteriosus is caused by the flow of blood from the high-pressure aorta into the low-pressure pulmonary artery. It is maximal in the left second intercostal space or under the left clavicle. It increases in intensity throughout systole, is maximal at the time of the second heart sound, and diminishes during diastole (Fig. 4.8F). It often has a 'machinery' or whirring quality. Similar murmurs are caused by systemic, pulmonary and coronary arteriovenous fistulae, and by rupture of an aneurysm of a sinus of Valsalva (see p. 343).

Pericardial friction (or rub)

As roughened visceral and parietal layers of pericardium slide over one another, they produce a harsh creaking sound which may be likened to the noise made by two pieces of sandpaper rubbing together. As the movement occurs during ventricular systole, ventricular diastole and atrial systole, the rub may be present at one or all of these times. It may be heard all over the precordium, or only at a localized site. It usually sounds superficial and can be accentuated by leaning the patient forward or by pressing the stethoscope diaphragm firmly on the chest. It can occur in acute pericarditis of any cause, as well as in uraemic pericarditis and during the course of acute myocardial infarction. In the latter condition, it is often evanescent, lasting for only a few minutes or hours.

GENERAL EXAMINATION OF PATIENTS WITH CARDIAC DISEASE

In addition to a detailed examination of the heart, a more general examination may reveal useful additional clues regarding underlying cardiac problems. The systemic manifestations of cardiac disease are considered later in the relevant chapters, but include:

- cyanosis and clubbing in congenital heart disease (Chapter 15);
- splinter haemorrhages, clubbing, Osler's nodes and splenomegaly in patients with subacute bacterial endocarditis (Chapter 14);
- xanthelasma and tendon xanthomata in patients with hyper-lipidaemia (Chapter 7).

The general examination of patients with cardiac disease should also include an assessment of additional features of right heart failure, assessing the presence of ankle oedema and hepatomegaly (Chapter 10).

Further reading

Boudreau Conover, M. & Tilkian, A. G. (1993) *Understanding Heart Sounds and Murmurs with an Intro-duction to Lung Sounds*. Philadelphia, Saunders.

Perloff, J. K. (1986) *Physical Examination of the Heart and Circulation*. Philadelphia: Saunders.

Turner, R. W. D. & Gold, R. G. (1984) *Auscultation of the Heart*. Edinburgh: Churchill Livingstone.

Non-invasive Investigation of the Heart

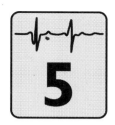

5

Cardiac investigations can be divided into those that necessitate the placement of catheters and other devices inside the heart ('invasive' investigations) and those that do not ('non-invasive' investigations). Currently, a great deal of both anatomical and physiological information can be gained from non-invasive investigations. Invasive investigations are still necessary to determine a patient's suitability for various interventions (such as cardiac surgery or coronary angioplasty) but are less commonly required to establish a diagnosis. Non-invasive investigations include electrocardiography (see Chapter 2), plain radiography, echocardiography, exercise testing, 24-h ECG monitoring, radionuclide imaging and magnetic resonance imaging.

Plain radiography

Plain radiographs are usually taken in postero-anterior and lateral views; oblique positions are sometimes used.

The normal cardiac contour

In the postero-anterior projection, the patient faces the X-ray cassette. In this view (Fig. 5.1) the right border of the heart consists (from above downwards):

- superior vena cava;
- ascending aorta;
- right atrium;
- inferior vena cava.

The left border of the heart is formed by:

- aortic arch;
- pulmonary artery and its left main branch;
- left ventricle.

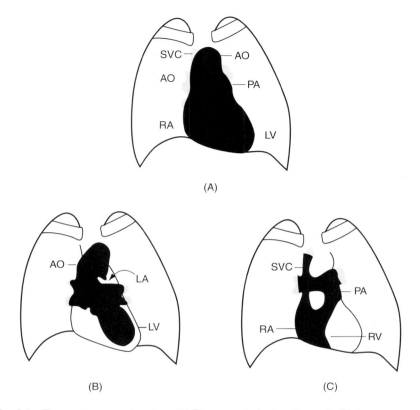

Fig. 5.1 The postero-anterior view. (A) The normal chest radiograph. (B) Appearances of the left side of the heart, after injection of radio-opaque material into the left atrium, showing the positions of the left atrium (LA), the left ventricle (LV) and the aorta (AO). (C) Appearances of the right side of the heart after injection of radio-opaque material into the superior vena cava (SVC). The positions of the right atrium (RA), the right ventricle (RV), and the pulmonary artery (PA), are shown.

Between the left ventricle and the diaphragm, there may be a small triangular shadow due to an epicardial fat pad. In this view, the maximum transverse diameter of the heart does not usually exceed 50% of the chest, measured from the inner aspects of the ribs, although 'cardiothoracic ratios' greater than this are sometimes seen in normal individuals.

In the lateral view (Fig. 5.2), the anterior border of the heart is formed by:

- pulmonary artery;
- right ventricle.

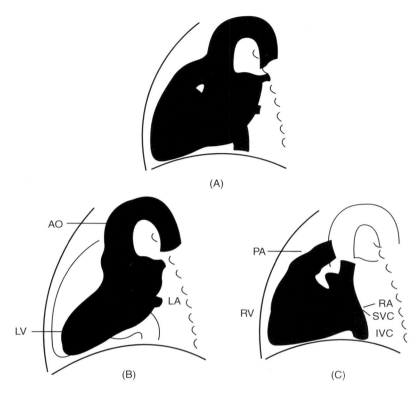

Fig. 5.2   The lateral view. (A) Normal chest radiograph. (B) Appearances of the left side of the heart, after injection of radio-opaque contrast medium into the left atrium, showing the positions of the left atrium (LA), left ventricle (LV) and aorta (AO). (C) Appearances of the right side of the heart after injection of contrast medium into the right atrium showing positions of superior and inferior venae cavae (SVC, IVC), right atrium (RA), right ventricle (RV) and pulmonary artery (PA).

The posterior border is formed by:

- left atrium;
- left ventricle.

Abnormalities of the cardiac contour

Enlargement of the left ventricle, which is most frequently due to hypertension, ischaemic heart disease, aortic valve disease and mitral regurgitation, produces depression and elongation of the cardiac apex (Fig. 5.3). Left ventricular enlargement is better seen in the lateral view.

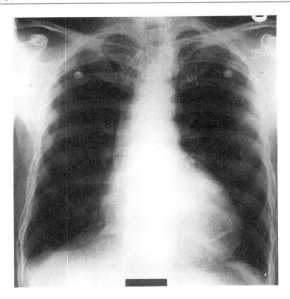

Fig. 5.3 Left ventricular enlargement. Depression and elongation of the cardiac apex in left ventricular enlargement.

A normal left ventricle may be displaced posteriorly by an enlarged right ventricle.

Right ventricular enlargement, usually the consequence of pulmonary hypertension or pulmonary stenosis, produces an elevation of the cardiac apex in the postero-anterior view, and in the lateral views of the heart makes the normally straight anterior border of the heart bulge towards or impinge on the sternum.

The body of the *left atrium* enlarges posteriorly and to the right, but its appendage protrudes to the left. Thus, in the postero-anterior view, the left atrial appendage is seen on the left border of the heart between the pulmonary artery and the left ventricle (Fig. 5.4), whereas the main body of the left atrium forms a dense shadow within the right atrial border, or protrudes to the right above the right atrium on the right side of the heart. Left atrial enlargement is best diagnosed in the lateral view, in which it can be seen displacing the barium-filled oesophagus posteriorly.

The *right atrium* enlarges mainly to the right and, in the postero-anterior view, makes the right border of the heart more prominent.

Enlargement of the *ascending aorta*, as from post-stenotic dilatation in aortic stenosis or from aneurysm of the ascending aorta, is seen as a projection to the right (Fig. 5.5). The sclerotic 'uncoiled' aorta of the elderly produces a loop above the heart shadow (Fig. 5.6).

A *pericardial effusion* causes generalized enlargement of the cardiac silhouette, with both lateral borders being smoothly convex (Fig. 5.7).

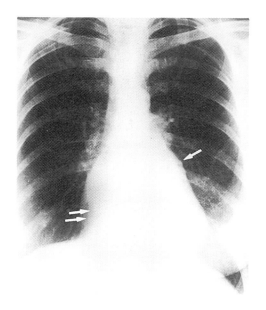

Fig. 5.4 Left atrial enlargement. The bulge produced by the left atrial appendage (arrowed) is seen on the left border of the heart between the positions of the pulmonary artery and left ventricle. This results in 'straightening' of the left heart border. Enlargement of the left atrium causes a double shadow to appear in the right heart border (arrows).

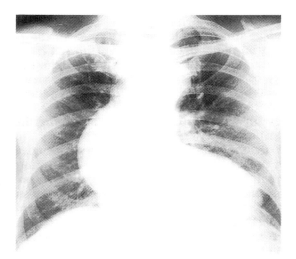

Fig. 5.5 Dilatation of the ascending aorta. Ascending aortic dilatation causes expansion of the upper right heart border. This example is due to the presence of a syphilitic aneurysm in the ascending aorta.

Calcification within the heart can sometimes be suspected on a plain radiograph (Fig. 5.8), but more specialized investigations are necessary for confirmation. Calcification in the mitral valve, which is usually rheumatic, is best visualized in the lateral view in which it is seen in the posterior third of the cardiac mass. The aortic valve is located more

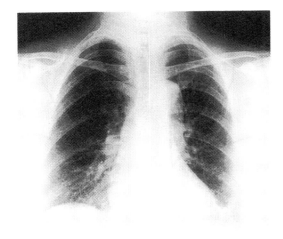

Fig. 5.6 Unfolded aorta.

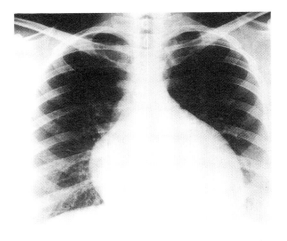

Fig. 5.7 Gross cardiac enlargement due to a pericardial effusion. Both lateral borders of the heart are smoothly convex.

in the centre of the heart; in the postero-anterior view it is situated just to the left of the spine. Calcification of the pericardium is best seen in a penetrated lateral view (Fig. 5.9).

Abnormalities of the pulmonary circulation

The plain chest radiograph is of great value in demonstrating abnormalities of the pulmonary circulation.

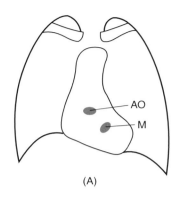 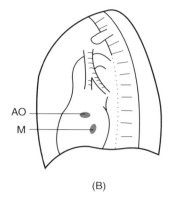

(A)   (B)

Fig. 5.8   The position of the aortic (AO) and mitral (M) valve calcification in the postero-anterior view (A) and lateral view (B).

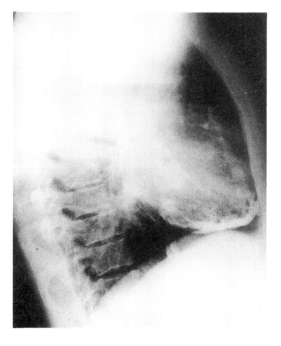

Fig. 5.9   Pericardial calcification. Lateral chest X-ray. A 'shell' of calcium is present outlining the inferior aspect of the ventricles.

Pulmonary venous hypertension, as occurs in left ventricular failure and mitral stenosis, is revealed by:

- *dilatation of the pulmonary veins*, particularly those draining the upper zones (upper lobe venous diversion);

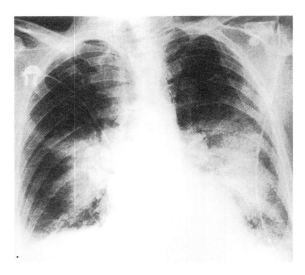

Fig. 5.10 Pulmonary oedema. Chest X-ray of a patient with severe pulmonary oedema following myocardial infarction. Widespread opacification is evident throughout the lung fields due to alveolar oedema.

- *interstitial oedema* causing thin horizontal lines at the bases (Kerley's lines), due to fluid in the interlobular septa and distended lymphatics;
- *alveolar oedema* causing a fluffy opacification (Fig. 5.10) spreading out from the hilar region, often providing a 'butterfly' appearance. The oedema can occasionally be unilateral.

In moderate pulmonary arterial hypertension, the main right and left pulmonary arteries are enlarged, although the more peripheral arteries may be normal. In severe pulmonary hypertension, the major pulmonary arteries, which are greatly dilated, contrast with narrowed peripheral pulmonary arteries; the major arteries appear to be 'cut off'.

When there is increased pulmonary blood flow, as in atrial septal defect, ventricular septal defect and persistent ductus arteriosus, both main and peripheral pulmonary arteries are dilated (Fig. 5.11). Fluoroscopy may show a vigorous pulsation (the 'hilar dance').

When the pulmonary blood flow is decreased, as in pulmonary stenosis, the pulmonary arteries are poorly seen. However, the main and left pulmonary arteries may be dilated by the jet of blood emerging from the stenosis.

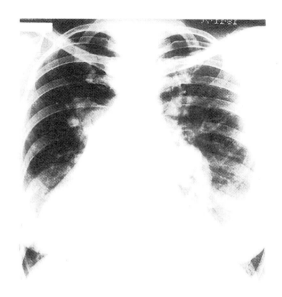

Fig. 5.11 Atrial septal defect. There is marked dilatation of the pulmonary conus and proximal pulmonary arteries. In this patient there is 'pruning' of the distal pulmonary markings due to the development of pulmonary hypertension.

Echocardiography

Modern echocardiography machines utilize ultrasound waves in four different ways to derive information about the structure and function of the heart. These are:

- M-mode echocardiography;
- two-dimensional echocardiography;
- Doppler ultrasonography (pulsed wave and continuous wave);
- colour flow mapping.

The first two modalities (M-mode and two-dimensional echocardiography) provide anatomical information about the heart. This includes the dimension of cardiac chambers, the thickness of the cardiac walls and the structure of the heart valves. Doppler ultrasonography and colour flow mapping provide functional information about the direction and velocity of blood flow through the heart.

M-mode echocardiography

A piezo-electric crystal, which acts as both a transmitter and receiver, is used to generate high-frequency pulses of short duration. These travel through body tissues at a known velocity but some are reflected back at boundaries between tissues that have different acoustic densities. Measurement of the time taken for the signal to be reflected back to the crystal allows the machine to calculate and display the distance from the crystal to the various boundaries crossed by the ultrasound beam. This is demonstrated in Fig. 5.12.

Two-dimensional echocardiography

In two-dimensional echocardiography, multiple M-mode beams are 'fired' in an arc to allow real-time planar imaging of the heart. The 'firing' of multiple M-mode beams can be achieved either with a single crystal which rotates within the transducer (so-called mechanical transducer) or with multiple crystals in the transducer which are electronically switched in sequence. Two-dimensional echocardiography can be used to 'position' the M-mode cursor for specific measurements (Figs 5.13 and 5.14). Used together, M-mode and two-dimensional

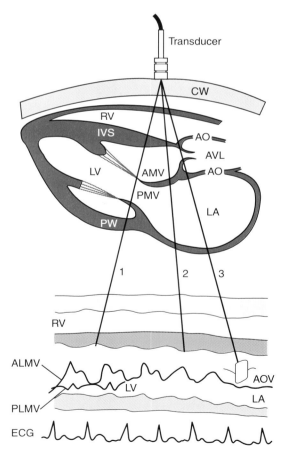

Fig. 5.12 The transducer is angled in different directions to permit study of the various cardiac structures. (1) The beam traverses the right ventricle (RV), interventricular septum (IVS), and anterior and posterior leaflets of the mitral valve (ALMV and PLMV). These leaflets separate abruptly as the blood flows rapidly from the left atrium to the left ventricle. As the flow decreases they approximate only to be separated again when atrial contraction propels more blood into the ventricle. (2) Provides good views of the RV, septum, ALMV and left atrium. (3) Shows separation of the aortic valve cusps in systole.

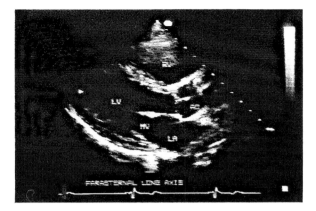

Fig. 5.13 Normal echocardiogram corresponding to Fig. 5.12, showing right ventricle (RV), left ventricle (LV), left atrium (LA), mitral valve (MV) and aortic valve (AO).

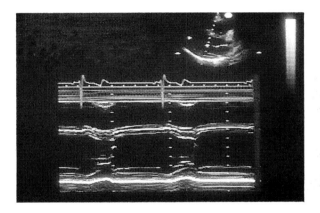

Fig. 5.14 Use of two-dimensional image to position the M-mode cursor. This allows measurement of the right ventricular and left ventricular diameters, the interventricular septal thickness and the left ventricular posterior wall thickness.

echocardiography are of great value in diagnosing and assessing the severity of the following conditions:

- mitral stenosis;
- aortic stenosis;
- left ventricular dilatation;
- right ventricular dilatation;
- left ventricular hypertrophy (Fig. 5.15);
- infective endocarditis;
- atrial myxoma;

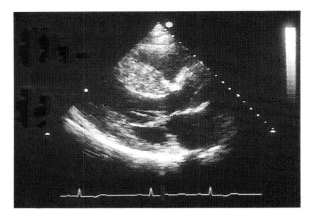

Fig. 5.15   Parasternal long axis showing marked thickening of the interventricular septum in a patient with hypertrophic cardiomyopathy.

- pericardial effusion and tamponade (Fig. 5.16);
- congenital heart disease.

Doppler examination

This technique makes use of the familiar phenomenon whereby the pitch of a sound appears to become higher as it moves towards an object and falls as it moves away. In the body, the red blood cells act as moving targets which reflect the ultrasound wave back to its source. Depending on the speed and direction of movement of the red blood cells, there will be a frequency shift in the returning ultrasound waves. If the red cells are moving away from the transducer, the reflected waves will have a lower frequency and longer wavelength; if blood is moving towards the transducer, the frequency of the reflected waves will be higher. This 'frequency shift' detected at the transducer can thus tell us about blood velocities within the heart. Two forms of Doppler examination are commonly used. These are termed pulsed-wave and continuous-wave Doppler ultrasonography.

Pulsed Doppler examination.   A single transducer is used, which first emits a brief ultrasound pulse and then switches to receive the return-ing signal. Because ultrasound has a constant velocity in the body, the depth of the target can be determined by the interval between emission and return of the signal. The time interval and, therefore, the depth of the target area being examined can be varied as required, and can be correlated with a simultaneously recorded cross-sectional echocardiogram, thus locating precisely the site of the area being exam-ined. Unfortunately, there is a limit to the rate at which pulses can be

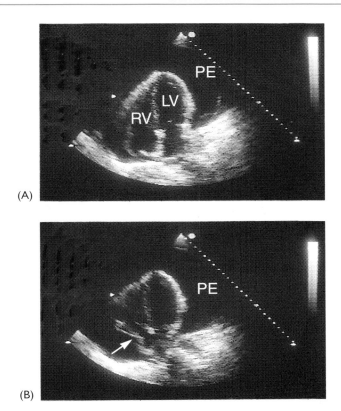

(A)

(B)

Fig. 5.16   (A and B) Massive pericardial effusion (PE) which appears as an echo-free space around the heart. (B) Diastolic 'collapse' of the free wall of the right atrium (arrowed). This is a sign of cardiac tamponade. Diastolic collapse of the right ventricle may also occur.

generated, because one wave may not have returned before the next is generated, leading to distortion (aliasing) of the signal. This prevents the recognition of high velocities. Pulsed Doppler, therefore, is used to sample blood velocities at specific sites within the heart, but cannot be used to measure the high velocities encountered with moderately or severely stenosed valves.

Continuous-wave (CW) Doppler examination. This enables high velocities to be recorded. In this technique, one transducer continuously emits ultrasound, which is detected by a separate receiver. Although continuous-wave Doppler ultrasonography can record high velocities, it cannot identify the depth at which the signal originated. Using continuous-wave Doppler, the pressure gradient across a stenotic lesion can be calculated from the Bernoulli equation:

Pressure gradient $= 4 \times (\text{Velocity})^2$

Doppler examination is particularly useful in assessing valvular stenoses.

Colour flow mapping

This technique essentially superimposes multiple Doppler signals on a two-dimensional echocardiographic image, allowing the direction and velocity of blood flow through the heart to be identified and displayed in colour.

Blood flow towards the transducer is conventionally known as red and that away from the transducer as blue. Very high velocities (for example, through stenotic or regurgitant valves or through small ventricular septal defects) usually appear as white or green 'plumes'.

Colour flow examination has proved of great value in identifying:

- mitral regurgitation;
- aortic regurgitation;
- ventricular septal defects and other congenital abnormalities;
- prosthetic valve dysfunction.

Transoesophageal echocardiography

In this technique, the ultrasound probe is mounted on a modified gastroscope and is passed into the oesophagus under light sedation. The technique is safe and usually achieves better images of the heart than the conventional transthoracic approach (Fig. 5.17). Transoesophageal echocardiography is particularly useful in the following circumstances:

- when conventional transthoracic imaging has failed to produce diagnostic information. This is common in obese patients or those with chronic lung disease in whom a suitable echocardiographic window cannot be identified;
- patients with suspected atrial masses not clearly seen on transthoracic echo (Fig. 5.18);
- patients with suspected atrial septal defects (Fig. 5.19);
- patients with suspected aortic dissection (Fig. 5.20);
- examination of the mitral valve with a view to mitral valve repair;
- identification of complications of infective endocarditis such as vegetations, aortic root abscess cavities, etc;
- intraoperative monitoring during cardiac surgery.

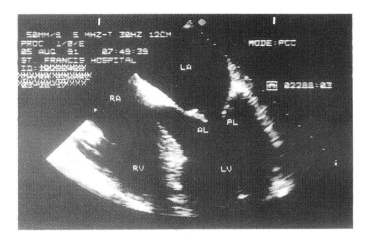

Fig. 5.17   Four-chamber view from the transoesophageal approach showing the left atrium (LA), left ventricle (LV), right atrium (RA) and right ventricle (RV). Note the close proximity of the probe to the anterior and posterior mitral valve leaflets (AL and PL), making transoesophogeal echocardiography an important investigation in patients with mitral valve disease.

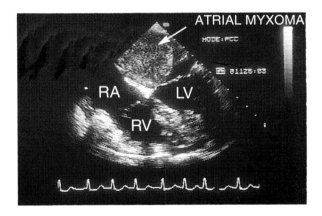

Fig. 5.18   A large left atrial myxoma seen on transoesophageal echo. This is attached to the inter-atrial septum and fills most of the left atrial cavity.

Exercise testing

Exercise testing is commonly used as a diagnostic test in patients with suspected angina but is also used for a number of other indications including:

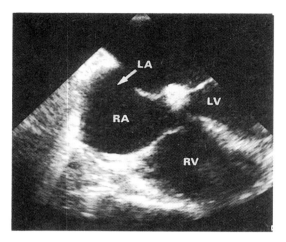

Fig. 5.19 Transoesophageal echo. The four chambers of the heart are shown. LA = left atrium, RA = right atrium, RV = right ventricle, LV = left ventricle. The patient has an atrial septal defect. The communication between the left atrium and right atrium is arrowed.

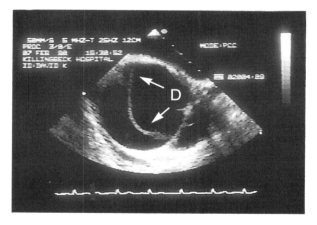

Fig. 5.20 Dissection of the ascending aorta. The dissection flap (D) is clearly visible.

- risk stratification following myocardial infarction;
- provocation of arrhythmias.

The patient is asked to exercise on either a treadmill or a bicycle. Several different exercise protocols exist of which the most widely used is the Bruce protocol. In this, the treadmill starts at a comfortable walking pace (approximately 3 miles per hour). The speed and incline of the treadmill are then both increased at 3-min intervals. A 12-lead

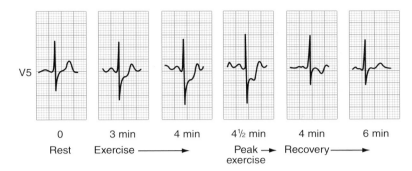

Fig. 5.21 Exercise ECG. The changes occurring in lead V5 throughout an exercise test are illustrated. During exercise there is a progressive depression of the ST segment, which returns to normal in the subsequent recovery period.

electrocardiogram is recorded throughout the test. The interpretation of the treadmill test depends on:

- the amount of exercise that the patients can achieve. This will depend on other factors such as age and fitness as well as the presence or absence of heart disease;
- whether or not the patient develops symptoms (such as chest pain) while on the treadmill;
- the presence or absence of ECG changes during the test or in the recovery period. Horizontal or down-sloping depression of the ST segment of 1 mm or greater is usually regarded as evidence of myocardial ischaemia (Fig. 5.21). Up-sloping ST segment depression is common in normal individuals and should not be regarded as pathological.

24-h ECG recording

With this technique, a continuous recording is made of two electrocardiographic leads for a period of 24 h. The patient has four electrodes attached which are connected to a device worn on a belt around the waist. The recording device weighs 1–2 lb and records the information either on an analog cassette tape or digitally in a solid-state system. This technique is particularly useful for patients with suspected paroxysmal arrhythmias. The patient can carry out normal activities during the recording period, and, indeed, should be encouraged to do whatever has provoked the symptoms in the past. An example of the usefulness of this type of investigation is illustrated in Fig. 5.22.

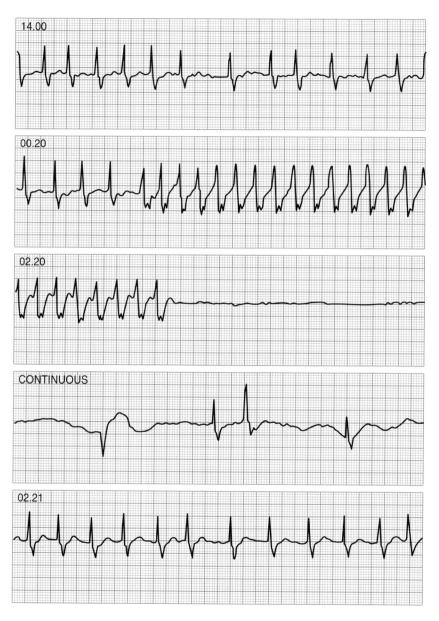

Fig. 5.22 The patient had a history of palpitations and syncope. On commencement of the tape (14.00) he was in atrial fibrillation. At 00.20 he developed sustained ventricular tachycardia. This lasted for 2 hours. On termination of the tachycardia (02.20) there was a prolonged asystolic pause followed by a ventricular escape beat. The patient subsequently continued in atrial fibrillation.

Radionuclide imaging

In radionuclide imaging, isotopes are injected through a peripheral vein. Depending on the isotope used, this may bind either to the myocardium or to the red blood cells. The radiation emitted is then detected by a gamma camera placed over the chest. These tests are usually employed in patients with coronary artery disease (or suspected coronary artery disease).

There are two types of radionuclide investigation:

Myocardial perfusion studies

Certain radiopharmaceuticals, of which thallium-201 is the most commonly used, are taken up into the myocardium in proportion to the regional blood flow. They therefore do not concentrate in areas of ischaemia or fibrosis. Thallium imaging has been found to be of greatest value in the detection of transient myocardial ischaemia in patients with suspected angina pectoris (Fig. 5.23). If the radio-isotope is injected intravenously during an exercise test at the time when the patient develops chest pain or ST depression, a 'cold spot' will be seen corresponding to the area of ischaemia, while the rest of the myocardium will take up the isotope. If nuclear imaging is repeated some 4 h later, when no ischaemia is present, the 'cold spot' will be seen to have disappeared. A reversible defect, therefore, provides evidence of impaired myocardial perfusion, raising the possibility that the patient might benefit from a revascularization procedure, either coronary artery bypass grafting or angioplasty. An area of previous myocardial infarction will also appear as a perfusion defect on the initial exercise scan, but the perfusion defect is irreversible and is still present on the resting scan 4 h later.

Thallium scanning is relatively sensitive and specific. However, because of the cost of thallium, it is frequently reserved as a second-line procedure to exercise testing. There are some situations in which a thallium scan is particularly useful:

- *in patients with an equivocal exercise ECG.* A thallium scan may clarify the diagnosis, without resort to coronary angiography;
- *to determine the functional significance of moderate coronary lesions.* Angiography in certain patients may demonstrate moderate coronary stenoses. If it is unclear whether such lesions are haemodynamically significant, then a perfusion study demonstrating reversible ischaemia in the appropriate territory may help in deciding whether the patient's symptoms are likely to benefit from some form of revascularization.
- *in patients incapable of performing an exercise stress test.* Many patients cannot perform a treadmill or bicycle exercise test adequately because of other medical conditions such as arthritis

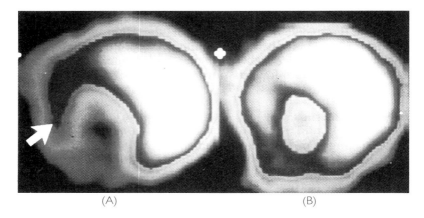

(A)   (B)

Fig. 5.23 Thallium scan. (A) Peak exercise. There is a defect in thallium uptake (arrowed), corresponding to an apical perfusion deficit. (B) After rest for 4 hours, uptake normalizes in this region. This reversible defect is indicative of ischaemia. A non-reversible, fixed defect would indicate infarction.

or intermittent claudication. In these circumstances, a thallium scan can be carried out with a pharmacological 'stress' to mimic exercise. The two most commonly used agents for this purpose are dobutamine and dipyridamole. Dobutamine mimics exercise by increasing the heart rate and blood pressure. Dipyridamole is a coronary vasodilator that produces greater dilatation in non-diseased than in diseased coronary vessels. As a result a 'coronary steal' phenomenon may occur, whereby blood flow increases in the non-diseased coronary segments at the expense of the diseased. Just as for exercise testing, this will show up as a perfusion defect on thallium imaging.

Thallium imaging is relatively sensitive and specific, but unfortunately the cost of thallium and the degree of skill and experience necessary for optimal interpretation limit its application.

Radionuclide ventriculography

The most common technique for the imaging of left ventricular function involves the use of technetium-labelled red cells so that the pool of blood in the left ventricle can be detected. By using the ECG to 'gate' the images ('gated pool scan'), segments of the cardiac cycle from successive beats can be superimposed. By obtaining 20 or more exposures during each cardiac cycle, it is possible to record the radionuclide equivalent of a cine-angiogram. This technique allows the evaluation of many aspects of left ventricular function including end-systolic and end-diastolic volumes from which the ejection fraction is calculated.

Regional wall motion abnormalities such as ventricular aneurysm can also be identified. As with myocardial perfusion imaging, radionuclide scans can be carried out during exercise or pharmacological stress. In normal individuals, the ejection fraction should increase during exercise and failure to do so usually indicates exercise-induced ischaemia. Careful examination of regional wall movement both before and during exercise can sometimes identify areas of local ischaemia, which will show normal movement at rest but will become akinetic during exercise.

Magnetic resonance imaging

This is a new and exciting imaging technique which is entirely non-invasive and does not require the use of contrast media. Like echo-cardiography, magnetic resonance imaging (MRI) can provide functional information related to the direction and velocity of blood flow in addition to anatomical information. Early interest has focused on imaging in congenital heart disease and in disease of the thoracic aorta. As technology advances, so imaging of smaller structures is likely to improve; one area currently being investigated is the use of MRI to detect patency of coronary artery bypass grafts.

Further reading

Campbell, R. W. F. & Murray, A. (1986) Dynamic Electrocardiography. Edinburgh: Churchill Livingstone.

Feigenbaum, H. (1986) Echocardiography, 4th edn. Philadelphia: Lea & Febiger.

Gerson, M. C. (Ed.) (1987) Cardiac Nuclear Medicine. New York: McGraw Hill.

Granger, R. G. & Allison, D. J. (Eds) (1986) Diagnostic Radiology. Edinburgh: Churchill Livingstone.

Jefferson, K. & Rees, S. (1980) Clinical Cardiac Radiology, 2nd edn. London: Butterworth.

Mendel, D. & Oldershaw, P. (1986) Cardiac Catheterization, 3rd edn. Oxford: Blackwell.

Popp, R. L. (1990) Echocardiography. New England Journal of Medicine 323: 101, 165.

Task Force on Assessment of Cardiovascular Procedures (1986) Guidelines for clinical use of cardiac radionuclide imaging. Circulation 74: 1469A.

Task Force on Assessment of Cardiovascular Procedures (1986). Guidelines for excercise testing. Circulation 74: 653A.

Invasive Investigations

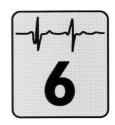

6

As a result of advances in non-invasive cardiac investigations, cardiac catheterization is now required less frequently to establish a diagnosis. However, the proliferation of interventional techniques for the treatment of heart disease (including cardiac surgery, coronary angioplasty, percutaneous balloon valvuloplasty) has meant that cardiac catheterization is now being performed more frequently than ever to assess the patient's suitability for all forms of interventional treatment.

Invasive diagnostic techniques can be considered under the following headings:

- right heart catheterization;
- left heart catheterization;
- coronary angiography;
- invasive electrophysiological studies.

Cardiac catheterization

Right heart catheterization

Under local anaesthesia, a catheter is introduced percutaneously into the femoral or basilic vein and advanced to the right atrium. It is manoeuvred under fluoroscopic control through the tricuspid valve to the right ventricle, thence to the pulmonary artery and finally wedged in a distal pulmonary artery. The pulmonary arterial wedge (pulmonary capillary) tracing so obtained is an indirect measurement of pressure in the left atrium (Fig. 6.1).

If appropriate radiological facilities are not available, a Swan–Ganz catheter with a balloon close to its tip may be used. If the balloon is inflated when the right atrium is reached, the tip will 'float' into a pulmonary artery. If the balloon is impacted in the artery, a pulmonary artery wedge tracing is obtained.

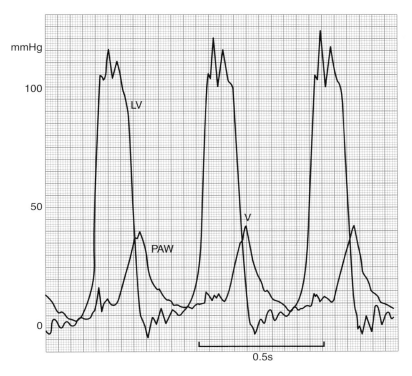

Fig. 6.1   Pulmonary artery wedge tracing. A pulmonary artery wedge tracing (PAW) is shown together with a left ventricular tracing (LV). There is a prominent V wave in the pulmonary wedge tracing due to mitral regurgitation.

If there is a septal defect, the catheter may be passed through this into the left side of the heart; if there is a persistent ductus arteriosus, this may be traversed.

The catheter can be used to record pressures in the different chambers of the heart and also to obtain blood samples from each vessel and chamber. Normal cardiovascular pressures are summarized in Table 6.1. Blood samples are usually taken for oxygen content or saturation. When a left-to-right shunt is present, the blood is found to be more oxygenated in the affected chamber and beyond than it is in the great veins:

- *persistent ductus arteriosus*, the oxygen saturation in the left pulmonary artery exceeds that in the right ventricle;
- *ventricular septal defect*, the oxygen saturation in the right ventricle and pulmonary artery is greater than that in the right atrium;
- *atrial septal defect*, the oxygen saturation in the right atrium exceeds that in the superior and inferior venae cavae.

Table 6.1 Normal cardiovascular pressures (mmHg)

	Mean	Range
Right atrium – mean	4	0–8
Right ventricle		
systolic	25	15–30
end diastolic	4	0–8
Pulmonary artery		
systolic	25	15–30
diastolic	10	5–15
mean	15	10–20
Pulmonary artery wedge – mean	10	5–14
Left atrium – mean	7	4–12
Left ventricle		
systolic	120	90–140
end diastolic	7	4–12
Aorta		
systolic	120	90–140
diastolic	70	60–90
mean	85	70–105

The presence of valve stenoses can be demonstrated:

- pulmonary stenosis can be confirmed by showing a systolic pressure difference between the pulmonary artery and right ventricle. This can be distinguished from infundibular stenosis in which the pressure gradient lies within the outflow tract of the right ventricle;
- tricuspid stenosis is present if the diastolic pressure in the right atrium is higher than that in the right ventricle.

Cardiac output can also be measured during right heart catheterization. The most commonly used method for measuring cardiac output utilizes a Swan–Ganz catheter with two separate lumens, one opening into the right atrium and the other to the pulmonary artery. This technique is based on the principle that the concentration of an injected substance is dependent on the volume injected and the volume of blood into which it is diluted. In this technique, cold saline of known volume and temperature is injected via the catheter into the right atrium. The temperature is then sampled in the pulmonary artery as the cold saline, diluted in the blood, passes the thermistor at the catheter tip. The transient fall in blood temperature is, therefore, indirectly related to the cardiac output, i.e. the greater the fall in temperature, the lower the cardiac output for a given volume of saline injected.

Left heart catheterization

Under local anaesthesia, a catheter is introduced into the femoral or brachial artery and advanced retrogradely until it reaches the aortic valve. The catheter can then be manipulated across the valve and into the left ventricle. The catheter is used to measure pressures or to deliver contrast injections (angiography).

Pressure measurements. Pressure gradients across the aortic and mitral valves can be measured in suspected aortic and mitral stenosis respectively, but these diagnoses are now more commonly made by echocardiography.

- *aortic stenosis* is assessed by pressure difference between the left ventricle and the aorta. This can be distinguished from cases of sub-aortic stenosis or hypertrophic cardiomyopathy, in which the pressure drop lies within the cavity of the left ventricle;
- *mitral stenosis* is assessed by the pressure difference between the pulmonary artery wedge and left ventricular pressures;
- measurement of the left ventricular end-diastolic pressure may be useful as an indicator of *left ventricular function.*

Ventriculography and aortography

The rapid injection of 30–40 ml of contrast medium by a power injector can be used to demonstrate the anatomy of the chambers of the heart and to look for evidence of valvular regurgitation. The images can be stored either on cine film at 25 to 50 frames per second, on analog video cassette, or digitally. Injection into the left ventricle (left ventricular angiography) is used to assess left ventricular function (Fig. 6.2) and also to look for mitral regurgitation. If the mitral valve is competent, there should not be any contrast leakage from the left ventricle into the left atrium. Similarly, injection of contrast into the ascending aorta will demonstrate whether or not there is significant aortic regurgitation.

Coronary angiography

This is by far the most commonly performed invasive cardiac investigation in Western countries. It is used both to establish whether or not a patient has significant coronary artery disease and to determine their suitability for interventional treatment including percutaneous transluminal coronary angioplasty and coronary artery bypass surgery. The procedure is carried out under local anaesthesia and often as a day case. After administering a local anaesthetic, fine plastic catheters (approximately 2 mm in diameter) are introduced. The most commonly used catheters are the Judkins shapes which are designed to be used from the femoral artery. Different catheters are generally used to cannulate the left and right coronary arteries (Fig. 6.4), although it is often

(A)
(B)

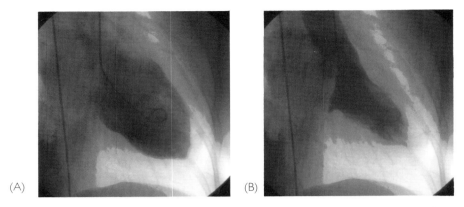

Fig. 6.2 Angiography demonstrating normal left ventricular function in a patient with competent mitral valve. (A) shows a frame taken at the end of diastole when the left ventricle is full of contrast. (B) shows a frame at the end of a systole when the ventricle has contracted and ejected blood into the aorta.

(A)
(B)

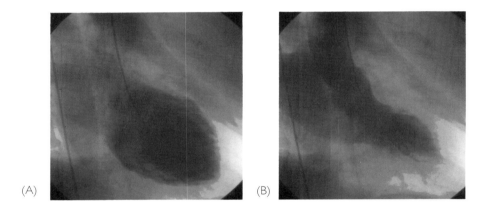

Fig. 6.3 (A) Left ventricular angiography in a patient with mitral valve regurgitation. Note the large amount of contrast medium which refluxes into the left atrium particularly during systole. This should be compared with the normal angiogram (B) in a patient with a competent mitral valve.

possible to cannulate both coronary vessels using a single catheter from the brachial approach. Multiple views are taken of both coronary arteries from different angles to ensure that all proximal segments of the arteries are adequately visualized. For each view, 5–10 ml of contrast medium is injected by hand and the films are recorded on to cine

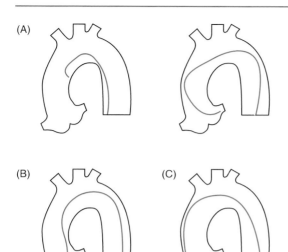

Fig. 6.4 Cardiac catheters. (A) A Judkins left coronary catheter advanced around the aortic arch to engage the left coronary artery. (B) Judkins right coronary catheter. (C) Pigtail catheter in aortic root.

film, video cassette or digital storage system. Examples of abnormalities seen at angiography are shown in Figs 6.5, 6.6 and 6.7.

Selective angiography is also the investigation of choice when re-examining patients who have recurrent symptoms following coronary artery bypass surgery. Specially shaped catheters are used to obtain views of the aorto-coronary vein grafts and also of the left internal mammary artery if this has been used as a conduit at the time of surgery.

All invasive procedures carry some risk for the patient but the risk of diagnostic coronary angiography with currently available equipment (soft-tipped catheters, non-ionic contrast media) should be very low. Most series report mortality rates of around 1 per 1000, with a risk of non-fatal stroke or myocardial infarction of 1 in 2000. Local femoral artery complications, such as haematoma or arterial dissection, are more common but are not usually severe.

Invasive electrophysiological studies

It is possible to position electrodes in various parts of the heart, having introduced them percutaneously through a peripheral vein (or rarely an artery). Thus, electrodes may be placed in juxtaposition to several sites in the atria and ventricles, and also adjacent to the bundle of His (Fig. 6.8). The sequence of activation of the heart may then be determined, and specific sites found where conduction is accelerated (as in the Wolff–Parkinson–White syndrome) or delayed (as in heart block).

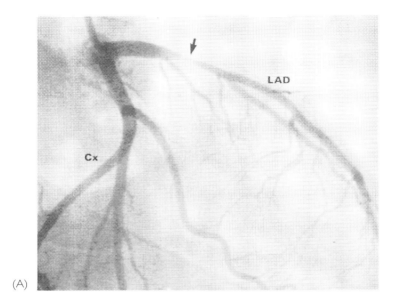

(A)

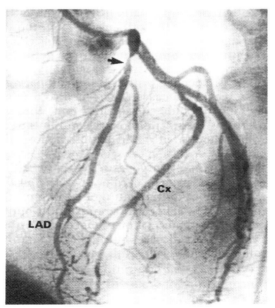

(B)

Fig. 6.5 Coronary angiography. Contrast medium has been injected into the left coronary artery. (A) Right anterior oblique projection. (B) Left anterior oblique projection. The left coronary artery divides into left anterior descending (LAD) and circumflex (Cx) branches. A stenosis in the proximal LAD is arrowed.

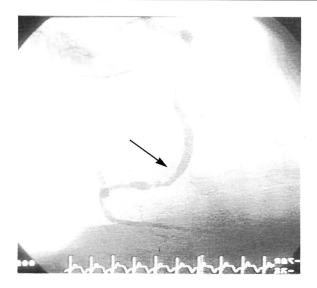

Fig. 6.6 Angiogram of a right coronary artery demonstrating a ruptured atheromatous plaque (arrowed).

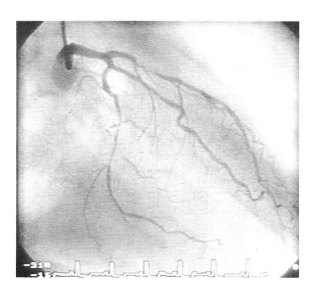

Fig. 6.7 Angiogram of a left coronary artery showing diffuse disease with multiple areas of narrowing (stenoses).

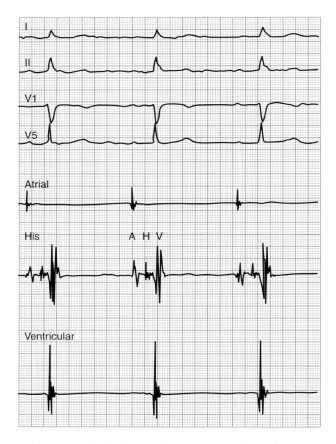

Fig. 6.8 Invasive electrophysiological testing. The traces show (from above downwards) four surface ECG channels, atrial, His bundle and ventricular intracardiac electrograms. The His bundle recording shows three wave forms, A, H and V corresponding to atrial, His and ventricular excitation respectively.

Furthermore, by introducing stimuli at an appropriate time and place, an arrhythmia may be triggered in susceptible patients, and the effect on it of various pharmacological and electrical measures assessed. This technique is particularly valuable in:

- *arrhythmia diagnosis*, e.g. distinguishing the mechanisms of supraventricular tachycardias;
- identification of the origin of a ventricular arrhythmia or of the site of a bypass tract in Wolff–Parkinson–White syndrome;
- assessing the efficacy of antiarrhythmic therapy. This is of particular value in patients with malignant ventricular arrhythmias. If a

drug is successful in preventing arrhythmia induction, this indicates that it is also likely to be successful in preventing spontaneous occurrences of the arrhythmia;

- *ablation* of accessory pathways or of the AV node using radio-frequency current (see p. 214).

Diseases of the Coronary Arteries – Causes, Pathology and Prevention

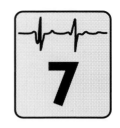

THE CORONARY CIRCULATION

There are two major coronary arteries – right and left (Fig. 7.1). The right coronary artery arises from the right coronary sinus of Valsalva and runs down in the groove between the right atrium and the right ventricle. In most hearts, its branches supply the sinus node, the atrio-ventricular node and bundle, the right ventricle and the inferior part of the left ventricle. The left coronary artery, which arises from the left coronary sinus of Valsalva, soon divides into two large branches: the anterior descending branch which runs down between the two ventricles anteriorly, and the left circumflex branch which passes around in the groove between the left atrium and the left ventricle. The anterior descending artery supplies the interventricular septum and the anterior wall of the left ventricle. The circumflex supplies the lateral and posterior aspects of the left ventricle. The major vessels traverse the external surface of the myocardium, sending branches perpendicularly

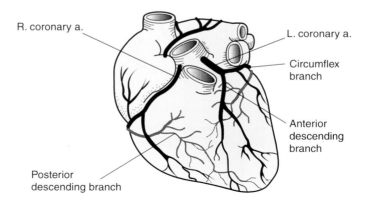

Fig. 7.1 The anatomy of the coronary arteries (see text).

into the muscle mass. There are normally many small anastomoses between the coronary arteries, but these are of no functional importance. When an area of the heart becomes ischaemic, the anastomoses enlarge and then provide a collateral blood supply to the affected muscle which is often vital for its survival.

The arteries divide to form arterioles and capillaries similar to those elsewhere in the body, and the venules and veins join to form larger venous channels. Virtually all the blood from the left coronary artery eventually drains into the coronary sinus; that from the right coronary artery drains mainly into the anterior cardiac veins. From these veins the blood passes into the right atrium.

The blood flow in the coronary arteries resembles that in other regions in being dependent on the blood pressure and on the vascular resistance of the arteries and arterioles. A distinctive feature of the coronary circulation is that the arteries are compressed by the contracting myocardium during systole so that the resistance to flow at that time is sharply increased. Consequently, coronary blood flow occurs mainly during diastole. Flow is largely determined by the calibre of the small coronary arteries. Certainly, the aortic diastolic pressure is also a determinant of coronary flow, but, according to Poiseuille's equation, flow is dependent directly on pressure differences but related to the fourth power of the radius. Therefore, a doubling of aortic diastolic pressure doubles coronary flow, whereas a doubling of the radius of the coronary arteries leads to a 16-fold increase in flow. In health, variations in coronary blood flow are mainly due to changes in impedance in the small coronary arteries; these dilate in response to as yet uncertain metabolic signals from the myocardium, but they are also under the influence of neurohumoral agents. A further influence is the flow-related release of endothelium-derived relaxing factor (identified as nitric oxide). Variations in tone also occur in the large coronary arteries but these affect blood flow only if these vessels are narrowed by disease or if they are extreme (spasm).

In the normal resting heart, almost all the oxygen is extracted during its passage through the capillaries; coronary sinus blood is therefore almost completely desaturated. Unlike other organs, the heart cannot call upon a venous oxygen reserve when faced by increased demands, and is largely dependent upon the ability of the coronary arteries to increase their diameter.

CORONARY ARTERY DISEASE

Coronary artery disease is the commonest cause of heart disease and the most important single cause of death in the affluent countries of the world. In the overwhelming majority of cases, disease of the coronary arteries is due to atherosclerosis.

However, the coronary arteries may also be involved in other disorders:

- congenital abnormalities such as arteriovenous fistulae and anomalous origin from the pulmonary artery;
- coronary embolism associated with thrombosis arising in the left atrium or ventricle, or from mitral or aortic valve prostheses, or from infective endocarditis;
- syphilitic aortitis involving the coronary ostia;
- occlusion of a coronary artery due to dissecting aneurysm;
- polyarteritis and other connective tissue diseases;
- coronary artery spasm which may affect both diseased and otherwise normal vessels (p. 95).

Definitions

Atherosclerosis has been defined (by a World Health Organization study group) as 'a variable combination of changes of the intima of arteries (as distinguished from arterioles) consisting of a focal accumulation of lipids, complex carbohydrates, blood and blood products, fibrous tissue and calcium deposits, and associated with medial changes'. It is synonymous with *atheroma* but not with *arteriosclerosis*, which is a less specific term used to describe hardening of arteries and arterioles.

Coronary artery disease. This term is used to describe coronary arteries that are affected by a pathological process. Coronary artery disease usually exists for many years before a disorder of myocardial function develops. It is, therefore, not synonymous with coronary (or ischaemic) heart disease.

Ischaemic heart disease is cardiac disease resulting from myocardial ischaemia. Although myocardial ischaemia also occurs in such conditions as aortic stenosis, the term 'ischaemic heart disease' is generally applied only to cases of atherosclerotic origin.

Coronary heart disease and **atherosclerotic heart disease** are synonymous with ischaemic heart disease.

Coronary thrombosis refers to occlusion of a coronary artery by thrombus. This may or may not lead to myocardial infarction.

Coronary occlusion. This term is used to describe occlusion of the coronary artery by any cause. Again, this may or may not cause myocardial infarction.

Myocardial infarction is necrosis of a portion of heart muscle as a result of inadequate blood supply.

Silent ischaemia is ischaemia in the absence of symptoms. The term is applied particularly to episodes of ST elevation or depression unaccompanied by pain.

Vasospastic angina (Prinzmetal's angina)

This term is used to describe a syndrome of which the essential features are angina pectoris due to an increase in coronary vasomotor tone and ST elevation in the ECG. The angina is attributable not to an increase in myocardial oxygen demand, as it is in classical angina, but to a transient reduction in coronary blood flow. The disorder may occur either in otherwise apparently normal coronary arteries or in atherosclerotic vessels. In the former case, the increase in tone must be extreme (spasm), but in severely stenotic arteries, even physiological changes in tone can produce a critical reduction in blood flow. The mechanism for coronary spasm is unknown, but it may be provoked by certain drugs, notably ergometrine.

The clinical picture is typically one of anginal pain occurring at rest, particularly in the early morning. The attacks are usually self-limiting, but the pain may be severe; they very seldom lead on to myocardial infarction. Nitrates and calcium antagonists are effective both in the treatment of individual episodes and when used prophylactically.

Coronary atherosclerosis

Pathology of coronary atherosclerosis and its complications

The atherosclerotic process probably starts with the 'fatty streak'. Fatty streaks are a common finding in the intima of young people; macro-scopically, they appear as yellow patches within the arterial wall. They are mainly composed of lipid-laden foam cells which are derived from macrophages and, to a lesser extent, from smooth muscle cells. Depending upon their location and the presence of the relevant risk factors, the fatty streak may progress to the characteristic lesion of atherosclerosis – the fibro-lipid plaque (Fig. 7.2). The major com-ponents of the plaque are lipid and arterial smooth muscle cells and their products, such as fibrous proteins and complex carbohydrates. Plaques vary from one another in their composition. At one extreme are fatty plaques, containing a large pool of cholesterol and its esters, separated from the lumen by a thin fibrous cap. At the other extreme are solid plaques, consisting of smooth muscle cells and connective tissue. Calcification may be superimposed. These deposits are focal and are most commonly located at the bends and bifurcations of arteries.

The atheromatous plaque, which is produced by this process, may itself narrow the lumen of the artery. The fibrous cap is prone to frac-ture, allowing the necrotic core to ulcerate and trigger off platelet aggregation and fibrin deposition. This is a repetitive process and leads to further narrowing, which may proceed to complete occlusion.

Necropsies on patients who have experienced *angina pectoris* usually reveal widespread but patchy coronary atherosclerosis and

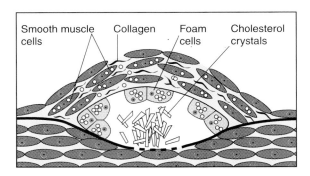

Fig. 7.2 A diagrammatic representation of an atheromatous plaque showing outer cap containing collagen and smooth muscle cells, and inner core showing foam cells and extracellular cholesterol crystals. (With permission from G.R. Thompson, *A Handbook of Hyperlipidaemia*, Current Science, 1989).

myocardial fibrosis. Evidence of old coronary occlusion and myocardial infarction is common. The basic pathological cause for the angina is the coronary arterial narrowing which has reduced the lumen of at least one of the three main coronary arteries by 75%. In most cases, two or all three of these arteries are affected.

Sudden death is often attributed to coronary artery disease when widespread coronary atherosclerosis is present. Recent coronary occlusion or myocardial infarction can be demonstrated in only a minority of cases but plaque rupture and non-occlusive thrombus are common. In most instances, it is probable that acute myocardial ischaemia has provoked fatal ventricular fibrillation.

The essential pathological feature of *acute myocardial infarction* is myocardial necrosis. This is usually, but not always, the consequence of total occlusion of a coronary artery. Plaque rupture is commonly found at necropsy; plaques that rupture are typically rich in lipid and have only a thin cap. There is often evidence of an inflammatory state with many macrophages and T lymphocytes within the plaque. Disruption of the cap allows blood to enter the lipid pool; collagen, crystalline cholesterol and oxidized low-density lipoproteins trigger the formation of a platelet-rich thrombus within the intima. A fibrin-rich thrombus may become superimposed and project into the lumen. It may further expand as many red cells infiltrate the network of fibrin to cause total occlusion. The thrombus will usually lyse spontaneously in the days after infarction but the process can be greatly accelerated by thrombolytic drugs.

If death occurs soon after the onset of myocardial infarction, there may be no gross changes in the myocardium, but enzyme-staining reactions and electron microscopy will reveal evidence of damage. Later, the infarcted area appears pale and is surrounded by a reddish area due to hyperaemia. Microscopically, the muscle cells lose their nuclei and, subsequently, necrotic changes take place in adjacent connective tissue and blood vessel walls. Leucocytic infiltration occurs at the edges of the infarct. The removal of necrotic muscle starts about the third day and continues for about 2 weeks. At the same time, granulation tissue containing blood vessels and fibroblasts invades the necrotic area. Finally, the infarct zone is replaced by scar tissue over a period lasting between 2 and 8 weeks. If the infarction involves the endocardial surface, a mural thrombus may develop; if it affects the epicardium, there may be pericarditis.

The location and size of a myocardial infarct depend upon the artery that is occluded and the collateral blood supply. In some cases, the infarct extends from the endocardium to the epicardium (transmural infarction); in others, only the subendocardial territory is involved. If the left anterior descending artery is occluded, the infarction involves the anterior wall of the left ventricle and may involve the septum. If the left circumflex is occluded, the infarction affects the lateral or posterior walls of the left ventricle. If the right coronary artery is occluded, the infarction chiefly affects the inferior (diaphragmatic) surface of the left ventricle but also the septum and right ventricle. Coronary artery occlusion may not lead to myocardial infarction if the area supplied by the occluded artery has an adequate collateral supply from adjacent arteries.

The infarcted tissue may thin and stretch in the days after infarction, particularly if this has been anterior. It is due to a combination of stretching of the tissues and the sliding of muscle bundles over each other. This process, known as infarct expansion, has adverse effects on left ventricular shape and contractile ability and is probably an important component of subsequent cardiac failure. It may be preventable if the load on the left ventricle is minimized in the early post-infarction period, as by the use of angiotensin-converting enzyme inhibitors.

The pathogenesis of atherosclerosis

Atherosclerosis results from interactions between the arterial wall and the constituents of the blood. A number of elements play important roles:

- the endothelium;
- monocytes/macrophages;
- smooth muscle cells;
- platelets;
- blood lipids.

The endothelium is composed of a single layer of cells that acts as a barrier, albeit a highly selective one, between the components of the blood and the arterial wall. Endothelial cells are also metabolically active, generate vasoactive substances, and present a non-thrombogenic surface (because they can form prostacyclin and because they have a coating of heparan sulphate). They can form the mitogen (i.e. growth factor) platelet-derived growth factor (PDGF) and produce endothelium-derived relaxing factor (EDRF) which causes relaxation of the underlying smooth muscle. The loss of integrity of the endothelium is of critical importance in the development of atherosclerosis. Very often the endothelium is denuded over plaques. Even when it is not, there is endothelial dysfunction.

Macrophages, which are derived from circulating monocytes, secrete several biologically important substances, including a number of growth factors (such as PDGF) and toxic oxygen metabolites. They also have receptors for oxidized low-density lipoprotein (IDL), which they ingest and degrade. They are the major source of foam cells in the fatty streak and the fibro-lipid plaque, and play a key role in connective tissue proliferation.

Smooth muscle cells, derived originally from the media, change their characteristics when they migrate to the intima. Instead of being primarily contractile, they take on many secretory functions. They also become responsive to growth factors (such as PDGF) and are then able to proliferate. They are an essential component of advanced atherosclerotic lesions, in which they accumulate lipid and form foam cells.

Platelets are crucially involved in the complication of thrombosis but also play a major role in the development of atherosclerosis. When activated, they release vasoconstrictor substances and growth factors which can stimulate virtually all the cell types found in the tissues.

Lipids are important components of most plaques, and affect the function of the endothelium, smooth muscle cells and macrophages. They contribute to the formation of foam cells, but there is also a considerable amount of free cholesterol in the tissues of many lesions. Much of the lipid that is taken up is in chemically altered form, having been modified by oxidation or acetylation. Modified LDL is a powerful chemoattractant for monocytes, and macrophages take up LDL avidly in the modified but not in the unmodified form.

'Response to injury' hypothesis

There is still much to be learned about the genesis of atherosclerosis, but current thinking is best integrated under the *'response to injury'* hypothesis. This proposes that the initial lesion is one in which the endothelium is 'injured' in some way, although the term 'injury' is used to cover functional disorders as well as physical disruption. Chronic hyperlipidaemia, with an increase in circulating LDL, leads to changes in the function of monocytes and platelets, as well as in the endothelial cells. The monocytes adhere to the endothelium, and are attracted to migrate into the subendothelial layer, where they become macrophages and take up lipid. These macrophages may secrete free oxygen radicals that further damage the endothelium; they also secrete growth factors that stimulate the migration and proliferation of smooth muscle cells. Damage to the intima may lead to exposure of platelets to the underlying connective tissue and foam cells, with consequent adherence, aggregation and thrombus formation. Mural thrombi may become incorporated into the plaque and contribute to progression of the atherosclerotic process.

Incidence and prevalence of ischaemic heart disease

The incidence of ischaemic heart disease varies greatly between countries and within them, but in all, the mortality from this cause rises rapidly with age. Few females, however, suffer from coronary disease under the age of 45; indeed under the age of 65, more than three times as many men die from coronary disease as do women. In the older age groups the incidence is approximately equal in the two sexes.

Myocardial infarction was seldom recorded as a cause of death until the 1920s, but subsequently the number of deaths attributed to coronary heart disease rose rapidly in Western countries, particularly after the Second World War. It peaked in the United States and Australia in the 1960s; subsequently the mortality in these countries has virtually halved (Fig. 7.3). Mortality from the disease rose until the 1970s in the UK, since when there has been a modest fall of about 25% for men and 15% for women. Within the UK, at least twice as many people die from coronary heart disease in parts of south-west Scotland as in south-east England. United Kingdom residents of South Asian extraction have substantially higher rates than the UK population as a whole.

The reasons for the differences in incidence and the remarkably changing mortality rates are not well understood, but probably relate mainly to diet and smoking behaviour.

Risk factors for ischaemic heart disease and their control

Epidemiological studies and clinical trials have provided valuable information about the risk factors associated with the development of coronary disease and the ways in which the risk of the disease can be reduced. The best identified risk factors are cigarette smoking, high lipid levels and hypertension but several others have been implicated. These include physical inactivity, diabetes, insulin resistance, genetic inheritance, and homocysteinaemia. These risks are multiplicative so that the possession of several factors greatly increases the chance of developing coronary heart disease.

Lipid disorders. There is much circumstantial evidence to incriminate lipid abnormalities in the genesis of atheroma. Thus, there is a strong and graded relationship between plasma cholesterol and the risk

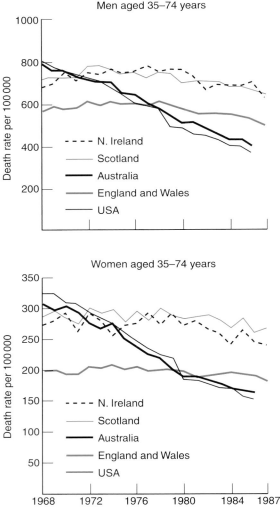

Fig. 7.3 The changing mortalities in different countries. (With permission from Julian and Marley, *Coronary Heart Disease: The Facts*, Oxford: Oxford University Press, 1991).

of subsequent coronary heart disease. Furthermore, clinical trials have demonstrated that the reduction of cholesterol by the use of lipid-lowering regimens reduces the risk of myocardial infarction and death from coronary heart disease.

There are several lipid fractions which have different relationships to coronary heart disease. About two-thirds of plasma cholesterol is transported as LDL and it is this that has been most strongly correlated with subsequent disease. By contrast, high-density lipoprotein (HDL) appears to be protective, because it transports lipid out of the arterial wall. The higher the plasma HDL concentration, the lower the risk of disease. There is less certainty about the role of triglycerides, although they appear to increase risk further when the LDL concentration is raised and/or the HDL level is low.

In countries, such as the United States and the UK, in which the average plasma cholesterol level of the community is relatively high, there is a much higher incidence of coronary artery disease than in countries (such as Japan and China) in which hypercholesterolaemia is rare. The cause of the high cholesterol levels is not yet fully established, although it seems likely that it is related in part to dietary factors. A high content of saturated fat (mainly of animal origin) in the diet is particularly suspect but a relative deficiency of polyunsaturated fats may also be important. In some countries, such as France, coronary heart disease is relatively rare in spite of lipid levels that are not greatly different from those in the UK. It is probable that a high intake of fruit and vegetables is protective because of their anti-oxidant effects.

Certain metabolic and endocrine disorders that disturb lipid metabolism are associated with a high incidence of coronary disease. These include hypothyroidism and diabetes mellitus. Women who have had bilateral oöphorectomy are liable to develop hypercholesterolaemia and premature coronary disease.

The *detection* of hyperlipidaemia depends upon blood sampling. Cholesterol estimates can be undertaken in the non-fasting state, but some other lipid measurements, such as triglyceride, require that the subject is fasting. Single measurements may be misleading both because of inaccuracy of the method and because of variability in the cholesterol level from time to time. Therefore, if a high level is suspected a repeat measurement should be obtained and, particularly if drug treatment is contemplated, a full lipid profile (to include HDL) obtained.

The significance of a particular cholesterol level depends upon many factors, such as age, sex and the presence of other risk factors such as cigarette smoking and hypertension. Thus a cholesterol level of 6.0 mmol/litre without other risk factors is associated with a good prognosis, while a much lower value is associated with a high risk of disease if the subject smokes and has a high blood pressure. The risk is particularly high in those with manifest coronary disease and the indications for lipid lowering are very strong in this context. Thus, the decision of how to treat an individual does not depend on the lipid level alone. A value of 6.5 mmol/litre has been suggested as a level at which vigorous intervention is required, using drugs only if diet fails, but in those with coronary heart disease an attempt should be made to reduce total cholesterol concentration to 5.0 mmol/litre or less.

Blood lipids should be measured in anyone with known ischaemic heart disease, diabetes or hypertension requiring drug treatment, or with a family history of hyperlipidaemia or coronary disease at a relatively young age (e.g. under the age of 55 years).

Treatment of hyperlipidaemia should start with dietary measures. Weight reduction alone substantially reduces hypertriglyceridaemia; alcohol restriction reinforces this. For hypercholesterolaemia, total fat should be reduced to 25–30% of food energy, polyunsaturated fatty acids, especially linoleic acid, providing 7–10%.

Several types of drug are used to correct hyperlipidaemia:

- *bile acid sequestrants* are anion exchange resins, which are not absorbed. Cholestyramine 8–12 g twice daily is effective in hyper-cholesterolaemia, but is unpleasant to take, and may cause dyspepsia and constipation. A large trial with this drug showed a reduction in myocardial infarction but no effect on total mortality;
- *nicotinic acid* reduces triglycerides and, to a lesser extent, cholesterol. The most troublesome side-effect is flushing, which can be diminished by aspirin. Treatment should start with 100 mg three times daily, and rise slowly to 1–2 g three times daily;
- *fibrates* reduce triglycerides and, to a lesser extent, cholesterol. Trials with fibrates have shown a reduction in coronary events, including myocardial infarction and death, but not in overall death rate;
- *HMG CoA reductase inhibitors* ('statins) block cholesterol synthesis in the liver by inhibiting the enzyme 3-hydroxy-3-methy-glutaryl coenzyme A reductase. They reduce plasma cholesterol by 25% or more. Large clinical trials have confirmed not only their effectiveness in reducing mortality and morbidity rates from coronary heart disease, but the absence of serious side-effects. They are indicated if diet fails to improve the lipid profile adequately. The most impressive results are seen in those who have angina or have had a myocardial infarction. In such patients, the aim should be to reduce cholesterol to below 5 mmol/litre. Expense limits their use in patients at lower risk, but they are indicated for those without manifest coronary heart disease if they have high lipid levels together with two or more other risk factors.

Dietary fat and ischaemic heart disease.   Major differences in lipid levels in different communities can be largely accounted for by diet. The LDL cholesterol level in the blood is determined chiefly by the intake of saturated fat, which is converted into cholesterol by the liver. There is relatively little cholesterol in the diet, so that the control of saturated fat is more important than limiting cholesterol intake. Polyunsaturates lower LDL cholesterol; monounsaturates also do so if they are substituted for saturates. The ratio of polyunsaturated fat to saturated fat in the diet is known as the P/S ratio; there are wide variations between P/S ratios in different countries, being high (about 1.0) in Japan and about 0.37 in the UK. Most of the saturated fat is derived from dairy products and fatty meat; a substantial impact on the P/S ratio can be made by substituting skimmed or semi-skimmed milk for the full fat form, a polyunsaturated margarine for butter, olive or polyunsaturated oil for saturated oils, and lean meat, chicken or fish for fatty meat.

Other dietary factors.   Epidemiological studies show that those who eat five or more helpings of fruit and vegetables a day have a lower prevalence of coronary heart disease. It is not clear whether this is due to the presence of high levels of the antioxidant vitamins A, C and E; it is therefore recommended that, rather than vitamin supplements, the public should be advised to consume more fruit and vegetables.

Hypertension.   The higher the blood pressure, whether systolic or diastolic, the greater is the risk of developing ischaemic heart disease. Hypertension may contribute to its development in two ways: by accelerating the development of arterial disease and by increasing the work load of the left ventricle. Evidence from clinical trials suggests that antihypertensive agents lower coronary mortality only moderately – less than one might have anticipated. This may be because the trials have been short-lived, or because the agents used have had adverse effects that counteracted the benefit of lowering blood pressure (see Chapter 16).

Obesity is common in patients with ischaemic heart disease, but is often associated with other risk factors such as diabetes, hyperlipidaemia and hypertension. It is probably an independent risk factor, particularly in women. A high waist-to-hip ratio (common in South Asian men) has been linked to coronary disease. Weight loss is to be encouraged as a way of diminishing risk.

Family history. Coronary artery disease often occurs in several members of the same family. While this may indicate a genetic factor, a shared environment (e.g. diet and smoking) may partially explain it, but it is likely that both genetic and environmental factors are involved. The inherited tendency is usually mediated through hyperlipidaemia (see p. 101) or hypertension. Although nothing can be done to correct the family history, it is important to recognize that those with familial disorders are very susceptible to environmental influences. The other risk factors should be attended to particularly diligently.

Cigarette smoking.   Heavy consumption of cigarettes is associated with a high incidence of myocardial infarction and sudden death. The association is particularly striking in the younger age groups, but applies at all ages. Giving up smoking reduces the risk, but the full effect may take some years to achieve. The avoidance of smoking is perhaps the most important single preventive measure in Western countries.

Physical activity. Physical exercise appears to have a protective effect. Its mechanism is not clear, but it may increase HDL levels, reduce blood clotting and, perhaps, encourage the enlargement of the coronary arteries and their anastomoses. Everyone who can do so should exercise regularly. Simple forms of physical activity such as brisk walking, cycling and swimming are adequate if performed for at least 20 min three times a week. The middle-aged, if unfit, should take up exercise gradually and should avoid the most vigorous competitive games such as squash.

Mental stress. It is widely believed that stress contributes to the development of coronary disease. This may well be so, but convincing evidence is not, as yet, available, perhaps because it is a very difficult area to study. There is no doubt, however, that stress can aggravate the symptoms of those with heart disease.

Diabetes. Ischaemic heart disease develops more frequently and at an earlier age in those with diabetes.

Insulin resistance. Many individuals with ischaemic heart disease who are not frankly diabetic are insulin resistant, i.e. they require a higher insulin level than others to maintain a normal blood glucose level. Obesity and physical inactivity seem to be important factors in its occurrence.

Haemostatic factors. It has recently been shown that individuals with high levels of factor VII activity and fibrinogen have an enhanced risk of coronary events.

Alcohol and coffee. Alcohol in moderation (e.g. 1–2 glasses of wine a day) is associated with a reduced incidence of ischaemic heart disease, but heavier drinking leads to hypertension and an increased risk. The consumption of more than six cups of coffee has also been linked to a higher risk.

Public health approaches to prevention of ischaemic heart disease

Changes in lifestyle are clearly important in the prevention of coronary disease, and these to a large extent are the responsibility of the individual. However, health professionals and the Government also play an important role.

Two strategies have been suggested to prevent coronary disease: a 'high-risk' strategy, involving the identification and treatment of those at high risk, e.g. hyperlipidaemic individuals, or a 'population' strategy, aimed at reducing risk factors in the community at large. The two approaches are not incompatible and both should be pursued, because whilst the high-risk patients are those most likely to benefit, they are relatively few in number and constitute only a small proportion of those who develop coronary disease.

Those at high risk can be identified on the basis of a family history of hyperlipidaemia or of coronary disease at a young age, or by a combination of risk factors such as hypertension, smoking and diabetes. Such individuals should have their lipids checked; they require skilled advice on the control of their risk factors. The population at large needs advice about a healthy diet and not smoking, the need for exercise and for having their blood pressure taken at least every 5 years. Both doctors and the Government need to be involved in providing such information; national food and taxation policies can strongly influence behaviour.

Futher reading

Fuster, F., Badimon, L., Badimon, J. J. & Chesebro, J. H. (1992) The pathogenesis of coronary artery disease and the acute coronary syndromes. *New England Journal of Medicine* **326**: 242, 310.

Pyörälä, K., De Backer, G., Graham, I. *et al.* (1994) Prevention of coronary heart disease in clinical practice. *European Heart Journal* **15**: 1300.

Scandinavian Simvastatin Survival Study Group (1994) Randomised trial of cholesterol lowering in 4444 patients with coronary heart disease: the Scandinavian Simvastatin Survival Study (4S). *Lancet* **344**: 1383.

Coronary Heart Disease – Angina and Unstable Angina

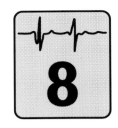

8

Definition

Angina pectoris is a discomfort in the chest and adjacent areas due to a transiently inadequate blood supply to the heart. As originally described by Heberden, it was only a symptom complex; there was no implied association with the heart. Today, the term is still used to describe a symptom, but its relationship to myocardial ischaemia is an essential component of the definition. As discussed on p. 95, there are many causes but coronary atherosclerosis is much the commonest. Almost invariably, at least one of the major coronary arteries has a reduction in luminal diameter of 70% or more; frequently two or three major arteries are involved. In most patients, there is a clear relationship to exercise, but the threshold for this may vary.

Characteristics of angina pectoris

Anginal pain has four major characteristics:

- its location;
- its character;
- its relation to exercise;
- its duration.

The location of angina pectoris. Angina pectoris is most often felt behind the middle or upper third of the sternum. Even when the discomfort may be more obvious in another area, the sternal region is usually involved to some extent. Angina may also be felt in the lower sternal or xiphisternal region, over both sides of the chest, more commonly the left, in the neck and lower jaw and in both arms, again particularly the left. It may affect only the upper arm, but often reaches the elbow, the wrist or the fingers. In some patients the elbow region escapes and the patient is aware of discomfort in the upper arm and a tingling feeling in the fingers. Rarely, it may radiate through to the left scapular region. It is very unusual for the pain to be located predominantly under the left nipple and virtually never is it confined to this area.

The character of angina pectoris.   Angina pectoris is most frequently likened to a pressing feeling, a tight band, or a heavy weight. Many patients deny actual pain and refer only to a sense of discomfort. It is not usually severe but can cause much anxiety and distress. It is not stabbing in quality, but the terms 'sharp' (meaning intense rather than knife-like) and 'burning' are sometimes used. The sensations in other areas are often different in character. In the neck, it is frequently described as 'choking'; in the lower jaw it may be 'like toothache'. The feeling in the arms is usually one of numbness, heaviness or tingling.

The relationship of angina pectoris to exercise and other provoking factors.   Angina pectoris is usually provoked by exertion, nearly always that of walking, particularly uphill. The amount of exercise required to produce angina varies from time to time in any individual, but it is more readily provoked after a heavy meal or in cold weather. There is also a diurnal variation. Patients often describe angina provoked by minimal exertion (such as washing or dressing) after rising from bed in the morning but are able to undertake much more strenuous activities later in the day without symptoms. This presumably reflects changes in coronary vasomotor tone. Emotion is also an important provoking factor; it may be readily induced by anger and irritation. Angina often develops during sexual intercourse.

Some patients experience nocturnal angina, which wakes them up. In some cases this may be due to dreams, but it is probable that increased coronary artery tone, which is maximal in the early morning, is often responsible.

Angina pectoris may be provoked by several different types of tachycardia, particularly paroxysmal tachycardia associated with very rapid ventricular rates. Anaemia also contributes to its development, although it is unusual for it to do so in the absence of coronary atherosclerosis.

The duration of the attack.   Most attacks last 1–3 min. Their duration is seldom less than 30 s or more than 15 min, although a vague sensation of discomfort may persist after the pain has stopped.

Other symptoms and signs of angina pectoris.   Some patients complain of breathlessness accompanying the anginal pain. Other symptoms include flatulence, feelings of faintness and acute anxiety. Tachycardia and a rise in blood pressure may be noted during an attack but there are usually no abnormal signs.

The electrocardiogram

Between attacks of angina pectoris, the ECG is usually normal. There may, however, be evidence of old myocardial infarction, or non-specific changes such as flattening or inversion of T waves, or signs of bundle branch block or left ventricular hypertrophy. If the patient is seen during an attack there are usually well-marked abnormalities which take the form of a horizontal or downward sloping depression of the ST segment (Fig. 8.1). Similar changes may be provoked by an exercise test (see below).

Diagnosis

By definition, angina is a symptom complex with a pathophysiological basis of myocardial ischaemia. The diagnosis must, therefore, depend on the history, combined with evidence of inadequate coronary blood flow.

There is usually no problem in determining the location of the pain and the factors that provoke it, but patients often find it difficult to find the words to describe the sensation they experience and estimates of the duration of the attack are often inaccurate. Most weight must therefore be placed on the first two elements. If the pain is located solely in the left sub-mammary region, or if it lasts for only a few seconds, it is almost certainly not ischaemic. Angina is seldom associated with tenderness of the chest wall, although it may occasionally be so. It is usually, but not always, relieved by glyceryl trinitrate. Angina pectoris is unlikely if walking is not a provoking factor, but some patients take so little exercise that the symptom arises only on emotion or at night.

Physical examination is of comparatively little value except for the exclusion of such causes as aortic stenosis and cardiomyopathy. However, because angina pectoris is often associated with hypertension, with diabetes and with aortic valve disease, the characteristic findings of these conditions may be observed.

Evidence of myocardial ischaemia is provided by the presence of characteristic ST segment changes during an attack. As spontaneous attacks are seldom witnessed, it is usually necessary to carry out an exercise test. The patient may be made to exercise on a bicycle

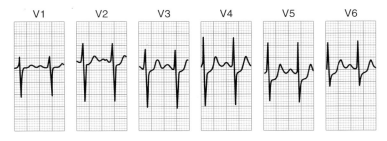

Fig. 8.1   ST depression during myocardial ischaemia. The chest leads are shown during an episode of angina. Extensive ST depression is evident, most marked in leads V5 and V6.

ergometer or a treadmill, preferably until chest discomfort is provoked. Standard and chest lead ECGs should be obtained during exercise and during the first 10 min of rest (see Fig. 5.21). A positive exercise test is one that shows a horizontal downward sloping ST depression of 1 mm or more. ST segments that slope upwards from the J point should not be regarded as evidence of ischaemia as they are often seen in normal individuals with tachycardia.

Even after careful history taking and ECG examination, the diagnosis may remain uncertain. Radionuclide studies with thallium-201 may be helpful, but it is often necessary to carry out coronary angiography to confirm or refute the diagnosis of coronary artery disease (see Chapter 6).

Differential diagnosis

Although the diagnosis of angina can usually be established on the basis of the history and ECG, there are a number of other conditions that have to be considered in the differential diagnosis. Perhaps the most common difficulty arises with musculoskeletal pains in the chest wall. Frequently no cause is found for such pains which are often associated with tenderness and usually located on one side of the chest rather than centrally. These pains are most likely to be provoked by such actions as lifting and pulling, which produce tension of the muscles attached to the ribs. Amongst identifiable musculoskeletal conditions may be included Tietze's syndrome (in which there is an inflammation of one or more costochondral junctions), a slipping rib cartilage, fractured ribs, or metastatic lesions in ribs. In these conditions, unlike angina, there is tenderness and the symptoms may be aggravated by inspiration. The pain of cervical spondylosis is sometimes most severe in the upper chest region and accompanied by discomfort in the shoulders and arms.

Stabbing pains under the left breast and persistent aches in the same region are common and are most unlikely to be due to ischaemic heart disease. It is often not possible to establish their cause, but these symptoms are very common in those with anxiety neurosis.

Disorders of the gastrointestinal tract may be difficult to differentiate from angina pectoris. Oesophageal reflux, often associated with hiatus hernia, gives rise to a central chest pain, but this seldom radiates to the arms, is of a more burning or bursting character, and is more readily provoked by stooping or lying flat, although it may be produced by exercise. The pain of peptic ulcer is usually situated in the epigastric region, and is associated with tenderness. It is related to food rather than to exertion and is usually relieved by alkalis or milk and not by glyceryl trinitrate. Cholecystitis and cholelithiasis may give rise to pain in the lower sternal region, but there is usually tenderness either in the epigastrium or in the right subcostal area; there is frequently associated nausea, and the pain is not related to exertion. It is important to recognize that these gastrointestinal conditions, particularly hiatus hernia and cholecystitis, are common in patients with ischaemic heart disease, and the presence of one of these disorders does not preclude the coexistence of angina pectoris.

Prognosis

Most patients who develop angina pectoris live a normal or nearly normal life for many years. Symptoms are liable to vary from time to time, becoming worse in winter and improving the subsequent summer. They may disappear altogether for months or years.

It is difficult to give an accurate prognosis for any individual, but the outlook is relatively unfavourable if there is associated hypertension, advanced age, cardiac failure or preceding myocardial infarction. Coronary angiographic studies have shown that the prognosis is good if disease is confined to one artery. By contrast, severe narrowing of the left main coronary artery and diffuse lesions of all three arteries are associated with a high risk of early death.

Most patients live for 5 years and about one-third for 10 years or more. The risk of sudden death or acute myocardial infarction is always present; before such events occur, there is frequently an exacerbation of the angina.

Treatment

The general management of angina pectoris is of great importance. The anxiety that the diagnosis arouses may cause incapacity, and it is important to emphasize the relatively good prognosis. Intense cold, walking into a wind or unnecessarily uphill should be avoided if they provoke the pain, as should taking large meals. Patients quickly learn to avoid activities that are likely to provoke episodes of angina. Usually, the patient can continue his or her occupation. Driving is permitted for patients with stable angina but the diagnosis of angina may have serious consequences for 'vocational' drivers (i.e. heavy goods vehicle drivers and coach drivers) as well as for airline pilots. Physical exercise is to be encouraged provided it does not induce discomfort, as it increases the threhold at which angina develops, but sudden strenuous effort should not be undertaken.

Risk factor modification

All modifiable risk factors should be addressed in the patient with angina. Cigarette smoking should be strongly discouraged and guidance given about weight reduction. The blood pressure should be recorded and, if necessary, treated. Blood cholesterol should be measured; if the level is above 5.5 mmol/litre on two occasions, then treatment with an

HMG CoA reductase inhibitor (such as simvastatin or pravastatin) should be commenced. This treatment is likely to be for life.

DRUG TREATMENT OF ANGINA

Aspirin

All patients with coronary artery disease, unless there are strong contra-indications, should be commenced on treatment with aspirin for life. The dose should be 75 or 150 mg once daily. The ideal dose is not known but there is no evidence of any additional benefit from doses exceeding 150 mg once daily.

Nitrates

Nitrates have been in use in the management of angina for more than 100 years, but they remain the first-line treatment.

The major pharmacological effect of nitrates is the relaxation of smooth muscle, which seems to result from an increase in intracellular cyclic guanosine monophosphate (cGMP) levels. Dilatation occurs in the coronary arteries, the peripheral arteries and the veins. Coronary artery dilatation leads directly to an increase in coronary blood flow, arterial dilatation leads to a fall in afterload, and a reduction in venous tone causes pooling, with a diminished venous return and preload. The relative importance of these different effects varies from one patient to another. Thus, the coronary vasodilator action is of particular value when an increase in coronary artery tone is an important component of angina, whereas it may have little influence in an artery with a fixed stenosis. In the latter situation, it is probably the venodilator action that is most relevant.

Most nitrates undergo extensive first-pass metabolism in the liver; this may be overcome by administering large doses, but the effects are rather unpredictable. Alternatives are to use *isosorbide mononitrate* which does not undergo first-pass metabolism, or to bypass the gut by sublingual, buccal or transdermal administration.

Nitrates have relatively minor side-effects, but headache is very common. This tends to diminish with continued use, but some patients find it even more distressing than the angina. Nitrates (particularly glyceryl trinitrate) may cause hypotension and syncope; patients should be advised to take at least their first dose sitting down.

A problem with continuous nitrate therapy is the development of tolerance. This can be avoided by a regimen that ensures a period in the day with little or no nitrate in the blood.

Glyceryl trinitrate (nitroglycerin, trinitrin) is standard therapy in angina pectoris. It is given sublingually either in tablet form or as an aerosol spray. The dose is usually 0.2–0.5 mg. It will stop an attack of angina in about 2 min, but is particularly effective if given prophylactically. Patients should, therefore, be encouraged to take a tablet or use the spray when they anticipate an attack; they should also be advised that the drug is not addictive, as many fear that they will become drug dependent.

Long-acting oral nitrates are effective if given in sufficient dosage, but headache is a common problem, and the regimen should ensure a nitrate-free period. Sustained-release once-daily preparations of isosorbide mononitrate (as 25, 50 or 60 mg preparations) appear to be more effective than smaller doses given at frequent intervals and do ensure a nitrate-free interval. The same considerations apply to transdermal patches.

Beta-adrenoceptor blocking drugs

These are now given routinely to most patients with angina unless there are contra-indications to their use. They block the action of catecholamines in increasing heart rate, blood pressure and cardiac contractility and thereby limit the myocardial oxygen needs during exercise. Beta-blockers have been shown to reduce the frequency of angina, to reduce the consumption of glyceryl trinitrate, to prolong exercise time during treadmill testing and to reduce ECG evidence of myocardial ischaemia at a given workload. Beta-blockers may exacerbate congestive cardiac failure and airways obstruction and should be avoided in patients with overt heart failure or with asthma. When given to patients free of heart failure or a history of asthma, the main side-effects of beta-blockers are fatigue and cold extremities, both of which disappear on stopping the drug.

In general, the choice of a particular beta-blocker is not of importance, but compliance is more likely to be achieved if a preparation that requires only once or twice daily administration (such as atenolol or bisoprolol) is used.

Calcium antagonists

Currently available calcium antagonists fall into two main groups, the dihydropyridines and the phenylalkylamines. The phenylalkylamines (verapamil and diltiazem) have potent depressant actions on the myocardium and the conducting system. They slow the heart rate both at rest and during exercise and are useful anti-anginal agents when beta-blockers are contra-indicated. These drugs can be combined with beta-blockers but this combination may lead to excessive bradycardia or to heart block. A usual dose is 60 mg three times daily for diltiazem and 80 mg three times daily for verapamil, although long-acting once-daily preparations of both drugs are now available. Side-effects with diltiazem are rare and the only commonly reported problem with verapamil is constipation.

The dihydropyridine calcium antagonists (nifedipine, nicardipine and amlodipine) have little effect on the myocardium and conducting tissue; their main action is to dilate the peripheral arteries and to reduce the workload on the heart. Used alone, they often cause a reflex tachycardia which can be avoided by concomitant use of a beta-blocker. Side-effects are common and include headache, facial flushing and ankle swelling. The usual dosage for nifedipine is 30–60 mg daily in divided doses or as a single slow-release preparation. The dose for nicardipine is 5–30 mg three times daily and for amlodipine is 5–10 mg once daily.

Calcium antagonists can worsen cardiac performance in those with poor left ventricular function, and generally should be avoided in patients with cardiac failure.

INTERVENTIONAL TREATMENT FOR PATIENTS WITH ANGINA

Percutaneous transluminal coronary angioplasty (PTCA)

In coronary angioplasty, a non-elastic balloon mounted close to the tip of a specially designed catheter can be passed to the site of a coronary stenosis and inflated there. This process produces clefts in the atheromatous lesion, compression and redistribution of its contents, endothelial desquamation, and stretching of the media. In most cases, this results in a substantial increase in the arterial lumen. This process is shown schematically in Fig. 8.2. Figure 8.3 demonstrates the improvement in calibre seen after coronary angioplasty.

The procedure is carried out under local anaesthesia and the patient is usually fit to be discharged home the following day. Coronary angioplasty was first performed in 1977 and its use spread rapidly in Europe and in North America over the following 10 years. Indeed, the total number of angioplasty procedures came to exceed the total number of coronary bypass procedures in the United States in 1988. During this period, two major complications of PTCA emerged. The first, abrupt vessel closure, usually occurred in the catheter laboratory and was caused by extensive dissection of the artery and the formation of an intimal flap which prevented antegrade flow. This usually resulted in chest pain with impending infarction and often led to emergency coronary artery bypass surgery. The second complication of conventional angioplasty was late restenosis. Here, the initial PTCA procedure usually resulted in an acceptable angiographic result and an improvement in the patient's symptoms. Within 6 months, however, symptoms returned in 25–35% of patients and repeat angiography showed restenosis. Histologically, this was caused by hyperplasia of the smooth muscle cells.

New developments in coronary angioplasty

Several novel approaches to coronary angioplasty have been developed over the past 10 years in the hope of reducing the rate of restenosis. Of

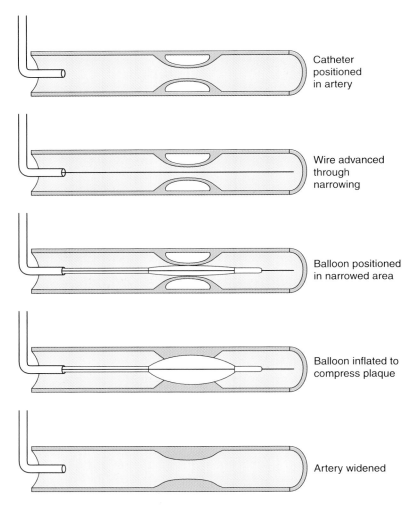

Catheter
positioned
in artery

Wire advanced
through
narrowing

Balloon positioned
in narrowed area

Balloon inflated to
compress plaque

Artery widened

Fig. 8.2 Percutaneous transluminal coronary angioplasty. (With permission from Julian and Marley, *Coronary Heart Disease: The Facts*, Oxford: Oxford University Press, 1991).

these, by far the most successful development has been the advent of coronary artery stents (Fig. 8.4). These are usually made from stainless steel but may be made from other metals. The most commonly used stents are mounted in a collapsed form on a deflated angioplasty balloon. The balloon is then passed to the stenosis and inflated in the lesion, thus expanding and deploying the stent. The balloon is then deflated and removed, leaving the stent as a scaffolding within the artery. Stents have proved extremely successful both in the

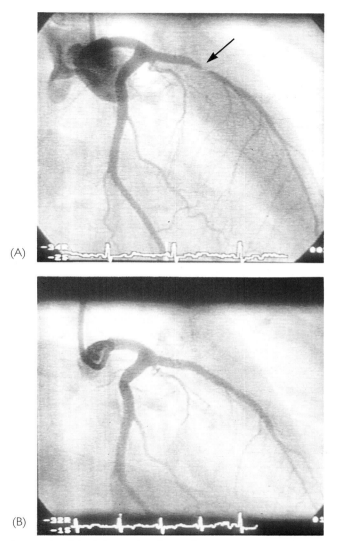

Fig. 8.3 A stenosis of the left anterior descending coronary artery (arrowed) before (A) and after (B) coronary angioplasty.

emergency treatment of abrupt closure, where they can often obviate the need for emergency bypass surgery, and in reducing the rate of late restenosis.

Furthermore, the development of coronary artery stents has allowed expansion of the indications for coronary angioplasty. In several clinical settings, coronary artery stenoses or occlusions can now be dilated

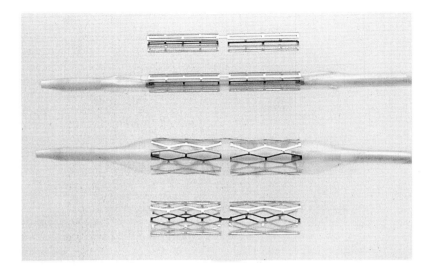

Fig. 8.4 Example of a coronary artery stent. From top to bottom: stent before insertion; stent crimped on a deflated angioplasty balloon; stent being expanded by inflation of the balloon; fully deployed stent.

and stented in greater safety and with a higher chance of long-term patency than was possible with conventional balloon angioplasty. The expanding indications for PTCA with stenting include:

- long coronary stenoses (Fig. 8.5);
- stenoses in vein grafts (Fig. 8.6);
- total coronary occlusions (Fig. 8.7).

Other angioplasty techniques have not been shown to reduce late restenosis but may be useful in certain situations. These include the following:

- *rotational atherectomy.* This device comprises an olive-shaped burr with multiple tiny diamonds embedded in the burr. This is rotated at high speed, resulting in emulsification of the atheroma. This device appears to be useful in patients with diffuse coronary atheroma.
- *directional atherectomy.* As its name implies, this device has a cutter that can remove and retrieve atheromatous lesions. This technique may be useful in eccentric stenoses.
- *laser angioplasty.* Laser energy is transmitted through multiple optic fibres to cut through stenotic or occluded coronary lesions.

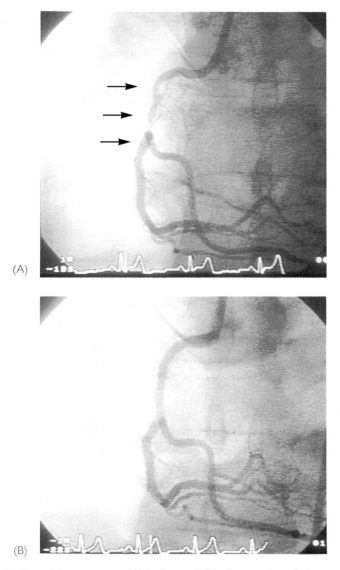

Fig. 8.5   Angiographic appearance (A) before and (B) after stenting of a long stenosis of a right coronary artery (arrows).

Coronary artery bypass surgery

The narrowed segments of coronary arteries can be bypassed using a length of saphenous vein taken from the leg. One end of the vein is

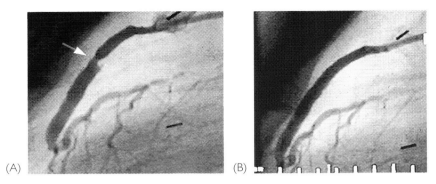

Fig. 8.6   Stenosis of a vein graft to the left anterior descending artery (arrowed) (A) before and (B) after coronary stenting.

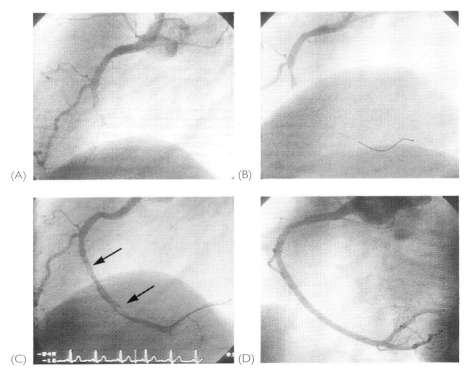

Fig. 8.7   Re-opening of a totally occluded right coronary artery. (A) Occlusion of a right coronary artery; (B) a guidewire has been passed through the occluded segment and into the distal right coronary artery; (C) after multiple balloon dilatations, the artery is now patent although there are areas of arterial dissection (arrowed); (D) two arterial stents have been positioned in the right coronary artery establishing a smooth line with good flow.

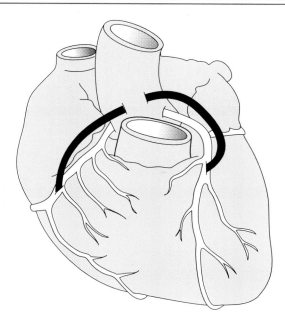

Fig. 8.8   Two saphenous vein bypass grafts, from the aorta to the anterior descending and right coronary arteries, respectively. (With permission from Julian and Marley, *Coronary Heart Disease: The Facts*, Oxford: Oxford University Press, 1991.)

attached to the ascending aorta and the other to the affected artery beyond the most distal obstruction as demonstrated by coronary arteriography (Fig. 8.8). Surgeons are increasingly trying to use lengths of artery instead of vein. The most commonly used artery for this purpose is the left internal mammary artery. In this case, the proximal end of the vessel is not detached from the left subclavian artery; the artery is, however, mobilized, its major side branches are tied off and the distal end is anastomosed to the coronary artery (most commonly the left anterior descending artery). Other arteries can be used in this way, including the right internal mammary artery and the gastro-epiploic artery. Recently, free arterial grafts (such as an excised radial artery) have also been utilized.

Grafts may, if necessary, be inserted into all the three major arteries, and into their larger branches. Provided left ventricular function is not severely impaired, the mortality rate of the operation is less than 1% in most centres. A small proportion of grafts close shortly after insertion. Approximately 50% will remain patent for at least 5 years with much higher patency rates (of around 90%) if an arterial conduit has been used. It has been found that antiplatelet therapy (e.g. aspirin 150 mg once daily) is helpful in maintaining patency, and lipid-lowering drugs should be given to all patients with cholesterol level greater than 5.5 mmol/litre.

The results of surgery are usually very satisfactory, at least for 5–10 years. Angina is abolished in at least 50% of cases, and greatly improved in a further 30%. As well as relieving angina, coronary artery surgery benefits the prognosis of patients with disease of the left main coronary artery, and also those who have disease of the three major vessels, together with left ventricular dysfunction, provided this is not too severe. Late deterioration may be due to graft closure, or to progression of the disease in the ungrafted vessels.

Surgery is indicated for those whose angina is not adequately relieved by full medical treatment, but it should also be considered as a measure to improve prognosis, even in the absence of symptoms, in certain groups of patient (see below).

Most centres carry out coronary artery bypass grafting under cardiopulmonary bypass after a sternotomy with full exposure of the heart and great vessels. Recent interest has focused on coronary artery bypass surgery without the need for cardiopulmonary bypass or sternotomy (so-called minimally invasive approaches). The safety of these techniques when compared with conventional coronary artery bypass grafting has yet to be established but this is certain to be a major interest in cardiac surgery over the next 10 years.

Unstable angina

Angina is regarded as being unstable if it has developed for the first time recently, or if pre-existing angina has worsened for no apparent reason. The pathophysiology of unstable angina is much more closely related to that of acute myocardial infarction than to stable angina. Several mechanisms may be involved, which include rupture of an atheromatous plaque (Fig. 8.9), with or without superimposed thrombosis, and coronary spasm. The clinical picture is very variable, ranging from relatively mild attacks of pain on exertion to recurrent attacks of severe pain at rest which are unresponsive to full medical treatment. During the episodes of pain, there are usually transient ECG changes, such as ST depression or elevation, or T wave abnormalities. The chief concern in unstable angina is the substantial risk of progression to myocardial infarction in the ensuing days or weeks.

Patients with rapidly worsening angina, and especially those with rest pain, should usually be admitted to hospital. Treatment should include aspirin and intravenous heparin, both of which have been shown to reduce the risk of myocardial infarction. If the patient is still in pain, or if pain recurs while in hospital, the addition of intravenous nitrates is often effective. Nitroglycerin should be given initially in a dosage of 5 µg per min; the dose may be increased each 5 min by 5 µg, and later by 10 µg per min, as necessary, with very careful observation of the blood pressure. Isosorbide dinitrate therapy may be started at 20 µg per min, and increased by steps of 20 µg. Beta-blockers should also be given. The role of calcium antagonists in unstable angina is less clear, although diltiazem may be useful in patients who have contra-indications to beta-blockade.

If a prompt response to rest and medical treatment is not achieved, it is best to proceed without delay to coronary arteriography, and then to angioplasty or coronary artery bypass surgery if these seem indi-cated.

Choice of treatment for the individual patient with angina

In the patient with stable angina, treatment should include aspirin and a beta-blocker together with identification and treatment of any modi-fiable risk factors such as hypercholesterolaemia or hypertension. Although there are no large-scale mortality studies looking at the effects of drug treatment on prognosis in angina, beta-blockers have been shown to reduce mortality if given early during the course of myocardial infarction. In the absence of other data, therefore, it seems logical to treat patients with angina with a beta-blocker, as they are at risk of myocardial infarction at some time. If the patient's symptoms are not controlled, a long-acting nitrate and/or a calcium antagonist can be added.

The decision as to when to undertake invasive investigations with a view to either PTCA or coronary artery bypass surgery varies widely from country to country and from region to region. In general, angiog-raphy should be undertaken if a patient's symptoms are not controlled on medical therapy or if an exercise test shows evidence of ischaemia at a low workload. This implies that most patients with angina should have an exercise ECG, not only to confirm the diagnosis of angina, but to help stratify the individual patient's risk of major adverse events such as myocardial infarction and death. This is necessary because the relationship between symptomatic status and the extent of coronary disease at angiography is often poor. In certain groups of patients, such as those with stenosis of the left main stem or stenoses of all three major coronary vessels and reduced left ventricular function, coronary bypass surgery has been shown to improve both symptoms and prog-nosis. It follows that patients with a strongly positive exercise test should be considered for angiography even if their symptoms are mild or absent. The decision as to whether or not an individual patient should undergo angiography will be influenced by other factors such as the patient's age and the presence of other medical conditions that might increase the risk of any interventional treatment.

If revascularization is warranted, this may take the form of either PTCA or surgery. In general PTCA (with or without coronary artery stenting) is preferred for patients with one- or two-vessel disease, and coronary artery bypass surgery is preferred for those with triple vessel disease, left main stem disease or diffusely diseased arteries. There are, however, no hard and fast rules and clinical practice will vary depending on local expertise. Several studies have compared the outcome of coronary surgery and PTCA in patients with multi-vessel disease; no significant differences have been demonstrated in major events such as death and myocardial infarction. If the initial treatment is PTCA, however, the patient should accept that reintervention (in the form of further PTCA or surgery) is more likely than if the initial treatment is surgical.

Further reading

Bain, D. S. (1992) Coronary angioplasty as a treatment of coronary artery disease. New England Journal of Medicine **326**: 56.

Guidelines and indications for coronary bypass graft surgery (1991) Journal of the American College of Cardiology **17**: 543.

Hirsh, J. (1991) Oral anticoagulant drugs. New England Journal of Medicine **324**: 1865.

Julian, D. G. (1985) Angina Pectoris, 2nd edn. Edinburgh: Churchill Livingstone.

Parker, J. O. (1987) Nitrate therapy in stable angina pectoris. New England Journal of Medicine **316**: 1635.

Coronary Heart Disease – Myocardial Infarction

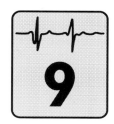

Myocardial infarction is the term applied to myocardial necrosis secondary to an acute interruption of the coronary blood supply. The pathological changes underlying myocardial infarction are described in detail in Chapter 7 (p. 92). Rupture of an atheromatous plaque leads to deposition of intra-coronary thrombus, which leads in turn to coronary occlusion. The term myocardial infarction refers to the consequent necrosis of myocardium. The morbidity and mortality of infarction arise from the resultant arrhythmias and loss of pump function.

The management of myocardial infarction has been transformed in the past decade. Whereas in the past management was largely reactive, treating complications as they arose, recent advances have led to a proactive approach, addressing the underlying pathological processes. This proactive approach to myocardial infarction is one of the success stories of modern cardiology. Large clinical trials have shown that the use of aspirin and thrombolytic therapy can reduce the mortality rate from acute infarction by almost 50%. Furthermore, in the recovery phase after infarction, intervention with beta-blockers and angiotensin-converting enzyme (ACE) inhibitors offer further substantial reductions in mortality.

It is reasonable to anticipate, therefore, that with current therapies the long-term mortality rate after infarction can be reduced by over 50%.

Clinical features

The common presenting symptom of myocardial infarction is severe chest pain. This is predominantly in the sternal region, but may radiate to both sides of the chest, to the jaw, to the shoulders and to one or both arms. It is usually described as tight, pressing, heavy or constricting. Sometimes the patient may deny 'pain' and describe a discomfort, not amounting to pain, in the centre of the chest. Although it can be brief, the pain usually lasts for more than half an hour and may continue for several hours. Unlike the pain of angina, it is seldom associated with exertion and is not relieved by rest or glyceryl trinitrate. The pain may be maximal at the onset, but often increases in intensity for a period of minutes or hours and then remains constant until it gradually recedes. Frequently, the patient gives a history of the recent onset of angina or the exacerbation of pre-existing angina in the preceding days or weeks.

The pain may be overshadowed by other symptoms, such as breathlessness or syncope. Occasionally, it is obscured because the infarction develops during anaesthesia or at the time of a cerebrovascular accident. Rarely, infarction may be truly pain-free.

Once the pain has been controlled, the patient may remain free of symptoms and make an uninterrupted recovery. However, complications develop in a substantial proportion of cases. The most important of these are:

- arrhythmias;
- cardiogenic shock;
- left ventricular failure.

These complications, which will be considered in detail later, are the common causes of death and are responsible for many of the abnormal physical signs that may be observed.

Physical signs

During the earliest stages of the attack, patients are obviously distressed and may be sweaty and cold. The general appearance improves when the pain is controlled and often, within a few hours, the patient looks well.

The pulse may be normal in volume and rate, but in severe attacks it is small and fast. Arrhythmias or bradycardia are also common.

The blood pressure usually falls progressively over a period of hours and days, reaching its minimum some time during the first week, and returning towards normal slowly over the next 2–3 weeks. There may, however, be a sharp fall in blood pressure at the onset of the infarction, which may progress to the severe hypotension of cardiogenic shock, or may resolve. Transient hypertension, perhaps resulting from intense pain, is sometimes observed.

The jugular venous pressure is usually normal or slightly elevated early in the course of acute myocardial infarction; it is seldom markedly elevated due to right-sided heart failure.

The apex beat, which is often difficult to feel, may be displaced outwards. Between the apex and the left sternal edge a systolic pulsation may be detectable, due to a protrusion of the infarcted anterior wall of the heart.

The first and second heart sounds are often soft. A fourth (or atrial) sound can be heard in most cases; a third heart sound is common when there is heart failure or shock.

A soft pansystolic murmur at the apex is not uncommon and is caused by mitral regurgitation either as a result of papillary muscle malfunction or secondary to dilatation of the left ventricle. Rarely, a loud systolic murmur may develop at the left sternal edge, due to a rupture of the ventricular septum, or at the apex, due to rupture of a papillary muscle. A transient pericardial rub occurs in some patients, usually on the second or third day.

Pulmonary crepitations are common but of little importance unless they are widespread and numerous because of pulmonary oedema.

Most of the abnormal physical signs described disappear within a few days of the onset of infarction, except in the most severely affected patients.

A fever, seldom exceeding 38°C, usually commences within the first 24 h and subsides in under a week.

There is often a slight leucocytosis and an increase in the erythrocyte sedimentation rate (ESR). The pyrexia, leucocytosis and raised ESR represent a reaction to myocardial necrosis.

Investigations

The electrocardiogram

The ECG is virtually always transiently or permanently abnormal after acute myocardial infarction. Because the ECG diagnosis of infarction depends upon the observation of a sequence of changes with time, serial records are vital.

The characteristic abnormalities (Fig. 9.1) are:

- pathological Q waves;
- ST segment elevation;
- T wave inversion.

Although the precise mechanisms responsible for these ECG changes are not yet determined, it is probable that the Q wave changes are the result of muscle death, that the ST abnormalities are due to muscle injury, and that the T wave abnormalities are due to ischaemia.

Classically, the earliest change in acute myocardial infarction is ST elevation. This occurs within minutes of arterial occlusion and represents transmural ischaemia in the territory of the infarct. Q waves, by contrast, arise due to myocardial necrosis and take some hours to develop fully (Fig. 9.1). The ST segment progressively returns to normal to be succeeded by T inversion in the first 24–48 h after infarction. Over a time course of weeks and months the T wave generally becomes

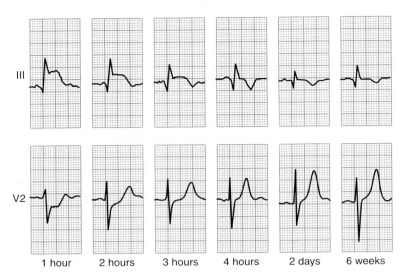

III

V2

1 hour   2 hours   3 hours   4 hours   2 days   6 weeks

Fig. 9.1   Progression of ECG changes in myocardial infarction. The progression of ECG changes during and after an inferior infarct is shown. Lead III (upper series) faces the area of infarction. V2 (lower series) demonstrates reciprocal changes. The time of each ECG from onset of symptoms is shown. The patient received thrombolytic therapy on initial presentation at 1 hour. In lead III, early ST elevation rapidly resolves, to be succeeded by a biphasic T wave and subsequently by T wave inversion. A Q wave develops over several hours. In the remote lead, V2, there is initial ST depression. This resolves with the disappearance of ST elevation in lead III.

less inverted and may even normalize. This is in contrast to Q waves, which usually persist indefinitely.

The time sequence of ECG changes in acute infarction is of importance in relation to thrombolysis. Firstly, patients seen in the earliest phase of infarction may not have developed Q waves. It is entirely appropriate in such cases to base the decision to commence thrombolytic therapy on the presence of ST elevation alone. Secondly, the rapidity of resolution of ST elevation provides a rough guide to the success of reperfusion: ST segments show rapid resolution in patients achieving successful reperfusion, compared with a more gradual resolution in those failing to reperfuse. As a rough guide, if ST segments have resolved by 50% or more within 90 min of the commencement of thrombolytic therapy, this indicates successful reperfusion. Finally, with the advent of reperfusion therapy, a greater proportion of infarcts may be 'arrested' in the course of development before the development of Q waves and fall into the category of 'T wave infarcts'. T wave infarcts are in general smaller than those resulting in the development of Q waves.

Pathological Q waves.   As Q waves represent a long-term marker of previous infarction, distinguishing pathological from physiological Q waves is of some importance.

Q waves may take several hours to develop after the onset of infarction. They usually persist indefinitely because the scar tissue that replaces the infarcted muscle is similarly uninvolved in electrical activation. Normally, Q waves in leads facing the left ventricle do not exceed 2 mm in depth or 0.03 s in width. Q waves and QS waves are normal in aVR, and are commonly found in V1 and V2. Deep Q waves are often also seen normally in lead III. The Q wave in lead III should be considered definitely abnormal only if it exceeds 0.03 s in duration, and if it is accompanied by Q waves in either lead II or aVF. The 'normal' Q wave in lead III usually diminishes or disappears on deep inspiration, whereas the 'pathological' Q wave persists.

Persistent ST elevation.   The ST segment generally returns to normal within 24–48 h of the onset of infarction. Persistent ST segment elevation suggests the possibility of a ventricular aneurysm.

Left bundle branch block may also obscure the changes of infarction, because in this disorder the septum is depolarized from right to left; this produces an initial R wave in left ventricular leads, preventing the appearance of a Q wave. The diagnosis can sometimes be made from ST and T wave changes.

Distribution of ECG changes in infarction.   The leads in which the infarct patterns are seen depend upon its location:

- *Anteroseptal* infarction produces changes in one or more of the leads V1 to V4 (Fig. 9.2).
- *Anterolateral* infarction produces changes from V4 to V6, and lead I and aVL.
- *Anterior* infarction is indicated by more widespread changes including most of the leads from V1 to V6, as well as lead I and aVL.
- *Inferior* (or diaphragmatic) infarction is registered by changes in leads II, III and aVF (Fig. 9.3).
- *Strictly posterior* myocardial infarction does not produce Q waves in the standard 12 leads. However, the loss of electrical activity from the posterior part of the left ventricle, leads to a tall R in V1, because the forces depolarizing the right ventricle are unopposed (Fig. 9.4).
- *Right ventricular* infarction (which is almost always associated with inferior infarction) produces transient ST elevation in V4R (Fig. 9.3B).

Further leads may be required for infarcts in unusual sites, V7 and V8 being helpful in lateral infarcts, and leads in the second or third intercostal spaces for high anterior and lateral infarcts.

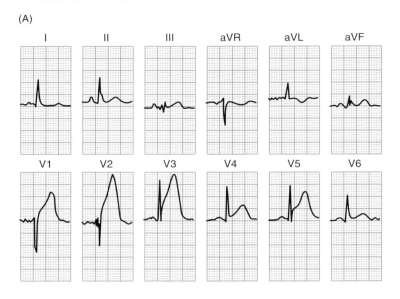

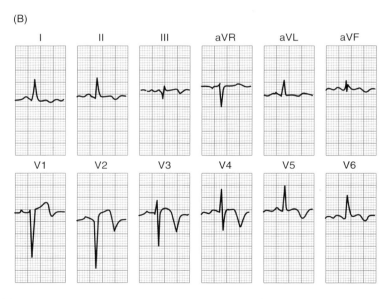

Fig. 9.2 Anteroseptal myocardial infarction. (A) 12-lead ECG recorded within one hour of onset of symptoms. Hyperacute changes are evident with marked ST elevation across the anterior chest lead. Tall peaked T waves are present in lead V2 and V3. (B) 12 hours later the acute ST changes have largely resolved, and have been succeeded by T wave inversion. A deep Q wave is present in lead V2.

Serum enzymes (Fig. 9.5)

Certain enzymes, present in high concentration in cardiac tissue, are released by necrosis of the myocardium. Their activity in the serum, therefore, rises and falls after myocardial infarction. The amount of enzyme released roughly parallels the severity of myocardial damage.

Creatine kinase (CK). Creatine kinase, which occurs in heart, skeletal muscle and brain, rises within 6 h of the onset of infarction, reaching a peak in 18–24 h. It may become normal after 72 h. Apart from myocardial infarction, abnormally high levels occur in muscle diseases, in cerebrovascular damage, after muscular exercise and with intramuscular injections.

The MB isoenzyme of CK is virtually specific for cardiac muscle and is now widely used in the diagnosis of myocardial infarction. The assay is of particular value in patients who have sustained skeletal muscle damage as an additional or alternative cause of a rise in CK concentration, for example patients who have received a DC shock, intramuscular injections or external cardiac massage.

Serum glutamic–oxalo-acetic transaminase (SGOT) (also called aspartate transaminase) is found particularly in the heart, skeletal muscle, brain, liver and kidney. After infarction, the SGOT level rises in about 12 h and reaches its peak in 24–36 h, returning to normal from the third to the fifth day.

Serum lactate dehydrogenase (LDH) is found in the heart, but also in red cells. It rises relatively late after infarction, reaches its peak 24–48 h

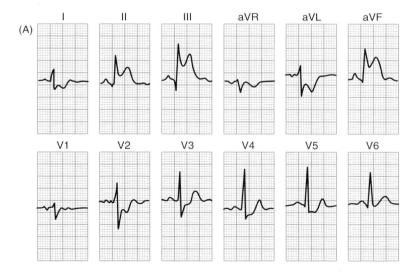

Fig. 9.3 (see caption on page 130)

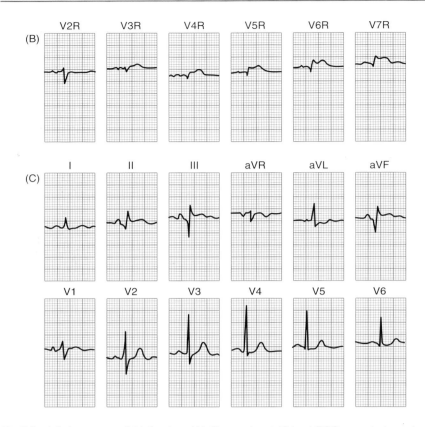

Fig. 9.3   Inferior myocardial infarction. (A) Conventional 12-lead ECG recorded one hour after the onset of symptoms showing ST elevation in leads II, III and aVF. There is reciprocal ST depression across the anterior chest leads, extending into leads I and aVL. (B) Right-sided chest leads recorded simultaneously. ST-elevation is apparent in leads V3R to V7R, indicating right ventricular infarction. (C) Conventional 12-lead ECG recorded 12 hours later. The acute ST segment changes have largely resolved. There are now deep Q waves in leads II, III and aVF.

afterwards, and may remain abnormal for 1–3 weeks. Unfortunately, even slight haemolysis raises its level. Isoenzymes are more specific.

Other enzyme markers for acute myocardial infarction have become available in recent years. These include troponin subunits (troponin T and troponin I) and myoglobin. These markers may offer the advantage of more rapid release characteristics and hence more rapid diagnosis in the case of myoglobin or greater specificity in the case of troponin. Their value in routine clinical practice remains to be assessed.

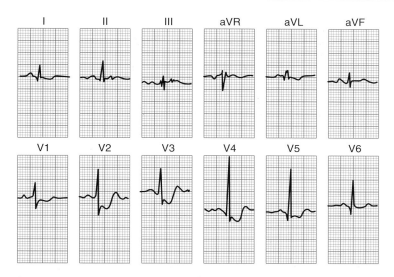

Fig. 9.4 Posterior myocardial infarction. Tall R waves are present in leads V1 and V2 accompanied by deep ST depression. These are reciprocal changes arising from a posterior infarction.

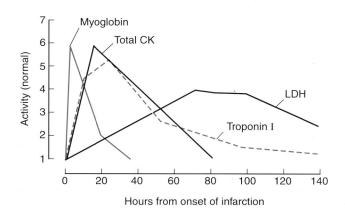

Fig. 9.5 Changes in serum enzyme activity following myocardial infarction are shown, demonstrating the differing rate of rise, peak level and direction of election for a number of enzyme reactors. (Adapted, with permission, from Antman, E.M. (1994) General hospital management. In Julian, D. L. and Brunwald, E. (eds) *Management of Acute Myocardial Infarction*, p. 63. London: WB Saunders Company.)

Diagnosis

In most cases, the diagnosis is suspected from the character, location and duration of the chest pain. The persistence of the pain beyond 15 min, its lack of relationship to exercise and the failure of glyceryl trinitrate to relieve it usually serve to differentiate it from angina pectoris. The development of abnormal physical signs and, more particularly, the appearance of arrhythmias, shock and failure also suggest that infarction has occurred. Fever, leucocytosis and raised ESR indicate necrosis rather than ischaemia. The definitive diagnosis depends upon the recognition of the ECG changes, supported by abnormal serum enzyme levels. Infarction is virtually certain if Q waves appear during the course of the illness, or if sequential ST and T wave changes are accompanied by transient but significant elevations of serum enzyme levels. Difficulties in diagnosis arise when the ECG or enzyme level changes are equivocal, or if serial ECG records or enzyme estimations are not made at appropriate times.

It is exceedingly difficult to differentiate some cases of acute myocardial infarction from unstable angina. This syndrome is characterized by attacks of ischaemic pain which are more prolonged and less related to exertion than are those of typical effort-induced angina pectoris, but there is no necrosis, nor are there the enzyme abnormalities of myocardial infarction. There may be ST elevation or depression but Q waves are not a feature.

The differentiation of myocardial infarction from massive pulmonary embolism may be difficult, but the chest pain of myocardial infarction is usually more severe and the breathlessness less marked. In pulmonary embolism, the ECG may be normal, or there may be characteristic abnormalities (see p. 347) and although there may be changes in LDH and SGOT, CK (and, more specifically MB–CK) is usually not raised. In cases of doubt, pulmonary angiography or radio-isotope scanning of the chest are helpful. Pulmonary infarction can be recognized by the location and pleural character of the pain and the radiographic appearances.

Acute pericarditis may produce symptoms and signs similar to those of an acute myocardial infarction (see p. 225). In many cases, the pericarditis is preceded by an upper respiratory infection and cough. The chest pain is more aching or stabbing in character, and is made worse by deep inspiration, movement or lying flat. Pyrexia often precedes the pain, whereas the temperature rise of myocardial infarction usually takes at least 12 h to develop. Although pericarditis may produce ST elevation and T wave inversion, the ST elevation is concave upwards (see Fig. 12.1) and is widespread rather than focal. Abnormal Q waves do not occur and enzyme changes occur only if there is accompanying myocarditis.

Dissecting aneurysm can cause severe central chest pain similar to that of acute myocardial infarction (see p. 338). The pain usually has a tearing quality, and tends to move into the upper dorsal spinal region and into the abdomen. The ECG does not show the changes of myocardial infarction, except when the dissection involves the origin of a coronary artery. In cases of doubt, the arterial pulses should be repeatedly checked, and a chest radiograph obtained to determine whether there is mediastinal widening. Trans-oesophageal echocardiography, computed tomography and magnetic resonance imaging are of diagnostic value.

TREATMENT OF ACUTE INFARCTION

Immediate treatment

The management of the early phase of myocardial infarction is critical; resuscitation from cardiac arrest is most often required at this time and interventions to limit infarct size should be administered as soon as possible. It is, therefore, of great importance that resuscitation and other relevant facilities should be available outside hospital. Depending upon local circumstances, these can be provided by suitably trained and equipped doctors or by paramedical personnel.

Usually, the most urgent measure is the relief of pain. When this is severe, opiates such as intravenous morphine sulphate (10 mg) or diamorphine (5 mg) are required and may have to be repeated. Unfortunately, these drugs may produce bradycardia, hypotension and respiratory depression, and it is advisable to combine them with atropine (0.6 mg) if there is bradycardia. Nausea and vomiting may occur and may require the administration of an intravenous anti-emetic such as cyclizine (50 mg). The inhalation of nitrous oxide 50% and oxygen 50% is useful if other analgesic measures are unavailable or have failed.

It is usual to admit all patients with suspected acute myocardial infarction to hospital. The main purpose of this is to ensure that intensive care is available in the first few unpredictable hours.

General management

The patient must be confined to bed immediately, but the degree of restriction depends upon the severity of the infarction. If this has been mild and there is no evidence of cardiogenic shock or cardiac failure, patients should be allowed to feed themselves, use a commode, and gently exercise their legs from the outset. Within 1–2 days it may be possible for them to sit out of bed. Mobilization thereafter is rapid and the majority of patients should be ready for discharge within 5–7 days. In patients with extensive infarcts or experiencing complications due to heart failure or arrhythmias, mobilization and discharge are necessarily slower.

One of the greatest dangers after a myocardial infarction is the development of an unwarranted anxiety. This can be prevented by encouragement and explanation from the onset; the patient must understand that there is a good chance of recovery and return to near normal activity. At every stage an optimistic attitude should prevail, and it should be apparent that the physician expects the patient to recover.

Coronary care

For the first few days after the onset of acute myocardial infarction, the risk of sudden and unexpected death is high. This is largely due to arrhythmias, which can be treated or prevented by appropriate therapy. Because of the close observation required at this time, and the need to have appropriate equipment and skills immediately available, intensive care of a special kind is required.

Coronary care of patients with myocardial infarction has three essential components:

- the concentration of patients at maximal risk in special areas;
- their care by nurses and doctors with specialized training;
- the immediate availability of apparatus for monitoring the ECG and for resuscitation.

Coronary care units should reduce anxiety; the patient should initially be reassured by the constant observation and the excellence of the medical and nursing care. Subsequently, when the most acute stage is over, they should be encouraged that close supervision is no longer necessary.

Drug management of acute myocardial infarction

Aspirin

Aspirin reduces the mortality rate of acute myocardial infarction by approximately 20%. Its benefits are additive to those of thrombolytic therapy. A 300 mg tablet of soluble aspirin should be given as early as possible in acute infarction, which may mean before admission or in the emergency receiving room, rather than delaying treatment until the patient has arrived on the coronary care unit.

All patients in whom myocardial infarction is a possibility should be considered for aspirin therapy. Unlike thrombolytic therapy, distinguishing cases of myocardial infarction from those with unstable angina is not crucial, as aspirin therapy is appropriate for both. Moreover, contra-indications to aspirin are encountered less often than

contra-indications to thrombolytic agents. In general a h
ulceration in the past should not be regarded as a cor
aspirin. Cases in which a contra-indication to ar
regarded as sufficiently strong to forego a 20% mortality
in acute infarction are rare.

Thrombolytic therapy

All patients with suspected myocardial infarction should be considered for thrombolysis. As in the case of aspirin, the reduction in mortality rate achieved with thrombolytic therapy has been of the order of
20%. However, unlike aspirin, the treatment carries significant risks,
and careful consideration needs to be given to the risks and benefits in
each individual patient. This will involve consideration of the extent
and site of infarction, the time delay from the onset of symptoms and
any possible contra-indications to thrombolysis.

In general, the larger the infarct the greater is the potential benefit of
thrombolytic therapy. Anterior infarcts are generally bigger than
inferior ones and are associated with a higher mortality rate. Patients
with anterior infarction, therefore, gain more in absolute terms from
thrombolysis than those with inferior infarction.

It is also possible to define extent of benefit in terms of ECG changes
on presentation. Two categories of patient have been shown to benefit
from thrombolysis and should be treated:

- patients with ST elevation;
- patients with left bundle branch block (LBBB).

The association of benefits of thrombolysis with LBBB may at first
seem surprising. However, in patients presenting with a history con-
sistent with infarction, the presence of LBBB suggests extensive
infarction and defines a group who stand to gain substantially from
thrombolysis.

By contrast, patients with ST depression or T wave inversion do not
benefit from thrombolytic therapy. These patients represent a heteroge-
neous group, some with unstable angina and others with smaller infarctions, in whom the risks of thrombolytic therapy outweigh the benefits.

Timing of thrombolytic therapy. The benefits of thrombolysis diminish rapidly with time and the goal should be to administer therapy as
early as possible. Candidates for thrombolysis should either be 'fast-
tracked' from the receiving room to the coronary care unit or should
have thrombolytic therapy commenced in the receiving room. In rural
communities with a substantial delay to hospital admission, out-of-
hospital thrombolysis should be considered as an alternative.

The time window during which the benefits of thrombolysis exceed the
risks is defined imprecisely. For the majority of infarcts, thrombolysis

should be considered in patients presenting within 6 h of the onset of symptoms. Treatment between 6 and 12 h is still likely to benefit high-risk groups, such as patients with large anterior infarcts. Treatment beyond 12 h is unlikely to be beneficial.

Complications of thrombolytic therapy. Not surprisingly, bleeding is the major complication of thrombolytic therapy. Of potential bleeding sites, by far the most significant is intracerebral haemorrhage. This occurs with a frequency of approximately 1 in every 200 patients receiving thrombolytic therapy and is very frequently fatal. Consequently, a history of previous intracerebral or subarachnoid haemorrhage should be regarded as an absolute contra-indication to thrombolytic therapy. A history of recent head injury or cerebrovascular accident (whether embolic or haemorrhagic) should similarly be regarded as a major contra-indication.

Recent severe gastrointestinal bleeding must also be regarded as a major contra-indication. Other contra-indications are relative. These are summarized in Chapter 22 (see Table 22.1). The significance of these relative contra-indications must be considered in relation to the potential benefit of treatment. In patients with a high systolic blood pressure, this should first be controlled with intravenous nitrates, before commencing thrombolytic treatment.

The hazards of thrombolytic therapy tend to be greater in the elderly. However, the elderly are also at increased risk of dying as a result of infarction and, in general, the benefits of thrombolytic treatment out-weigh the risks.

Choice of thrombolytic agent. Three types of thrombolytic agent are licensed for use in acute infarction in the UK:

- streptokinase;
- anistreplase (a derivative of streptokinase);
- tissue plasminogen activator (tPA).

One major trial (ISIS-3 (International Study of Infarct Survival)) has found the three agents to be equally effective. An accelerated dosage regimen of tPA has been compared with streptokinase in a further trial (GUSTO II (Global Use of Strategies to Open Occluded Coronary Arteries)) and was found to confer a marginal advantage over a conventional streptokinase regimen. tPA is, however, substantially more expensive than streptokinase and selection of therapy should take into account a consideration of the cost–benefit ratio of each treatment.

Streptokinase stimulates antibody formation. For this reason repeated administration of streptokinase is best avoided, as the presence of antibodies is likely to neutralize the drug and prevent achieval of an adequate thrombolytic state. Streptokinase should not be reused within a time window of 5 days to at least 1 year. It may be wiser to extend this window to 2 years or even to avoid reuse altogether.

Anticoagulant therapy

The routine use of anticoagulant therapy with subcutaneous heparin has not been found to confer any advantage when applied globally to all patients following infarction. There remain, however, a number of situations in which anticoagulant therapy continues to be appropriate:

- to prevent reocclusion following thrombolysis with tPA, intravenous heparin should be administered for 24 h;
- to prevent deep vein thrombosis in patients with complicated infarction or with other reasons for immobility, heparin can be administered subcutaneously in a dose of 12 500 units twice daily;
- to prevent thromboembolism in patients developing atrial fibrillation or with early aneurysm formation, initial treatment with intravenous heparin can be followed by long-term oral anticoagulation with warfarin.

Beta-blockade

Early intravenous beta-blockade confers some marginal advantages in acute infarction. There is a small reduction in mortality, which reflects a decreased incidence of death due to left ventricular rupture. However, early intravenous beta-blockade has not gained wide acceptance in UK coronary care units. The reasons for this are unclear but may reflect a cautious approach based on the experience that treatment may exacerbate heart failure and bradycardia in some patients.

The use of early intravenous beta-blockade should be distinguished from the use of oral beta-blockers in the recovery phase post-infarction where benefits are unequivocal (see below).

Angiotensin-converting enzyme (ACE) inhibitors

The use of ACE inhibitors in the acute phase of infarction is controversial. While benefits of a global approach – treating all patients – have been demonstrated, it is unclear whether this confers any additional benefit over a delayed, selective approach, commencing ACE inhibitors in targeted patients a few days post-infarction (see below).

Other drugs

The value of various other drugs, which include lignocaine, nitrates and magnesium, in acute infarction has been addressed in other large studies. It has been concluded that a global approach to the administration of these drugs confers no overall benefit. This is not to deny a continuing value of these therapies in specific situations, such as the use of lignocaine or magnesium to treat arrhythmias or the use of nitrates to treat symptoms of continuing angina.

Prognosis

In about one-quarter of all episodes of acute myocardial infarction, death occurs suddenly within minutes of the onset. Such cases are seldom seen by a physician. The remainder of this discussion is concerned with the prognosis of those who survive this immediate period.

The overall natural mortality rate, excluding the very early deaths, is approximately 15–30%, but this has been greatly reduced by treatment so that the in-hospital mortality rate now averages about 10%. The risk of death depends upon many factors, including the age of the patient, previous myocardial infarction and the presence of other diseases, as well as the extent of the infarction.

The mortality rate of the acute attack rises sharply with age. Today the death rate is probably less than 5% in those under 50 years of age, but may rise to 20–30% in the elderly. Mortality is higher in women than in men, but this is largely accounted for by the fact that infarction occurs relatively uncommonly in the younger female. The mortality rate is greater in recurrent compared with first infarction, particularly when there has been preceding cardiac failure.

The risk of dying is highest in the first few hours and decreases rapidly thereafter. Some 60% or more of all deaths within 4 weeks occur within the first 2 days. During this time, prognostication is difficult because dangerous arrhythmias may develop unpredictably. At the end of 48 h, the assessment of the prognosis for the rest of the 4-week period is reasonably accurate if the blood pressure, the signs of cardiac failure and the occurrence of serious arrhythmias are taken into account. Cardiogenic shock carries a mortality rate of 80–90%. Persistent tachycardia, continuing gallop rhythm and the development of right-sided heart failure are unfavourable features. Ventricular tachycardia, bundle branch block and atrial fibrillation are associated with a high mortality rate. Death may occur unexpectedly, late in the course of acute myocardial infarction, from further myocardial infarction, rupture and pulmonary embolism.

COMPLICATIONS OF ACUTE MYOCARDIAL INFARCTION AND THEIR MANAGEMENT

Disturbances of rate, rhythm and conduction

These occur in 95% of patients with acute myocardial infarction. In about half of these, they are severe enough to be of clinical importance.

Ventricular arrhythmias

Ventricular ectopic beats are almost invariable in the early phase of infarction. They are generally of no consequence, but those of the R-on-T variety (Fig. 9.6) are of significance as they may be a prelude to ventricular fibrillation.

Ventricular tachycardia is more sinister both because of the haemodynamic compromise it may cause in its own right and because of the possible progression to ventricular fibrillation. Ventricular tachycardia complicating acute infarction is generally polymorphic and non-sustained, in contrast to ventricular tachycardias arising late after infarction, which are frequently sustained and monomorphic.

The general rule for the treatment of both ventricular ectopics and non-sustained ventricular tachycardia is to avoid treatment unlesss the arrhythmia is causing haemodynamic compromise. Hypokalaemia and hypomagnesaemia should be corrected. If treatment is necessary, then intravenous lignocaine is the treatment of choice.

Ventricular fibrillation is the most important single cause of death in acute myocardial infarction and occurs in 8–10% of hospitalized patients. In about half of these cases, there has been no preceding shock or cardiac failure and the ventricular fibrillation is 'primary'. In the remainder, it can be regarded as being secondary to these complications.

Ventricular fibrillation is best treated by immediate d.c. shock of 200 J (see p. 396). If a defibrillator is not immediately available, external resuscitation must be initiated and continued until the apparatus arrives. The prognosis of patients with ventricular fibrillation depends on their condition before the onset of this arrhythmia. If free of shock or cardiac failure, and if d.c. shock is immediately available, 90% have a chance of being alive 1 month later. If either of these complications has been present, the chances are approximately 25%.

Atrial arrhythmias

Atrial fibrillation and atrial flutter are relatively common following myocardial infarction. They generally indicate a substantial infarction

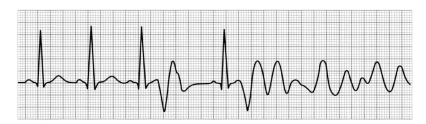

Fig. 9.6 Ventricular ectopic beats interrupting the T wave of preceding beats (R-on-T phenomenon). The second such beat initiates ventricular fibrillation.

causing significant ventricular dysfunction and as such are an adverse prognostic indicator.

Any underlying failure should be treated. Episodes of atrial fibrillation can be treated with either digoxin or amiodarone. Digoxin is a more conventional treatment, but its benefits are confined to limiting AV node conduction and hence ventricular response rate with no direct antifibrillatory action. Amiodarone offers the advantage of a class III antiarrhythmic action (see Chapter 11), with a direct antifibrillatory effect and so offers the haemodynamic advantage of restoration of sinus rhythm. On rare occasions it may be necessary to restore sinus rhythm quickly with a synchronized d.c. shock.

Bradyarrhythmias

Sinus bradycardia is common in the early phase of acute myocardial infarction, particularly in inferior and posterior infarcts. In some patients the bradycardia may be due partly to a vagal response to severe pain. Adequate pain relief may help to relieve the bradycardia. When sinus bradycardia does not result in haemodynamic compromise, no specific treatment is necessary. In cases of hypotension, intravenous atropine should be administered.

Junctional bradycardia is a frequent accompaniment of reperfusion and indeed can be used as a marker of successful reperfusion. Specific treatment is seldom necessary.

Heart block is a relatively common complication of inferior myocardial infarction, reflecting the fact that the right coronary artery provides the arterial supply to the AV node. All degrees of block may occur from PR prolongation to complete heart block, and transition between the phases of block is generally gradual. Second-degree block is common and is generally of Wenckebach (Mobitz I) type (see p. 203), with a gradually prolonged PR interval before the non-conducted P wave.

Pacing is seldom required in inferior infarction. Even if complete heart block ensues, there is generally a satisfactory escape focus ensuring the maintenance of an adequate heart rate. Pacing is indicated only in patients showing haemodynamic compromise. Complete heart block complicating inferior infarction generally resolves within a few days and permanent pacing is seldom necessary.

Complete heart block complicating anterior infarction is rare, but has a very different significance. It implies very extensive infarction, which of itself carries a poor prognosis. The site of block is more distal in the conduction system. As a consequence, block may occur suddenly or may be preceded by evidence of bundle branch block or Mobitz II second-degree block (see p. 203), but not by PR prolongation. As a further consequence the escape rhythm is unstable and has a wide QRS complex; temporary pacing is likely to be necessary. Permanent pacing may also be required, although whether this leads to any improvement in mortality in this very high risk group is unclear.

Bundle branch block

Block occurring lower in the conduction system will give the appearance of bundle branch block. This may involve any of the three subdivisions of the His–Purkinje system, the right bundle and either the anterior or the posterior division of the left bundle. If two fascicles are involved, this results in bifascicular block. All combinations are possible:

- left anterior and posterior fascicles (causing complete left bundle branch block);
- right bundle and left anterior fascicle (causing right bundle branch block and left axis deviation); and
- right bundle and left posterior fascicle (causing right bundle branch block and right axis deviation). This combination is rare.

When, in addition to the changes of bifascicular block, the PR interval is prolonged, this may indicate delay in conduction in the sole remaining fascicle. This is termed trifascicular block.

The development of changes of bundle branch block are indicative of a poor prognosis, which primarily reflects the extent of infarction rather than susceptibility to bradyarrhythmias. The role of pacing (temporary or permanent) is controversial.

Heart failure and cardiogenic shock

Left ventricular failure

This is seldom present at the onset, but develops within 48 h in perhaps one third of patients with acute myocardial infarction. It can be suspected from tachycardia, a third heart sound, widespread pulmonary crepitations and pulmonary venous congestion or oedema on the chest radiograph. Catheterization, using a Swan–Ganz or similar catheter, will show a pulmonary wedge pressure in excess of 20 mmHg.

Cardiogenic shock

The patient at the onset of infarction is often pale, distressed and hypotensive. This situation, which is often transient, may be attributed to pain and should not be described as cardiogenic shock. This term should be restricted to those patients who have the clinical picture of hypotension, with cold cyanosed extremities, sweating and mental torpor, which lasts at least half an hour, or who deteriorate rapidly until the blood pressure can no longer be recorded. There is a low cardiac output and a peripheral resistance insufficient to compensate for this, together with oliguria, hypoxia and acidosis. Arrhythmias and cardiac failure are frequently associated and the mortality rate is 80–90%

irrespective of treatment. Shock is largely the result of severe myocardial damage with more than 40% of the ventricular wall being infarcted. Occasionally, the shock picture is accounted for by arrhythmias such as ventricular tachycardia or complete heart block, in which case correction of the arrhythmia may result in recovery. In a few patients, particularly those who have been receiving diuretics, hypovolaemia may be a factor. In others, it is the consequence of right ventricular infarction. Rarely, a surgically correctable disorder, such as a ruptured papillary muscle or a ventricular septal defect, may be responsible (see below).

The most important single factor is the extent of myocardial damage sustained in the current and previous myocardial infarctions. Others, which are more amenable to correction, are:

- arrhythmias and conduction disorders;
- hypovolaemia, sometimes the consequence of previous treatment with diuretics, antihypertensives and pressor drugs;
- right ventricular infarction, which may produce a clinical picture of high venous pressure, with low systemic arterial and pulmonary wedge pressures;
- previous treatment with beta-adrenoceptor drugs;
- lesions such as a ventricular septal defect which are surgically correctable.

If possible patients with cardiac failure or shock should be categorized using the data available from intravascular monitoring with a Swan–Ganz catheter. Three major groups can be identified:

- those with 'backward' failure, i.e. with a cardiac index $> 2.21/min/m^2$ and pulmonary wedge pressure > 18 mmHg. Such patients maintain their blood pressure but have pulmonary oedema. Appropriate treatment includes diuretics and vasodilators (e.g. nitrates) and, possibly, digitalis;
- those with 'forward' failure, i.e. with a cardiac index $< 2.21/min/m^2$ and pulmonary artery wedge pressure < 12 mmHg. Such patients usually respond to the administration of plasma expanders;
- those with both pulmonary oedema and hypotension (cardiac output $< 2.21/min/m^2$ and pulmonary artery wedge pressure > 18 mmHg). The mortality rate in this group is very high, but an attempt should be made to improve left ventricular function by reducing afterload (with vasodilators) and increasing contractility with inotropic drugs (see also Chapter 10).

It is important neither to overload the circulation nor to lower the filling pressure of the left ventricle excessively. One should aim to keep the pulmonary artery wedge pressure between 15 and 20 mmHg.

The intra-aortic balloon pump (see p. 386) can produce temporary clinical improvement, but this is not maintained unless some major factor can be corrected, e.g. the surgical closure of a ventricular septal defect.

Right ventricular failure

It is important to distinguish right ventricular failure from other causes of heart failure following myocardial infarction as recognition can lead to appropriate corrective measures. Right ventricular infarction may occur in inferior and posterior infarcts. Typically patients have a depressed cardiac output or even cardiogenic shock in the presence of normal left ventricular filling pressures. The jugular venous pulse is characteristically raised, although the other classical features of right heart failure (ankle oedema and hepatomegaly) usually take several days to develop and are uncommon in the acute phase of infarction.

The ECG can be used to provide confirmation of right ventricular infarction. To do this, the right chest leads should be recorded, transposing the normal left precordial leads to the right precordium. Most patients with right ventricular infarction have ST elevation in lead V4R (right precordial lead in V4 position) (see Fig. 9.3B).

In patients with hypotension or cardiogenic shock due to right ventricular infarction, plasma volume should be expanded by administration of intravenous fluids to increase right-sided filling pressures. Pulmonary artery pressure monitoring may be of value in optimizing left heart filling pressures and is likely to be necessary in patients who have simultaneous left ventricular impairment.

Mechanical complications of infarction

A number of mechanical complications may occur giving rise to heart failure or cardiogenic shock. Their recognition is important as the conditions are potentially treatable.

Ventricular septal defect

This occurs in approximately 1 in every 200 patients with acute infarction. It results in the development of severe heart failure, and frequently leads to cardiogenic shock. Characteristically the patient suddenly deteriorates accompanied by the development of a pansystolic murmur, maximal at the left sternal edge. The differential diagnosis is papillary muscle rupture (see below). The two conditions can generally be distinguished by transthoracic echo. Alternatively, right heart catheterization can be undertaken to demonstrate a step-up in oxygen saturation at the right ventricular level.

Untreated, the complication is almost invariably fatal. Urgent surgical repair is generally indicated, although surgical mortality is high.

Papillary muscle rupture

Papillary muscle rupture is a second cause of acute haemodynamic deterioration after infarction, and is similarly accompanied by the development of a new pansystolic murmur. Echocardiography reveals the regurgitant jet across the mitral valve. Unlike ventricular septal defect, which generally complicates large infarcts, papillary muscle rupture may complicate relatively small infarcts. The treatment is surgical repair.

It is important to distinguish papillary muscle rupture from other causes of mitral regurgitation following myocardial infarction. Extensive left ventricular damage frequently results in functional mitral regurgitation. Treatment is the management of accompanying heart failure.

Cardiac rupture

Rupture through the wall of the left ventricle is responsible for about 10% of all deaths and particularly affects the elderly and the hypertensive. It is most likely to occur during the first few days and most commonly presents with the clinical features of cardiac arrest, but with continuing electrical activity in the electrocardiogram (electromechanical dissociation).

While rupture generally leads to immediate death, occasionally subacute rupture can occur, which may be amenable to surgical repair. Some cases of subacute rupture later give rise to the features of a pseudoaneurysm. In this condition organizing thrombus seals an area of left ventricular rupture, preventing the development of a haemopericardium. With time, the area of thrombus and the overlying pericardium may form a pseudoaneurysm, communicating with the left ventricular cavity.

Recurrent ischaemia and infarction

Following infarction, patients are vulnerable to recurrent ischaemia and extension of the original infarct. In addition, patients who have undergone successful reperfusion are vulnerable to reocclusion. In practice, it may be difficult to distinguish between infarct extension and reinfarction, and the two are best considered under the single term of recurrent infarction. Diagnosis is based on the development of additional ECG changes or a second peak in the level of cardiac enzymes.

Post-infarction angina is an indication for early coronary angiography with a view to coronary angioplasty or bypass surgery as appropriate. Patients developing further ST elevation should be considered for repeat thrombolysis or urgent angioplasty.

Miscellaneous complications

Pulmonary embolism and infarction.   Twenty or more years ago, pulmonary embolism caused death in about 3% of all patients admitted to hospital with acute myocardial infarction. It has become relatively rare, presumably because patients are now mobilized much earlier than they were. It is usually preceded by deep vein thrombosis in the legs, but this may not be clinically evident. Pulmonary embolism should be suspected if hypotension or right heart failure develop some days after the onset of myocardial infarction, and also when there is a pleuritic type of chest pain with or without haemoptysis.

Systemic arterial embolism.   Embolism may occur from mural thrombi situated in the left ventricle or left atrium. Hemiplegia is a common result, but there may be occlusion of any artery.

Cerebrovascular accidents.   Cerebrovascular accidents may precede, accompany or follow acute myocardial infarction. As mentioned, cerebral embolism is one cause, but cerebral infarction may develop, as may cerebral haemorrhage, particularly when thrombolytic drugs are used.

Pericarditis

The main differential of recurrent chest pain in the first few days after infarction lies between recurrent ischaemia/infarction and pericarditis. The diagnosis is generally a clinical one, based on the nature of the patient's discomfort. Characteristically pericarditic pain varies with inspiration and with body posture – worse on inspiration and alleviated by sitting up and leaning forward.

Treatment of pericarditic discomfort consists of aspirin. Non-steroidal anti-inflammatory agents and steroids are best avoided because of the concern that they may contribute to adverse ventricular remodelling and infarct expansion (see below). Caution is also advisable in the use of anticoagulants at this time because of the risk of haemorrhagic pericarditis.

LATE COMPLICATIONS OF INFARCTION

There are two main late consequences of myocardial infarction: impaired pump function and arrhythmias.

Infarct expansion

Ventricular impairment following myocardial infarction is due only in part to the myocardial necrosis that occurs at the time of the infarct. In the ensuing weeks and months ventricular remodelling occurs, which may lead to further deterioration in ventricular function. This secondary deterioration in ventricular function arises from expansion and thinning of the infarct zone (Fig. 9.7). This infarct expansion results in an increase in ventricular volume, which in turn causes an increase in wall tension. As a result a vicious circle may be established resulting in progressive ventricular dilatation.

ACE inhibitors reduce infarct expansion and help to prevent adverse ventricular remodelling. As a consequence, ACE inhibitors now have a major role in the management of patients after infarction (see below). Patients at increased risk of adverse remodelling include those with large infarcts, anterior infarcts and infarcts that have failed to reperfuse. ACE inhibitors are particularly indicated in these patient groups.

Ventricular aneurysm formation

Ventricular aneurysm formation represents the most extreme form of infarct remodelling. Although the prognosis in those affected is reasonably good, the area of paradoxically moving non-contractile myocardium leads to extra work for the remaining heart muscle. In some cases this contributes to cardiac failure together with a risk of embolism from mural thrombi. There is also an increased risk of serious ventricular arrhythmias. The presence of an aneurysm is suggested by a systolic pulsation of the anterior chest wall lasting more than

Infarct expansion

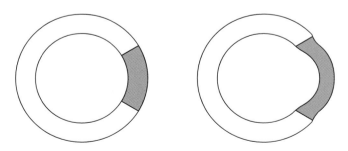

Fig. 9.7 Infarction thinning and elongation of the infarcted myocardium results in infarct expansion. This infarct expansion has an additional adverse effect on cardiac pump function.

3 weeks after the infarction. Other evidence includes persistent QS waves and ST elevation in the affected leads, an abnormal rounded protrusion from the left ventricular wall on the chest radiograph (Fig. 9.8), and paradoxical movement on fluoroscopy. These features are not always present. The aneurysm may be demonstrated by echocardiography, radionuclide studies and left ventriculography. If it is causing heart failure or serious arrhythmias, surgical removal of the aneurysm may be necessary. Anticoagulants reduce the risk of thromboembolism.

Late arrhythmias

The electrical changes occurring as a consequence of infarction lead to electrical instability and, in a small proportion of patients, to a long-term susceptibility to serious ventricular arrhythmias. In the majority of cases these arise from areas of electrically viable myocardium, separated by areas of fibrosis, which result in delayed conduction and create the re-entry circuits that give rise to ventricular tachycardia and ventricular fibrillation. Whereas ventricular tachycardia and fibrillation occurring within the first 24–48 h of infarction are due to the electrical instability of acute infarction, and do not imply a long-term

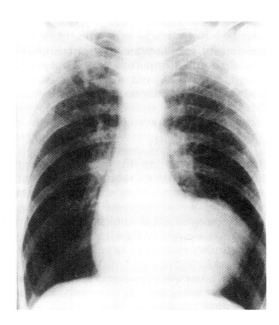

Fig. 9.8 Left ventricular aneurysm. An abnormal, rounded protrusion of the left heart border is apparent.

electrical instability, sustained ventricular arrhythmias occurring after this time are indicative of long-term electrical instability and a risk of sudden death. Such patients should be considered for electrophysiological investigations, anti-arrhythmic drug therapy or an implantable defibrillator (see p. 214).

RISK STRATIFICATION AT HOSPITAL DISCHARGE

In patients who have survived acute myocardial infarction, the outlook is better than is often appreciated. The prognosis is best in those who are free of hypertension, angina and cardiac failure. Overall, between 80 and 90% of patients survive at least 1 year, approximately 75% survive 5 years, and 50% 10 years and 25% 20 years. The risk of further infarction and sudden death persists but diminishes as time elapses.

Attempts should be made before discharge to identify patients at higher than average risk of recurrent infarction or death. Long-term prognosis is determined by three factors:

- left ventricular function;
- the extent of residual coronary disease;
- susceptibility to serious ventricular arrhythmias.

Assessment of ventricular function

Left ventricular function is the single strongest determinant of long-term outcome. This is most easily assessed by measuring left ventricular ejection fraction. This can be achieved by either echocardiography or radionuclide imaging. The relation between ejection fraction and prognosis (Fig. 9.9) is non-linear, mortality increasing markedly for values of ejection fraction below 30%.

Unfortunately the value of assessing left ventricular function as a determinant of prognosis has to be tempered by the limited ability to modify prognosis in patients with ventricular impairment.

Assessment of ischaemia

Estimating the risk of further infarction and appropriate intervention to reduce risk would be highly desirable objectives. There is, however, little clinical trial evidence defining an optimal approach to this problem, and clinical practice varies.

Coronary angiography offers the advantage of an accurate measure of the extent of residual coronary disease, but does not provide information on the functional severity of lesions. In many health care systems, offering coronary angiography to all patients recovering from infarction is not a feasible practical proposition.

Exercise testing is more generally applicable and enables a low-risk group not requiring further investigation to be identified. Exercise testing can be performed either before discharge using a relatively modest exercise protocol or after discharge using conventional submaximal testing. The former has the advantage of identifying high-risk individuals before discharge, while the latter offers the advantage of providing more complete diagnostic information. Once again, preference for pre- or post-discharge testing will depend on local circumstances.

Exercise testing following myocardial infarction fulfills a further most important objective: increasing patient confidence in their ability to resume a reasonably normal lifestyle and hence playing an important role in rehabilitation (see below).

Assessment of electrical instability

A number of non-invasive investigations have been shown to identify patients at risk of serious ventricular arrhythmias and sudden death following myocardial infarction. These include Holter monitoring, high-resolution electrocardiography, assessment of heart rate variability and measures of autonomic dysfunction. However, the tests have a relatively low positive predictive value. Moreover, at this time no simple drug treatment has been identified to improve prognosis. On this basis, screening methods for arrhythmia risk are still best considered a research tool rather than part of routine clinical practice.

DRUG TREATMENT AT DISCHARGE

A number of drug therapies have been shown to improve long-term prognosis after infarction and every patient post-infarction should be considered for these therapies. The therapies concerned are:

- beta-blockers;
- ACE inhibitors;
- statins;
- aspirin.

Beta-blockers

Long-term beta-blockade has been shown to reduce the mortality rate by about 25%. The benefit arises largely from a reduction in the number of patients dying suddenly. The potential benefits are greatest in those at greatest risk, particularly patients with more severely impaired ventricular function. This, of course, poses a problem in that beta-blockade may be poorly tolerated by these individuals. In many patients with mild to moderate heart failure, however, a beta-blocker can be introduced successfully. In such patients it is judicious to commence treatment with low-dose therapy and gradually to titrate dosage upwards.

ACE inhibitors

ACE inhibitors have also been shown to reduce long-term mortality following myocardial infarction. There is no general agreement as to when treatment should be started or as to which patients should be treated.

A global approach of treating all patients, starting therapy in the acute phase of infarction on the day of admission, has been shown to provide a small but statistically significant overall mortality benefit. An alternative approach is to wait until after the acute phase and commence treatment between days 3 and 5, targeting patients thought to be most at risk of infarct expansion (see p. 146). This selective approach is more cost-effective than a global approach to therapy. Using this selective approach, groups targeted for treatment might include:

- patients manifesting clinical or radiological evidence of heart failure;
- patients with a moderate or large anterior infarct;
- patients with significant left ventricular impairment as reflected by an ejection fraction of less than 40% or significant regional wall motion abnormalities on echocardiography.

Statins

Hypercholesterolaemia is a risk factor for further infarction, and lowering cholesterol levels has been shown to reduce recurrent coronary events after infarction. Patients with infarction have already identified themselves as at risk from coronary disease and an aggressive approach to cholesterol lowering is therefore justified.

The threshold cholesterol level for considering the addition of cholesterol-lowering drug therapy is uncertain. Benefits of statin therapy have been demonstrated in a population of post-infarct patients, irrespective of cholesterol levels at presentation, suggesting that whatever the initial cholesterol level the patient will benefit from having it lowered further. However, subgroup analysis suggests that benefits are modest when the initial total cholesterol concentration is less than 5.0 mmol/l, and in particular it may be reasonable to confine treatment to patients with a cholesterol level greater than this value.

Checking cholesterol levels in patients after infarction is problematic. In the first 24 h of infarction, values are representative of the patient's normal cholesterol level. Following this, cholesterol levels fall for several weeks and may give a falsely low estimate in comparison with long-term values. Ideally, therefore, samples for cholesterol estimation should be drawn within the first 24 h of infarction or else delayed to subsequent outpatient follow-up.

Aspirin

Aspirin is of proven benefit in the acute and subacute phases after myocardial infarction. In common with other patients with established coronary disease, it is conventional to continue with long-term aspirin therapy unless the drug is contra-indicated or the patient experiences significant side-effects relating to its use.

REHABILITATION

Although many patients make an initially satisfactory recovery following myocardial infarction, the longer term outcome in terms of return to normal activities, including work, and freedom from recurrences is often disappointing.

Failure to return to a normal life may be due to physical factors, but it is often the result of anxiety or inadequate instruction and rehabilitation. It is helpful if, in the milder case, a limited exercise tolerance test is carried out 1–2 weeks after the infarction in which the patient exercises until a heart rate of 120–130 is achieved. If such a heart rate can be attained without cardiac symptoms or ST depression on the ECG, the outlook is very good and the patient can be encouraged to return quickly to a near normal life. For example, 4–8 weeks after discharge, the individual should be walking out of doors and up hills and stairs, be able to return to car driving and sexual activity, and should go back to work, provided this is not physically strenuous, shortly thereafter. Patients whose exercise tolerance is less good require slower convalescence and more careful observation. If angina pectoris or dyspnoea are major symptoms, careful attention to drug therapy and consideration of angioplasty or surgery is necessary.

Many patients find a formal rehabilitation programme helpful in restoring confidence and physical well-being. The patient usually attends two or three out-patient sessions a week for a period of 3–6 months. A graduated exercise programme, tailored to the individual patient, is accompanied by counselling on lifestyle, and advice on preventive measures and relaxation techniques.

The stopping of smoking and the control of hyperlipidaemia, hypertension and diabetes are all important in the survivor of myocardial infarction and should be emphasised in the rehabilitation programme.

Further reading

Acute Infarction Ramipril Efficacy (AIRE) Study Investigations (1993) Effect of ramipril on mortality and morbidity of survivors of acute myocardial infarction with clinical evidence of heart failure. *Lancet* **342**, 821.

[Anonymous] (1992) How to anticoagulate. *Drugs and Therapeutics Bulletin* **30**: 77.

Antman, E. M. (1994) General hospital management. In Julian, D. L. and Brunwald, E. (Eds), *Management of Acute Myocardial Infarction*, p. 63. London: WB Saunders Company.

Fibrinolytic Therapy Trialists Collaborative Group (1995) Indications for fibrinolytic therapy in suspected acute myocardial infarction: collaborative overview of early mortality and major morbidity results from all randomized trials of more than 1000 patients. In Ball, S. G. (Ed) *Myocardial Infarction: From trials to practice*, p. 67. Petersfield: Wrightson Biomedical Publishing.

GUSTO Angiographic Investigators. The comparative effects of tissue plasminogen activator, streptokinase, or both on coronary artery patency, ventricular function and survival after acute myocardial infarction (1993) *New England Journal of Medicine* **329**: 1615.

Hirsh, J. (1991) Heparin. *New England Journal of Medicine* **324**: 1565.

ISIS-2 Collaborative Group (1988) Randomized trial of intravenous streptokinase, oral aspirin, both, or neither among 17 187 cases of suspected acute myocardial infarction. *Lancet* **ii**: 349.

ISIS-4 Collaborative Group (1995) Randomized factorial trial assessing early oral captopriol, oral mononitrate and intravenous magnesium sulphate in 58050 patients with suspected acute myocardial infarction. *Lancet* **345**: 669.

Julian, D. G., & Braunwald, E. (Eds) (1994) *Management of Acute Myocardial Infarction*. Philadelphia: Saunders.

Lindsay, H. S. J., Zaman, A. G., Cowan J. C. (1995) ACE inhibitors after myocardial infarction: Patient selection or treatment for all? *British Heart Journal* **73**: 397.

Pfeffer, M. A., Braunwald, E., Moye, L. A. et al. (1992) Effect of captopril on mortality and morbidity in patients with left ventricular dysfunction after myocardial infarction. *New England Journal of Medicine* **327**: 669.

Sacks, F. M., Pfeffer, M. A., Moye, L. A. et al. (1996) The effect of pravastatin in coronary event after myocardial infarction in patients with average cholesterol levels. *New England Journal of Medicine* **335**: 1001–9.

Wenger, N. K. (1986) Rehabilitation of the coronary patient. *Progress in Cardiovascular Diseases* **29**: 181.

Yusuf, S., Peto, R., Lewis, J. et al. (1985) Beta blockade during and after myocardial infarction: An overview of the randomized trials. *Progress in Cardiovascular Diseases* **27**: 335.

Heart Failure

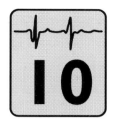

Failure in anything implies expectations unfulfilled, and one's definition of heart failure depends upon what one expects of the heart. No single definition suffices because the clinical and physiological criteria necessarily differ.

The clinician regards his patient as having heart failure when there are symptoms or physical signs attributable to inadequate cardiac performance. The physiologist regards the heart as failing when the contractility of the ventricles or the cardiac output falls outside the statistically defined normal range. There is no clear distinction between normality and abnormality; values in the 'abnormal' range may be found in normal hearts in the face of extreme demand, and 'normal' values may be encountered in diseased hearts when the demands are slight.

Cardiac failure, as it is understood in clinical practice, denotes the presence of one of the complexes of symptoms and signs associated with the 'congestion' of tissues and organs or attributable to the inadequate perfusion of tissues and organs:

- *pulmonary venous congestion* results from disordered function of the left ventricle or left atrium;
- *systemic venous congestion* is similarly due to disorders of the right ventricle and atrium, but is often the end-result of left-sided heart failure. The clinical features derive, in the main, from engorgement of the systemic veins and capillaries.

The heart has also failed when it cannot maintain an adequate blood pressure in spite of a peripheral vascular resistance that is normal or high but, by convention, this type of cardiac failure is referred to as acute circulatory failure or cardiogenic shock rather than heart failure.

THE PATHOPHYSIOLOGY OF HEART FAILURE

The causes of heart failure

The heart fails either because it is subjected to an overwhelming load, or because the heart muscle is disordered:

- *a volume load* is imposed by disorders which demand that the ventricle expels more blood per minute than is normal. Examples include thyrotoxicosis and anaemia, in which the total cardiac output is increased; and mitral regurgitation and aortic regurgitation, in which the left ventricle has to expel not only the normal forward flow into the aorta but also the large volume of regurgitated blood as well;
- *a pressure load* is imposed by disorders which increase resistance to outflow from the ventricles (typified by systemic hypertension due to increased impedance of the peripheral arterioles, and by aortic stenosis in which there is narrowing of the outflow orifice of the left ventricle);
- *disorders of myocardial function* result not only from diminished contractility but also from loss of contractile tissue, as occurs in myocardial infarction. This is the commonest cause of heart failure. An additional factor in this condition is a paradoxical movement of infarcted muscle which further increases the work of the remaining myocardium.

In many cases, a combination of mechanisms contribute to failure. For example in patients with rheumatic heart disease, myocardial damage, valve narrowing and regurgitation may all be contributory.

Cardiac and circulatory responses in heart failure

The heart at first responds to pressure and volume overloads in much the same way as it does to normal increases in demand, such as those imposed by exercise. As the disorder progresses, more cardiac and circulatory adjustments take place which, for a time, may maintain an adequate circulation but many of the so called 'compensatory' mechanisms are inappropriate. During evolution the circulatory system has had to evolve methods of combating blood loss and trauma rather than, for example, myocardial infarction, and the responses invoked are relevant to the former stresses rather than the latter. Indeed, the clinical manifestations of heart failure are largely the effects of 'compensatory' mechanisms which eventually embarrass the circulation.

Dilatation of the heart – increase in end-diastolic volume

In response to a volume load, the heart dilates, i.e. the ventricular volume is increased. Up to a point, dilatation is a normal and efficient response but it is abnormal when it cannot be wholly ascribed to the volume load. Pathological dilatation of this kind occurs when there is myocardial disease, when, because of decreased contractility, the ventricle must be stretched to a greater extent for a given stroke volume. Even in those cases in which dilatation may at first be regarded as a physiological response, it eventually becomes disadvantageous because, as the ventricle increases in size, greater tension is required in the myocardium to expel a given volume of blood. This is in accordance with the law of Laplace which indicates that the tension in the myocardium (T) is proportional to the intraventricular pressure (P) multiplied by the radius (R) of the ventricular chamber ($T \propto PR$). The greater tension results in increased oxygen requirements.

This sequence is a major contributory factor in the deterioration in ventricular function following myocardial infarction. Following infarction 'remodelling' of the ventricle occurs involving expansion and thinning of the infarct zone (Fig. 9.7). This infarct expansion causes an increase in the end-diastolic volume. In some patients this may help to compensate for the impaired contraction and to restore stroke volume to normal, but in others the resultant increase in wall tension causes progressive expansion, establishing a vicious circle of increasing wall tension and further expansion. In extreme cases this can lead to aneurysm formation.

Hypertrophy of the heart

When the ventricle has to face a chronic increase of pressure load, such as that imposed by arterial hypertension, aortic stenosis or pulmonary hypertension, the myocardium hypertrophies, i.e. it increases in weight as a result of an enlargement of individual muscle fibres. The process affects only those chambers upon which there are increased demands. The mechanism responsible for the development of cardiac hypertrophy is uncertain but it seems likely that it is a response to increased stretching or tension in muscle fibres which result from a raised diastolic volume or pressure. Hypertrophy may be regarded as a normal compensatory mechanism which permits the heart to cope with the increased demands, but becomes self-defeating when it is excessive. The thickening of the fibres increases the distance by which oxygen has to diffuse from the capillaries; eventually this leads to impaired oxygenation of the centre of the fibre. It is probable that this hypoxia is an important factor in the fibrosis which frequently develops in hypertrophied muscle.

Impaired myocardial contractility

In many types of heart disease, the major defect lies in the myocardium itself. This is the case in patients with myocarditis and cardiomyopathy. Myocardial involvement is often considerable in rheumatic heart disease.

Even when the primary disturbance is that of a volume or pressure overload, intrinsic myocardial function may eventually be affected adversely by dilatation and hypertrophy. Why the impaired myocardial contractility develops is uncertain, but it has been attrtibuted by some to overstretching of the sarcomeres (see p. 3). There may be a slowing up in the conversion of chemical energy into muscular work as a result of depression in the activity of ATPase, the enzyme responsible for the release of energy from ATP. Other possible contributory factors include depletion of noradrenaline (norepinephrine) stores in the myocardium.

The cardiac output in heart failure

By definition cardiac failure is present when the cardiac output is insufficient for the needs of the body, but some patients with an output in the normal range manifest the clinical features of cardiac failure, whereas other patients with low outputs are free of symptoms and signs. However, in cardiac failure, even if the cardiac output is normal at rest it usually responds inadequately to exercise. In conditions such as beri-beri and thyrotoxicosis, in which the cardiac output is abnormally high, it is still insufficient for the exceptional metabolic demands.

Neuroendocrine response to heart failure

Cardiac failure activates several components of the neuroendocrine system, which play an important intermediary role in its clinical manifestations (Fig. 10.1).

Sympathetic nervous system.   Activation of the sympathetic nervous system results in an increase in myocardial contractility, heart rate, and vasoconstriction of arteries and veins. Although this may be beneficial in maintaining blood pressure, it is adverse in so far as it increases preload, afterload, and myocardial oxygen requirement. There is also an increased plasma noradrenaline, but myocardial catecholamines are reduced.

Renin–angiotensin–aldosterone systems.   Both the fall in cardiac output itself and the increase in sympathetic tone reduce effective blood flow to the kidney and, consequently, increase renin secretion. Salt restriction and diuretic therapy also augment this. As a result, there is a rise in angiotensin II levels, which leads directly to vasoconstriction and indirectly, by stimulating aldosterone secretion, to sodium retention and the expansion of blood volume. This is advantageous in so far as increasing preload helps to maintain stroke volume by the Starling mechanism, but it does so at the expense of circulatory congestion.

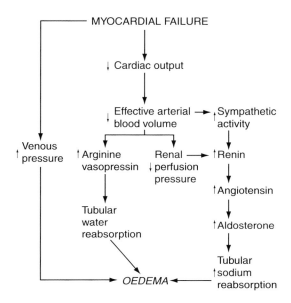

Fig. 10.1 Some of the neuroendocrine and renal responses to cardiac failure.

Arginine vasopressin (antidiuretic hormone). The reduced effective blood volume of heart failure stimulates the release of arginine vasopressin, leading to water retention. This is a feature of late, rather than early, cardiac failure.

Atrial natriuretic peptide. Distension of the atria leads to the release of this peptide which has natriuretic and vasodilator properties. Its role in cardiac failure is still unclear.

The regional circulations in cardiac failure

There is a redistribution of blood flow to different organs and tissues in cardiac failure, as there is on exercise. This redistribution is mediated through vasoconstriction in certain areas, notably the renal arterioles. The renal blood flow falls disproportionately, and may be reduced to one-quarter of normal. There is little reduction in the coronary or cerebral blood flow, but there is vasoconstriction of the skin and splanchnic vessels.

Salt and water retention

An almost invariable feature of cardiac failure is the retention of sodium and water. This leads to a substantial increase in extracellular and plasma volume and plays a large part in the production of the clinical features of cardiac failure. Some of the factors responsible for the fluid and salt retention are discussed above, but undoubtedly there are still undiscovered mechanisms.

Diminished glomerular filtration. Glomerular filtration is reduced in cardiac failure, although to a lesser extent than is renal blood flow. Diminished glomerular filtration may play some part in sodium retention, but it is probably not an important factor except when the failure is severe.

Increased tubular reabsorption. There is abundant experimental evidence that tubular reabsorption of sodium is increased in cardiac failure. There is no doubt that, in certain patients, there is increased aldosterone secretion, and that this hormone, by its action on the distal tubule, promotes the reabsorption of sodium whilst increasing the excretion of potassium and hydrogen. However, evidence of hyperaldosteronism is confined to advanced failure; aldosterone antagonists are relatively ineffective in the treatment of sodium retention in early failure. The enhanced tubular reabsorption of sodium found in cardiac failure seems to be mediated through some mechanism as yet undiscovered.

As mentioned, water retention in heart failure is usually secondary to sodium retention. In some patients with advanced cardiac failure, however, there is a disproportionate retention of water. In these patients, the kidneys can no longer excrete solute-free water and the serum sodium concentration falls as a result of dilution ('dilutional hyponatraemia').

Raised venous pressure in cardiac failure

When the left ventricle fails the pulmonary venous pressure rises, and when the right ventricle fails the pressure rises in the systemic veins. This can be largely explained by the inability of the failing ventricle to discharge the blood presented to it effectively. The increased blood volume resulting from sodium and water retention contributes to the venous return and is thus a factor in producing the raised venous pressure, as is venoconstriction.

The effect of left ventricular failure on the lungs

As explained above, when the left ventricle fails, the diastolic pressure in the left ventricle rises and with it the left atrial pressure. Since the pulmonary veins and capillaries are in continuity with the left atrium, the pressures in these vessels rise concomitantly. In mild left ventricular failure, the pressures in the left atrium and pulmonary veins are within normal limits at rest but rise on exercise. As failure advances, the left atrial pressure progressively increases from its normal level of 5–10 mmHg to one of 25–30 mmHg. The hydrostatic pressure in the capillaries is then close to that needed to overcome the osmotic pressure exerted by the plasma proteins and may lead to an exudation of fluid from the capillaries into the alveolar walls and alveoli. If the pressure in the atrium rises rapidly, there may be a sudden exudation of fluid into the alveoli. If this process takes place slowly, exudation may proceed gradually with a slow build up of tissue tension occurring in the alveolar wall. This restricts further exudation of fluid and limits the risk to the alveoli. In response to this process, some fibrosis may take place in the alveolar wall. The pulmonary congestion caused by the high pulmonary venous pressure and by the changes in the alveolar walls makes the lung more rigid (less compliant). As a result of this, more work must be done by the respiratory muscles to move a given volume of air.

Arrhythmias in heart failure

Patients with heart failure have a high incidence of sudden death. The majority of deaths are thought to be due to ventricular tachycardia or ventricular fibrillation.

A number of factors contribute to the occurrence of ventricular tachyarrhythmias in patients with heart failure. These include:

- high circulating catecholamine levels;
- electrolyte disturbance, particularly diuretic-induced hypokalaemia;
- proarrhythmic effects of inotropic drugs;
- stretch on the myocardium may result in arrhythmias through the process of 'contraction–excitation feedback'.

Arrhythmia prevention in patients with heart failure is a particular problem. The efficacy of antiarrhythmic drugs is reduced and there is, moreover, an increased incidence of proarrhythmic side-effects. In addition, most antiarrhythmic drugs have negative inotropic effects.

Although vasodilator treatment with angiotensin-converting enzyme (ACE) inhibitors has been shown to reduce mortality due to progression of heart failure (p. 166), it has not reduced mortality from sudden death, and this remains a major unsolved problem.

CLINICAL SYNDROMES OF HEART FAILURE

Left heart failure

Aetiology

The features of left heart failure develop when there is a major obstruction to outflow from the left atrium (e.g. mitral stenosis) or when the left ventricle can no longer cope with the demands upon it. The common causes of left ventricular failure are:

- myocardial infarction;
- systemic hypertension;
- aortic valve disease;
- mitral regurgitation;
- cardiomyopathy.

Clinical features

The clinical features of left-sided cardiac failure are largely the consequence of pulmonary congestion. The symptoms are:

- dyspnoea on exertion;
- orthopnoea and paroxysmal nocturnal dyspnoea;
- acute pulmonary oedema.

The physical signs of left ventricular failure may include:

- pulmonary crepitations;
- third heart sound;
- pleural effusion;
- pulsus alternans – alternate large and low volume pulse – this is an indication of severe left ventricular failure.

Investigations.   The chest radiograph shows:

- pulmonary venous congestion particularly of the upper lobe;
- interstitial oedema;
- alveolar oedema.

Some of these features are illustrated in Fig. 5.10.

The electrocardiogram may be of value although it does not provide direct evidence of left heart failure. For example, it is unusual for hypertension or aortic valve disease to lead to the symptoms of left heart failure without producing ECG evidence of left ventricular hypertrophy first. Again, it is unusual for coronary artery disease to lead to left heart failure if the ECG is normal. This is not, however, true of mitral regurgitation.

Echocardiography plays a particularly important role in the investigation of patients with heart failure. Typically left ventricular end-diastolic dimensions are increased and decreased systolic function is apparent. Echocardiography is also important in the exclusion of other potentially treatable causes of heart failure such as aortic stenosis or mitral regurgitation.

Differential diagnosis. The diagnosis of left heart failure is usually not difficult when there is progressive dyspnoea coupled with clinical evidence of advanced left-sided heart disease. However, this evidence may not always be unequivocal and there may be difficulty in distinguishing the symptoms of heart failure from those of pulmonary disease. The dyspnoea of left heart failure is more likely to be provoked by lying down flat. Patients with dyspnoea due to pulmonary disease usually have a history of asthmatic attacks or of chronic cough and sputum.

Paroxysmal nocturnal dyspnoea and acute pulmonary oedema may be difficult to differentiate from acute respiratory attacks. The latter are commonly associated with bronchospasm and purulent sputum. In contrast, the patient with acute pulmonary oedema is usually free of pulmonary infection, has fine crepitations rather than rhonchi and is liable to cough up pink frothy sputum. Furthermore, examination usually reveals the signs of left-sided heart disease. Correct diagnosis is of great importance because the therapy of the two conditions is different. For example, morphine may be lethal in respiratory failure, but invaluable in acute pulmonary oedema. Similarly, high concentrations of oxygen are useful in acute pulmonary oedema but may be dangerous in respiratory failure. The chest radiograph is also helpful in showing signs of oedema or infection. In cases of doubt, estimation of the arterial CO_2 tension is of value because this is usually low in acute pulmonary oedema and high in respiratory failure.

Right heart failure

Aetiology

Failure of the right side of the heart occurs when the right ventricle can no longer cope with the demands upon it, or when there is tricuspid stenosis. Common causes of right ventricular failure include:

- left ventricular failure with its consequent effects upon the pulmonary circulation;
- right ventricular infarction (see p. 143);
- pulmonary disease, particularly chronic bronchitis and emphysema;
- pulmonary hypertension (see p. 349);
- pulmonary valve disease;
- tricuspid regurgitation.

Clinical features

The characteristic features of right heart failure are:

- *elevated jugular venous pressure.* In the normal individual, the venous pressure in the internal jugular veins does not exceed 2 cm vertically above the sternal angle when the patient is reclining at 45°. In right heart failure this figure is exceeded. Even if normal at rest, it rises on exercise;

- *hepatomegaly.* If chronic, this may result in cirrhosis;
- *oedema.* This is of the dependent type and usually most evident in the pretibial and ankle regions;
- *ascites.* This may occasionally occur in patients with severe right heart failure.
- *tricuspid regurgitation.* This can occur in patients with severe or long-standing right heart failure, when right ventricular dilatation results in a functional incompetence of the tricuspid valve. A prominent V wave may be evident in the jugular venous pulse and a pulsatile liver edge may be palpable.

Differential diagnosis. In patients presenting with isolated signs of right heart failure, the possibility of pericardial constriction on tamponade should be considered as an alternative diagnosis (see Chapter 12).

Other clinical features of cardiac failure

There are a number of common but less specific features of cardiac failure. Fatigue is a frequent symptom which is difficult to evaluate.

The nutrition of patients with cardiac failure is often good in the early stages, but cachexia sets in as disability increases. In the very advanced case, cerebral symptoms may develop with dulling of consciousness, confusion or changes in personality. Patients with cardiac failure are prone to develop venous thrombosis and pulmonary emboli are common. Mild jaundice, due to hepatic congestion or cirrhosis, is quite frequent in right-sided heart failure. Proteinuria due to renal congestion is often present.

THE MANAGEMENT OF CARDIAC FAILURE

Ideally, the treatment of cardiac failure is the correction of the cause, but for a variety of reasons this may not be possible, at least initially. In some conditions, such as ischaemic heart disease and the cardiomyopathies, damage to the ventricular muscle may be irreversible and no currently available methods of treatment can correct the underlying muscle weakness. In other disorders, the radical treatment necessary for cure, such as major surgery, cannot be safely undertaken until cardiac failure has been corrected.

The principles of treating cardiac failure may be enumerated as follows:

- the correction or amelioration of the underlying disease;
- the control of precipitating factors;
- the reduction of demands on the heart by weight loss and the restriction of physical activity;
- pharmacological therapy to modify the heart failure state and, particularly, to reverse the adverse consequences of neuroendocrine and renal responses to heart failure.

The objectives of therapy are twofold: to alleviate the symptoms caused by heart failure and to improve the prognosis.

The correction or amelioration of the underlying cause

When heart disease is due to such causes as thyrotoxicosis or hypertension, corrective treatment can be started immediately. In congenital and rheumatic heart disease, surgical management is usually required, but this may have to be deferred until the maximum benefit has been achieved from medical treatment.

In the case of ischaemic heart disease, the cause of heart failure is generally previous myocardial infarction rather than ongoing ischaemia. Coronary revascularization procedures cannot ameliorate the damage caused by previous infarction and for this reason play little part in the management of heart failure.

The control of complicating factors

Cardiac failure is often precipitated or exacerbated by factors superimposed on the underlying heart disease. Amongst these are:

- arrhythmias;
- infections;
- pulmonary embolism;
- anaemia;
- excessive sodium intake;
- over-exertion.

The recognition of precipitating factors is of great importance in the management of heart failure, because the correction of these complicating conditions will often result in the abolition of symptoms.

Restriction of activity

Rest reduces the demands on the heart and leads to a fall in venous pressure and a reduction in pulmonary congestion. It allows a relative increase in renal blood flow and often leads to a diuresis. However, bed rest also encourages the development of venous thrombosis and pulmonary embolism.

The degree of physical restriction necessary depends upon the severity of the cardiac failure. When there is severe pulmonary congestion or peripheral oedema, a period of complete rest may be required. At this time, the patient is usually most comfortable propped up by two or more pillows in bed or in an armchair. Complete bed rest is seldom necessary for more than a few days, after which a gradual increase in activity should be encouraged, depending upon the response.

In patients with lesser degrees of heart failure, regular exercise should be encouraged. This should not be exhaustive, but the patient should aim to undertake regular aerobic activities such as walking or swimming. Isometric exercise, which is likely to increase peripheral resistance, is best avoided.

Pharmacological therapy

Two categories of drugs are commonly used in the management of patients with heart failure: diuretics and vasodilators. Other drugs that may have a role in particular patients include beta-blockers, digoxin and anti-arrhythmic agents.

MANAGEMENT OF SODIUM AND WATER RETENTION

Sodium and water retention are part of the neuroendocrine response to a fall in cardiac output in patients with heart failure (Fig. 10.1). Both may contribute to the patient's symptoms and hence both dietary sodium restriction and diuretics play an important role in the management of symptomatic heart failure.

Low salt diets effectively counteract cardiac failure. However, with the availability of potent diuretic drugs, no extreme limitation of sodium intake is usually necessary. Nevertheless, some restriction is desirable and inability to control cardiac failure is quite often due to the patient not reducing sodium intake sufficiently. All patients should be advised not to add salt at meals and to avoid obviously salty foods. Occasionally, a strict salt restriction must be applied. It is seldom necessary to practise water restriction, but in cases of dilutional hyponatraemia, a limitation of 1 litre per day may be helpful. These patients may be identified by a lack of response to conventional treatment for cardiac failure in association with a low serum sodium concentration.

Diuretics are valuable in the management of patients with symptomatic heart failure. Unlike vasodilator therapy (see below) there have been no studies to assess possible effects on prognosis, beneficial or adverse, and their role should be restricted to the treatment of symptomatic patients.

All the commonly used diuretics act by promoting sodium excretion, with enhanced urate excretion as a secondary effect.

The loop diuretics: frusemide, bumetanide

These drugs prevent reabsorption at multiple sites including the proximal and distal tubules and the ascending limb of the loop of Henle. They produce a profound diuresis with the excretion of large quantities of sodium and chloride. When given by mouth, action commences in about 1 hour and is complete in 6–8 hours. If given intravenously, the onset of action is almost immediate.

Thiazide diuretics

The many drugs in this group are essentially similar except in their potency and duration of action. Most of the thiazide diuretics act for 12–24 h whereas polythiazide and chlorthalidone exert their effect for 48 h or more. They may have several sites of action, but the main mechanism is the inhibition of sodium reabsorption in the distal convoluted tubule.

These diuretics are less potent than the loop diuretics, but are rather more likely to produce hypokalaemia. If the serum potassium is low, supplements of slow release potassium chloride should be used.

These drugs sometimes cause hyperglycaemia and hyperuricaemia, and may precipitate diabetes and clinical gout. Other occasional undesirable effects include agranulocytosis, thrombocytopenia, nausea, abdominal discomfort, impotence and skin rashes.

Thiazide and loop diuretic combinations.   Combination of a thiazide and loop diuretic is of value in patients with refractory oedema. A particularly vigorous diuresis may ensue, and it is advisable to reduce the dose of both drugs to guard against intravascular volume depletion, severe hypokalaemia and deterioration in renal function. Close supervision of such combination therapy is essential.

Potassium-sparing diuretics

This group comprises two classes of agent:

- *spironolactone.* This drug is an aldosterone antagonist;
- *amiloride and triamterene.* These drugs inhibit the collecting duct sodium conductance.

Potassium-sparing diuretics are relatively ineffective when used singly. Their chief value in the treatment of heart failure is in combination with either a loop or a thiazide diuretic, to reduce the potassium losses associated with these agents.

Hyperkalaemia is a potential complication, particularly in patients with impaired renal function.

VASODILATOR THERAPY

Constriction of the arterioles and veins is a characteristic feature of cardiac failure. In early cardiac failure, the reduction in vascular bed may be beneficial in ensuring an adequate venous return and maintaining the blood pressure, but frequently, particularly in more advanced failure, the arteriolar constriction imposes an excessive after-load and a venoconstriction too high a preload. Depending upon the pathophysiology of the individual case, it may be desirable to reduce preload or afterload or both.

Generally, in cardiac failure, it has been found that the optimal fill-ing (or end-diastolic) pressure of the left ventricle is between 15 and 20 mmHg. If the pressure is higher than this, pulmonary congestion will result. The administration of a venodilator will cause the filling pressure to fall, but the cardiac output either stays the same or increases. Ideally, before using a venodilator, the left ventricular end-diastolic pressure should be measured indirectly from a pulmonary wedge pressure recording. Venodilator drugs should not be given to patients with filling pressures of less than 15 mmHg; the admini-stration of venodilating drugs should be discontinued when such a pressure has been achieved.

The increased arteriolar resistance that results in excessive afterload imposes a burden on the heart which leads to a fall in cardiac output with or without a rise in end-diastolic pressure. Arteriolar vasodilators usually result in a brisk rise in cardiac output.

Vasodilators differ in their predominant site of action:

- *nitrates* act predominantly as venodilators;
- *hydralazine* acts predominantly as an arterial dilator;
- ACE inhibitors act as combined venous and arterial dilators.

ACE inhibitors

ACE inhibitors such as captopril and enalapril have a unique mecha-nism in that they block the enhanced activity of the renin–angiotensin system (see p. 157), but have additional vasodilator properties. They seem to be superior to other orally administered vasodilators in their effectiveness and, at low dosages, in their lack of side-effects.

ACE inhibitors are of value in improving symptoms in patients with heart failure. In addition, a number of large well-controlled studies have shown that ACE inhibitors improve prognosis in patients with symptomatic heart failure. In view of these mortality benefits, ACE inhibitors should be prescribed, unless contraindicated, in all patients with symptoms of heart failure. They may also slow progression to symptomtic heart failure in individuals with ventricular impairment who are currently free of symptoms.

Following myocardial infarction, ACE inhibitors are of particular value. They are indicated not only for the treatment of failure, but also for the prevention of adverse remodelling (see Chapter 9, p. 146). A number of studies have shown that ACE inhibitors improve survival following infarction in a spectrum of patients, ranging from those who are asymptomatic but show significant ventricular dysfunction, to those who have clinical evidence of ventricular impairment.

ACE inhibitors are also of value in treating heart failure arising as a result of ventricular dilatation associated with either mitral or aortic regurgitation. The drugs are, however, contraindicated in patients with significant mitral or aortic stenosis.

Two problems limit the use of ACE inhibitors in patients with heart failure, hypotension and renal impairment. As many patients with congestive heart failure have low blood pressure, this restricts the use of these agents. The problem of hypotension is particularly marked after the first dose. First-dose hypotension can be minimized by reducing the dose of the ACE inhibitor on commencing therapy and omitting diuretics for 1–2 days beforehand.

ACE inhibitors occasionally cause deterioration of renal function. They are contraindicated in patients with an initial creatinine level greater than 200 μmol/litre. Renal function should be checked routinely 1–2 weeks after commencing ACE inhibition.

Cough is a potentially troublesome side-effect, occurring in up to 10% of patients. The mechanism is unclear but may be due to inhibition of the metabolism of bradykinin in the lung. Switching to a different ACE inhibitor is rarely effective in alleviating the problem. Some patients will, however, respond to a reduction in dose.

Other vasodilators

The widespread applicability and indications for ACE inhibitors are reduced the importance of other vasodilators in the management of heart failure. Nitrate vasodilators remain of value in the management of acute left ventricular failure. Sublingual glyceryl trinitrate can be administered in the acute phase and can be followed by an intravenous infusion. Nitrates act predominantly as venodilators. Hydralazine, by contrast, is predominantly an arterial dilator. The two can be combined in the long-term management of patients with heart failure to achieve combined preload and afterload reduction. This combination has been shown to improve both symptoms and prognosis. However, it has been largely superseded by ACE inhibition, which offers greater prognostic benefit. A nitrate–hydralazine combination may, however, still be of benefit in patients in whom ACE inhibitors are contraindicated.

Beta-blockers

Superficially one might anticipate that beta-blockers would be contra-indicated in heart failure. This is undoubtedly the case for patients with severe heart failure in whom beta-blockers may lead to further deterioration of already severely impaired left ventricular function. There is, however, growing evidence that beta-blockers are of benefit in patients with features of mild to moderate heart failure. Increased sym-pathetic activity is part of the normal neurohumoral adaptive response to heart failure. The disadvantages of this increased adrenergic drive may, however, outweigh the advantages. The increased adrenergic drive is likely, for example, to increase susceptibility to arrhythmias and this may be reduced by beta-blockade. However, patients with severe heart failure may require their increased adrenergic drive to maintain a reasonable cardiac output and beta-blockers are contraindicated.

Great care is therefore necessary in determining which patients with heart failure should receive beta-blockers. Precise selection criteria are as yet unclear. When beta-blockers are used in this situation, they should be commenced cautiously with low doses and the dose gradu-ally titrated upwards.

Digitalis glycosides

These were, for many years, regarded as standard therapy for cardiac failure and are the only inotropic agents widely used in the long-term oral management of patients with heart failure. They are of undoubted value in the control of atrial fibrillation and if this is of importance in the genesis of cardiac failure, they will quickly relieve it. Their role in cardiac failure in sinus rhythm is less certain.

Mechanisms of action.   The inotropic action of digitalis is mediated through the sodium/potassium-ATPase (sodium) pump, to which it binds. The inhibition of this pump leads to an accumulation of intra-cellular sodium; because of the sodium–calcium exchange system, this results in an increase in the amount of calcium available to activate contraction. Digitalis also has sympathomimetic and parasympathetic (vagal) effects. The latter is clinically important, in that it causes slow-ing of the sinus rate and delays conduction through the atrioventricular node. Digitalis reduces the refractory period of atrial and ventricular muscle and, therefore, enhances the risk of ectopic rhythms.

Administration.   Digoxin is the most commonly used digitalis prepa-ration. Because oral therapy is safest, this route should be used if possible. The intravenous route should be employed only in cases of urgency and should always be avoided if a digitalis preparation has been administered within the previous week.

Intravenous digoxin produces an effect within 15 min and has peak activity in about 2 h. When given by mouth, the effects start in about 1 h and are maximal at about 6 h.

Digoxin is excreted in an unchanged form by the kidneys. This is normally complete in 4–5 days, but is delayed in the presence of renal failure. For this reason digoxin dosage should be reduced in patients with impaired renal function.

Drug interactions.   Digitalis glycosides may be involved in important drug interactions. Quinidine increases the plasma concentrations of digoxin, probably by displacing it from tissue sites. Amiodarone and verapamil have similar effects. When any of these drugs is added the dosage of digoxin should be reduced. Because hypokalaemia enhances digitalis toxicity, concomitant treatment with potassium losing diuretics must be cautious.

Toxicity.   The commonest toxic effects of digitalis therapy are malaise, anorexia, nausea and, later, vomiting. In some patients, there is excessive salivation, yellow vision or diarrhoea.

More serious than these symptoms are the many different types of conduction and rhythm disturbance that may occur:

- *ventricular ectopics.* These are generally well tolerated, but are an indication for reducing digitalis dosage;
- *ventricular tachycardia and ventricular fibrillation* may occur in cases of serious toxicity;
- *supraventricular rhythm disturbances* may be provoked, of which the most important is atrial tachycardia with block (p. 189);
- *atrioventricular dissociation* (p. 202) and junctional rhythms (p. 183) may occur. In more severe cases, complete heart block can develop.

Potassium depletion promotes the development of digitalis-induced disturbances of rhythm and conduction, and should be assumed to be present when these occur, in spite of a normal serum potassium. Digitalis should be discontinued immediately and potassium depletion corrected. It is important never to use d.c. shock therapy in the treatment of digitalis-induced arrhythmias.

Toxicity can usually be corrected by withholding the drug and, if indicated, giving potassium. Pacing may be required for heart block, and antiarrhythmic drugs for arrhythmias. In severe cases of digitalis poisoning, fragments of antidigoxin antibodies (Digibind) may be used to bind digoxin and rapidly reverse toxic effects.

Plasma digoxin levels.   Plasma digoxin levels are of limited value in assessing toxicity. Therapeutic and toxic ranges overlap and consequently a digoxin level which is therapeutic in one patient may be toxic in another. As a generalization, provided the serum potassium is normal, toxicity is unlikely with digoxin concentrations below 2 µg/litre and very likely with values greater than 4 µg/litre.

Digoxin estimation should only be undertaken when there is a definite indication. The mere fact that a patient is taking digoxin is not an indication for an assay, in the absence of other clinical indications. Appropriate indications include:

- suspected toxicity;
- changing renal function;
- subtherapeutic clinical response;
- potential drug interactions;
- suspected poor compliance.

It is essential that samples should be timed correctly – at least 6 h should elapse between the time of dosing and the time of sampling.

Indications.   Digitalis is indicated in cardiac failure for the control of atrial arrhythmias. Its role in cardiac failure in sinus rhythm remains uncertain. Recent studies have shown that digoxin improves symptoms of heart failure and reduces the incidence of death due to progressive heart failure. This is offset by an accompanying increase in arrhythmic deaths. As a consequence, overall effects on mortality are neutral.

Digoxin is most likely to be efficacious if there is cardiomegaly with a dilated ventricle and a third heart sound. It is unlikely to be helpful in cases of constrictive pericarditis or in mitral stenosis without atrial fibrillation. It is potentially dangerous in hypertrophic cardiomyopathy (p. 238).

Other inotropic agents

The long-term use of oral inotropic agents in the management of patients with heart failure has been largely discredited. The use of phosphodiesterase inhibitors, for example, is associated with an increased incidence of arrhythmias and increased mortality. Intravenous inotropic agents, however, still play an important role in the management of acute circulatory failure due to cardiogenic shock (see below).

ACUTE CIRCULATORY FAILURE (SHOCK)

The terms acute circulatory failure, low output state, and shock are used to describe a syndrome comprising arterial hypotension, cold, moist and cyanosed extremities, a rapid weak pulse, a low urine output and a diminished level of consciousness. This clinical pattern is common to a number of disorders such as severe blood or gastro-intestinal fluid loss, burns and acute myocardial infarction. As yet, physiological studies have not clearly defined the nature of the changes responsible for the clinical syndrome, but a common factor is a sudden fall in cardiac output associated with tissue hypoxia.

Causes of shock

There are a number of causes of shock:

- hypovolaemic shock. This is exemplified by haemorrhage and loss of fluid from burns, vomiting and diarrhoea;
- septicaemic shock;
- anaphylactic shock;
- acute pancreatitis;
- cardiogenic shock. Shock is described as cardiogenic when it is clearly cardiac in origin. This may be due to many different causes, including myocardial infarction, massive pulmonary embolism, dissecting aneurysm, pericardial tamponade, rupture of a valve cusp, and arrhythmias. In cardiogenic shock, the central venous pressure is usually raised, in contrast to hypovolaemic shock, in which it is characteristically low.

Although the fall in cardiac output and blood pressure is an essential feature of shock, these abnormalities are insufficient to account for the syndrome. Falls of the same magnitude may be seen in some patients in whom the clinical features of shock are not seen and in whom the prognosis is good. In the first stage of shock, there is a fall in cardiac output and blood pressure, due to either a diminution in venous return or to an inability of the myocardium to expel an adequate stroke volume. As a consequence of the hypotension, there is a fall in renal blood flow, with oliguria. Reflex tachycardia takes place. Compensatory mechanisms follow, with arteriolar constriction affecting particularly the kidneys, abdominal viscera, muscle and skin. Vasodilatation of the cerebral and coronary vessels permits the maintenance of a relatively good blood flow in these territories. If the vasoconstriction is sufficiently great, the blood pressure may be kept at or close to normal levels but at the expense of producing tissue hypoxia with consequent acidosis. If the underlying process can be corrected quickly, recovery may ensue, but if shock persists untreated for many hours, the stage of irreversibility may be reached. At this time, the correction of the original cause fails to prevent death. The nature of irreversible shock remains undetermined, but has been attributed to the production of endotoxins, and to irreparable cellular changes as a result of hypoxia in the liver, kidney, heart or brain.

Aetiological diagnosis

Although the condition responsible for shock is often obvious, there is sometimes no evident cause. In such cases, no effort must be spared in identifying it quickly, for successful therapy depends upon this.

Cardiac causes, provided they are thought of, can usually be recognized by a combination of clinical examination, ECG, X-ray and echocardiography. The cause of hypovolaemic shock may be difficult to establish; this applies particularly to intra-abdominal haemorrhage and to occult infection.

Treatment

General management

If the patient is in severe pain or distress, opiates should be given intravenously (provided there is no contraindication) and high-flow oxygen administered, preferably by a tight-fitting face mask making use of the Venturi principle, or by mechanical ventilation. Unless there is pulmonary oedema, the patient should be laid flat, with the legs slightly raised. A catheter should be introduced to measure urinary output. Arterial blood gases and pH should be monitored. Although central venous monitoring may be adequate for the less severe cases of traumatic shock, a Swan–Ganz balloon-tip catheter should be used to obtain pulmonary artery and 'pulmonary capillary wedge' pressures, particularly if a cardiac or pulmonary cause is known or suspected. As measurement of blood pressure by a sphygmomanometer is unreliable in severe shock, direct arterial pressure monitoring should be undertaken, when possible.

Correction of hypovolaemia

This is essential in shock which is not cardiogenic, but may also be of importance in myocardial infarction when prior diuretic therapy has caused fluid depletion, or in right ventricular infarction. One should aim to raise the central venous pressure to between 10 and 15 mmHg, and keep the pulmonary wedge (or pulmonary artery diastolic) pressure between 15 and 20 mmHg. Immediate replacement may be with saline; subsequently, the amount and nature of the fluid infused should be determined by estimates of that lost.

Inotropic agents

These drugs enhance myocardial contractility, but at the expense of increased oxygen consumption. The sympathomimetic drugs isoprenaline and noradrenaline were much used in the past, but they have been largely superseded by dopamine and dobutamine.

The effects of dopamine, a natural precursor of noradrenaline, depend upon the dose. Administered intravenously in a dosage of 2–5 µg/kg/min, it causes dilatation of renal and mesenteric vessels; at doses of 5–10 µg/kg/min, it increases myocardial contractility and cardiac output. At higher doses, it causes vasoconstriction (it should not be infused directly into a peripheral vein as leakage may cause local necrosis). Dopamine may induce nausea and vomiting, and can lead to an excessive tachycardia and arrhythmias.

Dobutamine is a synthetic sympathomimetic agent whose predominant action is one of stimulating β_1 activity. It is less likely to cause vasoconstriction or tachycardia than dopamine. It is given by intravenous infusion at a rate of 2.5–10 µg/kg/min.

Both these drugs need to be given with careful monitoring of intravascular pressures.

Mechanical support

The intra-aortic balloon pump is of value in acute myocardial infarction if shock has been caused by a surgically correctable lesion, such as a ventricular septal defect or papillary muscle rupture (see also p. 386).

CARDIAC TRANSPLANTATION

Cardiac transplantation is now well established in the management of refractory heart failure, not amenable to other forms of treatment. The prognosis of transplant recipients has dramatically improved, since the introduction of cyclosporin for immunosuppression. One-year survival is now approaching 90%, with a 5-year survival in excess of 60%.

In the majority of transplant recipients, the cause of heart failure is either cardiomyopathy or end-stage ischaemic heart disease. In both cases, the indication for treatment is severe symptoms, refractory to medical therapy and not amenable to other forms of surgery. Such patients have a very limited life expectancy, which is dramatically improved by transplantation.

Selection criteria for transplantation include:

- patients not amenable to conventional surgery;
- patients remaining severely symptomatic despite maximal medical treatment;
- poor prognosis without transplantation;
- freedom from other major diseases, particularly diabetes, peripheral vessel disease, renal impairment, malignancy and pulmonary hypertension;
- likelihood of good prognosis and quality of life post-transplant.

The timing of transplantation is difficult. On the one hand, the patient must have severe enough impairment of left ventricular function to warrant a transplant. On the other, if the operation is undertaken at a stage when the patient has end-stage heart failure, causing failure of other organ systems, the success of transplantation decreases dramatically.

The success of cardiac transplantation has meant that the number of patients who could potentially benefit from transplantation exceeds the number of donor hearts available. As a result, transplant waiting lists are relatively long and many patients die while awaiting a donor heart. In patients considered at high risk of arrhythmic death while awaiting a donor heart, the short-term use of an implantable defibrillator can be considered as a 'bridge to transplant'.

Immunosuppression

Immunosuppression is achieved by a combination of:

- cyclosporin;
- corticosteroids;
- azathioprine.

Using multiple therapy, successful immunosuppression can be achieved with lower doses of each agent. This minimizes the side-effects of each. The degree of immunosuppression needs to be greatest in the earlier stages after transplantation, but can subsequently be reduced to a low maintenance level. Patients remain susceptible to episodes of rejection, but these can be managed by increasing immunosuppressive therapy when they occur.

Rejection

The recognition of episodes of rejection is important in transplant patients. The patient is generally non-specifically unwell. Clinical features may include the development of a third heart sound and atrial arrhythmias. The ECG may show reduction in QRS voltages, but this is a relatively late finding.

Diagnosis is based upon cardiac biopsy and this should be undertaken on suspicion of rejection. This is a simple procedure performed under local anaesthetic using either rigid biopsy forceps introduced into the jugular vein in the neck or using a biopsy catheter introduced into the femoral vein.

Complications

In addition to rejection, heart transplant recipients are subject to a number of other problems.

Infection. This remains a major cause of death in transplant recipients. Viral infections, such as cytomegalovirus and Herpes zoster, which produce relatively trivial infections in normal individuals, can be life-threatening in immunosuppressed patients. It is important that even minor symptoms should be investigated to detect and treat any infective illness early.

Accelerated atherosclerosis. Heart transplant patients develop accelerated atherosclerosis. This occurs both in patients whose preoperative diagnosis was cardiomyopathy and in those with preoperative ischaemic heart disease. It is important that any contributory factor to atherosclerosis, such as hypercholesterolaemia, should be adequately controlled. Patients should also undergo regular assessment with coronary angiography.

Cyclosporin nephrotoxicity. Patients should be regularly reviewed with a check of their renal function and cyclosporin levels, to minimize the risk of nephrotoxicity.

Cushingoid features. The features of Cushing disease are, in general, less troublesome with the advent of cyclosporin and reduction in steroid dosage.

Malignancy. It is well recognized that there is an increased incidence of malignant disease, particularly lymphoproliferative disorders, in immunosuppressed patients.

Despite these difficulties, cardiac transplantation is a highly successful procedure, in patients fortunate enough to receive a transplant. The main limitation in the growth of transplantation continues to be availability of donor hearts.

Heart–lung transplantation

Heart–lung transplantation is still much less common than simple heart transplantation. Conditions requiring heart–lung transplantation include primary pulmonary hypertension and congenital cardiac abnormalities which have resulted in Eisenmenger's syndrome. These indications have now grown to include patients with end-stage pulmonary disease, particularly patients with cystic fibrosis.

The success rate for heart–lung transplantation is not yet as good as that for heart transplantation, with 1-year survival rates reported of approximately 70%.

Further reading

Chatterjee, K. (1996) Heart failure therapy in evolution. *Circulation* **94**: 2689.
Cleland, J. G. F. (1993) *The Clinician's Guide to ACE Inhibition.* Edinburgh: Churchill Livingstone.
Colucci, W. S. & Braunwald, E. (1996) Pathophysiology of heart failure. In Braunwald, E. (Ed.) *Heart Disease.* Philadelphia: Saunders.
Editorial (1992) The prevention of heart failure. *New England Journal of Medicine* **327**: 725.
Eichorn, E. J., Hjalmarson, A. (1994) Beta-blocker treatment for chronic heart failure. The frog prince. *Circulation* **90**: 2153.

Lant, A. (1985) Diuretics: clinical pharmacology and therapeutics. *Drugs* **29**: Part I: 57; Part II: 162.

Packer, M. (1993) The development of positive inotropic agents for chronic heart failure: How have we gone astray? *Journal of the American College of Cardiology* **22**: 119.

Parmley, W. W. (1989) Pathophysiology and current therapy of congestive heart failure. *Journal of the American College of Cardiology* **13**: 771.

Perlroth, M. G. & Reitz, B. A. (1996) Heart and heart–lung transplantation. In Braunwald, E. (Ed.) *Heart Disease*. Philadelphia: Saunders.

Smith, T. W. (1988) Digitalis: mechanisms of action and chemical use. *New England Journal of Medicine* **318**: 358.

Smith, T. W., Kelly, R. A., Stevenson, L. W. & Braunwald, E. (1996) Management of heart failure. In Braunwald, E. (Ed.) *Heart Disease*. Philadelphia: Saunders.

SOLVD Investigators (1991) Effect of enalapril on survival in patients with reduced left ventricular ejection fractions and congestive heart failure. *New England Journal of Medicine* **325**: 293.

Disorders of Rate, Rhythm and Conduction

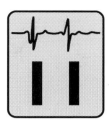

MECHANISMS OF ARRHYTHMIAS

As is discussed in more detail in Chapter 2, there are electrically two types of cell in the myocardium – the automatic and the non-automatic – the automatic cells having the capacity of self excitation. The group of automatic cells with the most rapid rate of spontaneous depolarization dominates the heart as the pacemaker. This is normally the sinus node, which is under the control both of the vagus and of the sympathetic nervous system. Ectopic rhythms, in which the heart is activated from a pacemaker other than the sinus node, arise from a variety of mechanisms:

- escape of lower centres;
- increased automaticity of other zones;
- re-entry.

Escape of lower centres

An increase in vagal activity reduces the rate of spontaneous depolarization of the sinus node and thereby slows the heart; another group of automatic cells may then exhibit a rate faster than that of the sinus node and become the pacemaker.

Increased automaticity of other zones

Increased sympathetic activity increases the rate of discharge not only of the sinus node, but also of other areas, including the ventricles. Ischaemia, digitalis intoxication and electrolyte disorders also enhance ventricular automaticity.

Re-entry

Re-entry arrhythmias arise due to a self-perpetuating 'circus' movement of the cardiac impulse. There are two requirements for re-entry:

- non-uniform refractoriness;
- slow conduction.

Non-uniform recovery of refractoriness is necessary to create an area of unidirectional conduction block (Fig. 11.1). Slow conduction is necessary to fulfil the fundamental requirement that conduction time over the re-entry circuit should exceed the longest refractory period of any point in the circuit.

For most re-entrant arrhythmias, the re-entrant conduction pathway cannot be defined anatomically. Re-entry occurs in small areas of atrial or ventricular muscle (micro re-entry). In some instances, however, the anatomical components of the re-entry circuit can be defined. The best

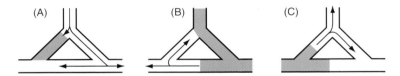

Fig. 11.1   The re-entry phenomenon. In (A) the impulse cannot enter a zone which is still in the refractory phase. In (B) this zone has become receptive as adjacent muscle becomes refractory. In (C) the impulse leaves the newly activated zone and re-enters the same tissue as was activated in (A) which has now recovered. The refractory zone is shown in red.

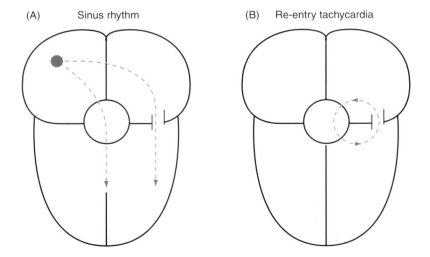

Fig. 11.2   Re-entry mechanisms: Wolff–Parkinson–White syndrome. (A) In sinus rhythm the ventricles are activated over two pathways, via the AV node and via an accessory pathway. (B) During the common form of re-entry tachycardia a re-entrant loop is established conducting antegradely via the AV node and retrogradely via the accessory pathway.

example of such a macro re-entry pathway is the Wolff–Parkinson–White syndrome, in which a slender bundle of myocardium forms a bridge between the atria and the ventricles, bypassing the atrioventricular node (Fig. 11.2). Re-entry tachycardias commonly arise by conduction of the cardiac impulse from atrium to ventricle through the AV node and from ventricle to atrium over the accessory pathway. Slow conduction through the AV node ensures that conduction time over the re-entry circuit exceeds the maximum refractory period in the pathway.

In most re-entrant arrhythmias, however, the pathways are less clearly defined.

DISTURBANCES OF RATE AND RHYTHM

Sinus node abnormalities

Sinus tachycardia

Sinus tachycardia is sinus rhythm at a rate faster than is normal (Fig. 11.3). In adults, this is commonly defined as being greater than 100/min. In children the heart rate, even at rest, frequently exceeds 100/min, and in infants may exceed 150/min. Amongst factors associated with disease which cause sinus tachycardia are:

- anaemia;
- hyperthyroidism;
- fever;
- blood loss and hypovolaemia;
- heart failure;
- drugs such as adrenaline, isoprenaline, ephedrine, propantheline, atropine and thyroxine.

Sinus tachycardia is seldom harmful and may be a compensatory mechanism.

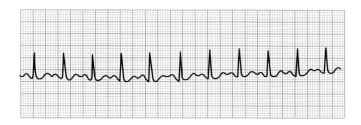

Fig. 11.3 Sinus tachycardia.

The patient with sinus tachycardia may complain of palpitation which is of gradual and explicable onset, unlike the abrupt and unexpected appearance of the symptom in paroxysmal tachycardia. The diagnosis is usually obvious when there is a regular pulse at a rate of more than 100/min. Frequently, the tachycardia subsides during the examination as anxiety diminishes. Carotid sinus pressure causes little slowing in contrast to its usually dramatic effect in atrial tachycardia or atrial flutter. The ECG shows P waves having a normal relationship to QRS complexes. The J point may be depressed; the ST then slopes upward.

Sinus tachycardia does not of itself require treatment although the underlying cause of tachycardia should be sought and, where necessary, treated.

Sinus bradycardia

Sinus bradycardia describes a slow heart in sinus rhythm (Fig. 11.4). This term is commonly applied to heart rates of less than 60/min, although such rates are frequently seen in healthy elderly people; in the highly trained athlete the heart rate may be less than 40/min. Amongst factors causing sinus bradycardia are:

- increased vagal tone (e.g. during carotid sinus massage);
- myxoedema;
- hypothermia;
- raised intracranial pressure;
- drugs including digitalis and the beta-adrenergic blocking agents such as propranolol.

Sinus bradycardia seldom gives rise to symptoms or undesirable haemodynamic effects but, occasionally, in the elderly and in acute myocardial infarction, cardiac failure or hypotension may develop if the stroke output cannot be increased to compensate adequately for the slow rate. The heart can be accelerated by atropine 0.6 mg subcutaneously or intravenously. Oral sympathomimetics, such as long-acting

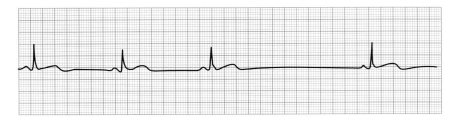

Fig. 11.4   Sinus bradycardia. A marked sinus bradycardia of 40 beats per minute is followed by a 2.7 second pause before the next sinus beat.

isoprenaline, can also be used to treat sinus bradycardia, but in general pacing is preferable.

Sick sinus syndrome

Sinus bradycardia is a component of the sick sinus syndrome, a relatively common condition amongst the elderly. The bradycardia may be complicated by paroxysms of atrial tachyarrhythmias (tachycardia, flutter or fibrillation), the so-called bradycardia–tachycardia syndrome (Fig. 11.5). Syncope may result either from too slow or too fast a heart rate.

Sick sinus syndrome is seldom life-threatening, but frequently causes distressing symptoms of palpitations, dizziness or syncope. These can be treated by implantation of a pacemaker. Tachyarrhythmias may require antiarrhythmic drug therapy combined with a pacemaker to guard against bradycardia.

Sinus arrhythmia (Fig. 11.6)

Normally, the sinus node does not discharge with absolute regularity owing to variations in vagal tone. These variations are related to respiration, and it is characteristic in the young to find acceleration of the heart during inspiration with slowing during expiration. This phasic change in the rhythm of the heart is known as sinus arrhythmia. It is

(A)

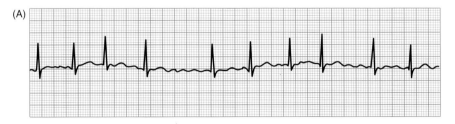

(B)

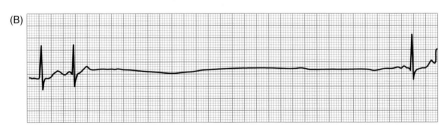

Fig. 11.5   Sick sinus syndrome with bradycardia and tachycardia. (A) Tachycardia due to atrial fibrillation. (B) Termination of atrial fibrillation is followed by a prolonged asystolic pause, eventually terminated by a sinus beat.

seldom clinically obvious in adults, but is occasionally seen in the healthy old person. It is of no clinical importance, but it must be differentiated from the other types of arrhythmia. Its relationship to respiration usually makes this easy.

Supraventricular arrhythmias

A variety of rhythm disturbances can arise in the atria and AV junctional area (that is, the AV node and adjacent specialized tissues). These may result from either increased automaticity or re-entry.

Atrial ectopic beats (atrial extrasystoles, atrial premature beats)

Atrial ectopic beats are common in normal individuals, but seldom give rise to symptoms, apart from an awareness of heart irregularity from time to time. They cause an occasional irregularity in an otherwise normal pulse, and are usually abolished by exercise. The diagnosis is readily confirmed from the ECG (Fig. 11.7) which shows a premature beat occurring earlier than the next anticipated sinus beat. The P wave differs in configuration from that of a sinus beat, because depolarization of the atria takes place in an abnormal direction. The

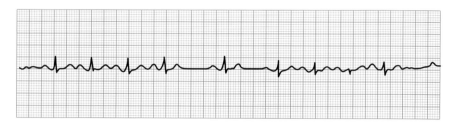

Fig. 11.6   Sinus arrhythmia. Acceleration of the sinus rate is evident during inspiration and slowing during expiration.

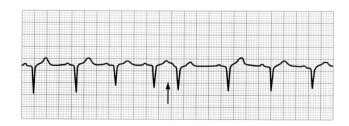

Fig. 11.7   Atrial ectopic beat. A premature P wave (arrowed) is followed by a QRS complex of normal appearance.

accompanying QRST complex is usually similar to that of previous beats of sinus origin because the pathway of ventricular depolarization is normal. Occasionally, the QRST complex is abnormally broad ('aberrant') because the impulse passes down only one of the bundle branches, the other still being refractory from the preceding beat. It then simulates the appearance of a ventricular ectopic beat (see p. 195) but is usually preceded by a P wave.

Atrial ectopic beats may presage the appearance of other atrial arrhythmias but they require no treatment.

Junctional (nodal) ectopic beats

Ectopic beats deriving from the junctional tissue are quite common and, like atrial ectopic beats, usually benign. They are responsible for an occasional irregularity in an otherwise regular pulse and cannot be diagnosed without an electrocardiogram, which shows the same features as with atrial ectopic beats except that the P wave is inverted in lead II and is either buried in the QRS complex, or precedes or follows it by a very short interval. No treatment is necessary.

Junctional (nodal) rhythm (Fig. 11.8)

In this condition the junctional tissue is acting as the pacemaker of the heart and the ECG appearance is that of a succession of junctional ectopic beats. It is usually a transient condition resulting from a depression of sinus node activity. It occurs in some normal individuals and may be provoked by digitalis or ischaemic heart disease. The heart rate is usually in the region of 50–60/min and no treatment is required. If the heart rate is undesirably slow, it can be accelerated by the use of atropine.

In patients with acute myocardial infarction treated with thrombolytic therapy, the occurrence of junctional rhythm is an indicator of successful reperfusion.

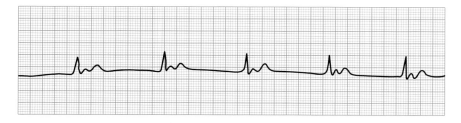

Fig. 11.8 Junctional rhythm. In this example retrograde conduction into the atria is relatively slow and a P wave can be distinguished after the QRS complex, interrupting the ST segment.

Paroxysmal supraventricular tachycardias (Fig. 11.9)

In its broadest sense, the term paroxysmal supraventricular tachycardia might refer to any recurrent supraventricular arrhythmias. However, arrhythmias originating within the atrium (atrial tachycardia, atrial flutter and atrial fibrillation) are generally excluded. The term encompasses a number of different arrhythmias, which share certain characteristics – starting abruptly, usually being regular at a rate of 140–220/min, and being associated with narrow QRS complexes, closely resembling those seen in sinus rhythm. Aberrant conduction with broadening of the QRS may, however, occur as may rates above and below those quoted.

The majority of arrhythmias are due to re-entry. In the commonest form, re-entry involves dual pathways within the AV node which have different rates of conduction and refractoriness. In other cases re-entry is dependent on the presence of an additional connection (accessory pathway), linking atrium and ventricle. The best recognized form is Wolff–Parkinson–White syndrome, which is characterized in sinus rhythm by a short PR interval and delta wave (p. 187). During the common form of tachycardia, excitation passes from atrium to ventricle over the AV node and from ventricle to atrium via the accessory pathway. As the ventricles are excited over the normal route QRS complexes are narrow. The absence of a delta wave during sinus rhythm does not exclude the possibility of an accessory pathway, as some pathways only conduct retrogradely from ventricle to atrium. These pathways are hence 'concealed' during sinus rhythm, but can still conduct retrogradely giving rise to a re-entrant tachycardia.

The attacks may last only seconds, but they often persist for minutes or hours or, much less commonly, for days. They may recur at short intervals or be separated from one another by weeks, months or even years. It is sometimes possible to identify provoking factors such as tobacco, coffee and alcohol. Paroxysms are most often encountered in otherwise normal people in whom they give rise to palpitation, but no serious haemodynamic effects. These tachycardias can, however, pro-

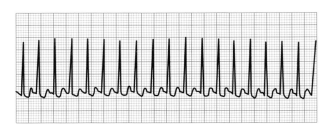

Fig. 11.9 Supraventricular tachycardia. Regular narrow QRS tachycardia at a rate of 220 beats/min.

duce cardiac failure and hypotension in the presence of heart disease because of the increased workload of the heart and the inadequate filling time during diastole.

The patient usually complains of attacks of rapid regular palpitation of abrupt onset, sometimes accompanied by dizziness or even syncope. When the attack is prolonged or when it occurs in those with heart disease, there may be dyspnoea and ischaemic chest pain. There may also be polyuria.

The episodes are often so brief and infrequent that no doctor ever sees them; if the patient is observed at the time, the pulse is found to be regular at a rate between 140 and 220. Carotid sinus massage frequently terminates the attack, but if it fails to do so, it has no effect upon the pulse rate. The ECG usually reveals QRST complexes of normal or near normal configuration occurring rapidly and regularly. The presence and timing of a P wave is of diagnostic value (Fig. 11.10):

- a P wave which is 'absent' (hidden in the QRS or in the terminal portion of the QRS) suggests AV node re-entry as the underlying mechanism of tachycardia;
- a P wave following the QRS suggests the presence of an accessory pathway.
- Atrial flutter with a 2:1 AV block should also be considered in a differential diagnosis (Fig. 11.10).

It is difficult to obtain conventional ECG recordings of the attacks because of their unpredictability and brevity; the documentation of episodes is aided by dynamic electrocardiography (Holter monitoring), and by patient-activated ECG recorders.

The ECG between attacks is usually normal, but the appearances of the Wolff–Parkinson–White syndrome, the 'short PR syndrome' (with a normal QRS), or other abnormalities of conduction may be seen.

Termination of the acute attack.   In the treatment of the individual attack, the patient may be taught to carry out the Valsalva manoeuvre and the doctor can use carotid sinus massage. If these procedures prove unsuccessful, drug treatment should be considered. As the majority of tachycardias arise by re-entry either within or involving the AV node, drugs slowing AV nodal conduction are indicated:

- intravenous adenosine causes a transient but profound inhibition of AV node conduction (for mode of use and contraindications see Chapter 22);
- intravenous verapamil is an alternative (5–10 mg intravenously over 30–60 s); verapamil should not be given if the patient is already receiving a beta-blocker.

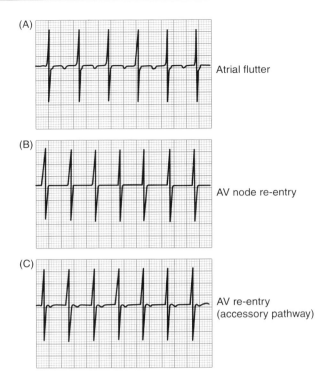

(A)

Atrial flutter

(B)

AV node re-entry

(C)

AV re-entry
(accessory pathway)

Fig. 11.10 Differential diagnosis of regular narrow QRS tachycardia. Schematic ECGs. (A) Atrial flutter with 2:1 AV block. Close examination of the trace reveals two flutter waves for every QRS complex. The second flutter wave is partly hidden in the terminal portion of the QRS complex. (See also Fig. 11.12.) (B) Atrioventricular nodal re-entry tachycardia. Atrial depolarization is generally synchronous with ventricular depolarization. The P wave is either lost within the QRS complex or is in the terminal portion of the QRS complex. (C) Atrioventricular re-entry tachycardia due to the presence of an accessory pathway. A P wave is evident after the QRS complex, reflecting retrograde atrial activation over the accessory pathway. (See also Fig. 11.11.)

In patients in whom the safety and efficacy of intravenous verapamil has been demonstrated, it is reasonable to provide the patient with a supply of oral verapamil to take a stat 120 mg dose in the event of an acute attack, hence avoiding the need for hospital attendance.

Prevention. Because of the repetitive paroxysmal nature of the tachycardia, prevention is often of greater importance than the treatment of the individual attack. When possible, a provoking factor such as strong coffee or tobacco should be identified and avoided. If episodes are infrequent and symptoms are not severe, drug treatment is not required and simple reassurance is all that is necessary. In other patients stat doses of verapamil as outlined above can obviate the need for continuous drug treatment. When drug therapy is required, a number of drugs can be considered. These include beta-adrenergic blocks and verapamil. Class I antiarrhythmic drugs such as flecainide are also effective for prophylaxis, but their long-term safety is in doubt and these drugs are best avoided if possible.

The advent of radiofrequency catheter ablation has revolutionized the treatment of patients with paroxysmal supraventricular tachycardia (see p. 214). Ablation offers a definitive cure to the problem and should be considered in patients with significant continuing symptoms despite drug therapy and in those intolerant of drug therapy or in whom drug therapy is contraindicated.

Pre-excitation (Wolff–Parkinson–White syndrome)

In this condition, an anomalous conduction pathway bypasses the AV node. This permits the abnormally early activation of part of one ventricle, the remaining ventricular muscle receiving its impulse normally. This leads to a short PR interval (less than 0.12 s) and a slurred upstroke and widening of the QRS (Fig. 11.11).

The normal and abnormal conduction pathways are able to form part of a re-entry circuit (Fig. 11.2) (p. 178). This facilitates the occurrence of paroxysmal tachycardia. In the common form of re-entry tachycardia the ventricles are excited normally through the AV node and His–Purkinje system. Consequently there is no pre-excitation during tachycardia and the delta wave disappears (Fig. 11.11B). On presentation, this narrow QRS tachycardia may be indistinguishable from other causes of paroxysmal supraventricular tachycardia.

Sudden death occasionally occurs in patients with Wolff–Parkinson–White syndrome. The danger lies not in re-entry tachycardia, but in atrial fibrillation (Fig. 11.11C). Normally in patients with atrial fibrillation, the ventricles are protected from the rapid rate of atrial depolarization by the gating effect of the AV node. In patients with an accessory pathway this protection is lost. If the refractory period of the pathway is short, impulses from the atrium can be conducted at very high rates to the ventricle and can result in ventricular fibrillation. Atrial fibrillation, complicating Wolff–Parkinson–White syndrome, should be treated with a drug acting selectively on the accessory pathway to abolish pre-excitation. Intravenous flecainide or intravenous amiodarone are the drugs of choice. Alternatively, the patient can be cardioverted to restore sinus rhythm.

In many patients, the identification of Wolff–Parkinson–White syndrome is an incidental finding at routine ECG. If the patient is asymptomatic, the risks of the condition are generally considered to be very low, and further investigation is generally unnecessary unless indicated on grounds of occupation or sporting activities. Information on

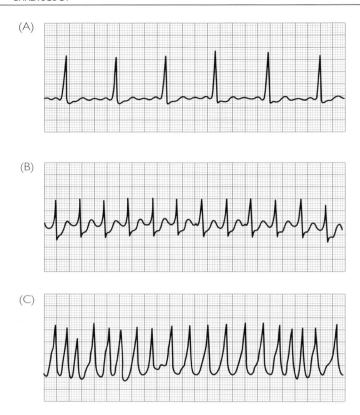

Fig. 11.11   ECG patterns in Wolff–Parkinson–White syndrome. (A) Sinus rhythm. A short PR interval and delta wave are evident. (B) Re-entrant tachycardia. This is the common form of re-entrant tachycardia conducting from atrium to ventricle over the AV node and retrogradely from ventricle to atrium over the accessory pathway. It results in a narrow QRS tachycardia with a loss of delta wave. (See also Fig. 11.2) (C) Atrial fibrillation. The characteristic features of atrial fibrillation in Wolff–Parkinson–White syndrome are apparent. I. Irregular QRS complexes. 2. Varying QRS morphology, reflecting different degrees of activation over the AV node and accessory pathway. 3. Some very short RR intervals (less than 200 ms), reflecting rapid conduction over the accessory pathway.

speed of pathway conduction can sometimes be derived from exercise testing – if pre-excitation disappears during exercise this indicates a relatively slow conducting pathway, and the patient would not be able to sustain very high ventricular rates if atrial fibrillation should develop.

In patients with symptomatic arrhythmias, the advent of radio-frequency ablation has revolutionized the treatment of the condition and in general radiofrequency ablation is the preferred option to drug therapy (p. 214).

Atrial tachycardia with block

This is a relatively rare arrhythmia, which is commonly due to advanced digitalis intoxication. There is nearly always cellular potassium depletion, but the serum potassium is not necessarily low.

The ventricular rate depends upon the degree of AV block. Commonly, this is 2:1 and there are no adverse haemodynamic effects as the ventricular rate is about 80–100/min.

The clinical recognition of this rhythm disturbance is virtually impossible and the diagnosis must be made from the electrocardiogram, in which P waves are seen to occur at a rate of 140–220/min; there is either a prolongation of the PR interval or some of the P waves are not followed by QRS complexes. Carotid sinus pressure produces a transient increase in the atrioventricular block with a corresponding fall in the ventricular rate – a response quite unlike that of paroxysmal supraventricular tachycardia (see p. 194).

Atrial tachycardia with block is seldom dangerous in itself and generally does not require specific treatment. Digitalis should be stopped and potassium supplements given. Electrical shock should not be used unless it is certain that digitalis intoxication is not responsible, as it may induce more serious arrhythmias.

Atrial flutter (Fig. 11.12)

In this arrhythmia, the atria beat regularly at a rate of 250–350/min – usually close to 300/min. In most cases the arrhythmia arises due to a re-entry circuit within the right atrium, due to an area of slow conduction in an isthmus of myocardium between the inferior vena cava, tricuspid valve and coronary sinus.

Some degree of AV block is almost invariable. In most instances the ventricles beat regularly because of a 2:1, 3:1 or 4:1 response to the regular atrial activity, but it is irregular if the degree of block varies from cycle to cycle. The commonest variety is that of 2:1 block which characteristically has a ventricular rate of 140–160. In cases with 2:1 block flutter waves are not always obvious. Any regular, narrow QRS complex arrhythmia in this rate band should be closely scrutinized for the presence of flutter waves (Figs 11.10 and 11.12).

Atrial flutter is commonly a complication of underlying organic heart disease, although it occasionally occurs as a primary condition in patients with no definable cardiac abnormality. Common associations include:

- rheumatic heart disease;
- ischaemic heart disease;

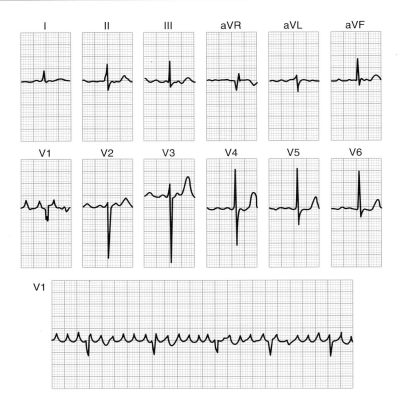

Fig. 11.12 Atrial flutter. Flutter waves are most readily apparent in the right-sided chest leads V1 and V2. They are also seen in inferior leads, III and aVF. A high degree of AV block is apparent with five to six flutter waves for every one QRS complex. Rhythm strip lead is V1.

- myocarditis;
- hyperthyroidism.

It may be persistent or occur in paroxysms which are usually self-limited to hours or days, but it may progress to atrial fibrillation. The symptoms resemble those of atrial tachycardia, with palpitation, dizziness or syncope. The arrhythmia often provokes cardiac failure.

The pulse is usually regular at a rate of 140–160/min. It may be possible to see venous 'flutter' waves in the neck. Carotid sinus massage leads to a transient increase in the atrioventricular block, with a slowing of the ventricular rate only as long as the pressure is maintained.

The electrocardiogram is diagnostic with 'flutter' waves of a sawtooth appearance, best seen in leads VI and III occurring at approximately 300/min. The sawtooth nature of the complexes may be obscured by the QRS complexes when there is 2:1 block, but it is readily revealed when carotid sinus massage is applied.

Drug treatment is seldom effective in restoring sinus rhythm. Digitalis increases the AV block, brings the heart rate under control, and sometimes abolishes the arrhythmia. Intravenous amiodarone is more likely to restore sinus rhythm, but requires a central line for its administration. Class I antiarrhythmic agents are best avoided because of the risk of slowing the flutter rate, enabling 1:1 conduction of the flutter waves into the ventricle, with consequent haemodynamic deterioration. Shock (d.c.) is indicated if immediate correction is necessary and is almost invariably effective (see p. 213).

In the patient liable to paroxysms of atrial flutter, beta-blockers, particularly sotalol, may be of some value. If this is ineffective, oral amiodarone is an alternative, but carries a risk of serious long-term side-effects (see p. 214). In some patients with refractory atrial flutter, radiofrequency ablation provides an alternative treatment strategy (see p. 214).

Atrial fibrillation (Fig. 11.13)

In this arrhythmia, irregular atrial impulses occur at rates over 300/min. It may be due to multiple foci of ectopic activity or to wavelets of excitation following variable courses through the atrial myocardium depending upon the location of patches of excitable and refractory muscle. Some degree of AV block is invariable; the ventricular rhythm is slower than the atrial but it is also irregular.

The presence of atrial fibrillation suggests that there has been either a pathological process involving the atria, as in rheumatic heart disease, or that there has been a rise in pressure with atrial dilatation secondary to mitral valve or left ventricular disease. Common causes of atrial fibrillation include:

- rheumatic mitral valve disease;
- ischaemic heart disease, particularly acute myocardial infarction;

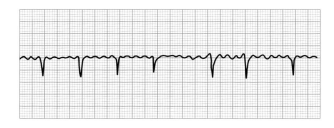

Fig. 11.13   Atrial fibrillation. The rhythm strip shows narrow QRS complexes which are irregularly irregular.

- alcohol;
- thyrotoxicosis;
- hypertension;
- acute infections, particularly when these affect the lungs;
- cardiopulmonary surgery.

It is a rare complication of many other types of heart disease. In a substantial proportion of patients, no evidence of organic heart disease can be found – 'lone' atrial fibrillation. The incidence of lone atrial fibrillation is greater amongst younger patients.

Atrial fibrillation may be paroxysmal, with attacks lasting for a few minutes or hours. This is particularly likely in acute myocardial infarction, in chest infections, and in the early stages of thyrotoxicosis and mitral valve disease. In rheumatic cases, the arrhythmia usually becomes established eventually and persists for the rest of the patient's life.

Atrial fibrillation leads to untoward effects for three major reasons:

- the ventricular response may be so fast that there is inadequate time for diastolic filling and the cardiac output falls;
- the atrial contribution to ventricular filling is lost;
- stasis in the ineffectively contracting atrium encourages thrombosis. As a consequence, embolism is common, particularly in patients with mitral valve disease. Emboli from the right atrium produce pulmonary artery obstruction; those from the left atrium may lodge in cerebral, renal or other peripheral vessels.

The first symptom may be that of irregular palpitations, but in many patients atrial fibrillation leads to the sudden development of left ventricular failure and pulmonary oedema. The onset may also be insidious with gradually increasing dyspnoea.

The diagnosis is usually easy because the arterial pulse is totally irregular. The ventricular response to atrial fibrillation appears random. Because of the varying times available for filling of the ventricles, the output of the heart and the volume of the pulse alter from beat to beat. This chaotic pulse serves to differentiate atrial fibrillation from atrial or ventricular ectopic beats, which are the arrhythmias most likely to be confused with it. In these latter conditions some periods of regularity are usually observed, and often the irregularity will be noted to occur every second, third or fourth beat. The venous pulse in atrial fibrillation is also irregular. The heart rate at the apex ('the apex rate') is usually higher than the radial pulse rate because the heart expels so little blood in some beats that no pulsation can be appreciated in the peripheral arteries.

In the ECG, the P wave disappears but atrial activity produces an irregular undulation of the base line (Fig. 11.13). The QRS complexes are totally irregular in timing, except in the rare situation of atrial fibrillation complicated by complete heart block. In most cases of untreated atrial fibrillation, the ventricular rate lies between 100 and 160/min, but rates above or below this are not uncommon.

Although patients with the arrhythmia may survive for many years with few symptoms, atrial fibrillation is frequently a serious complication because of the risks of heart failure and embolism.

Treatment. There are four aspects to the treatment of atrial fibrillation:

- the control of ventricular rate;
- the restoration of sinus rhythm;
- the maintenance of sinus rhythm;
- prevention of embolism.

Control of the ventricular rate. Control of the ventricular rate is a priority because it is the fast ventricular rate that is most deleterious, rather than the atrial fibrillation per se, and also because the arrhythmia may terminate spontaneously. Depending upon the severity of the clinical situation, digoxin or one of the other cardiac glycosides may be given intravenously or orally. In most cases, oral administration is satisfactory, and brings the heart rate under control within 2–3 h. When full digitalization has been achieved, the ventricular rate at rest should be held at about 70–80/min. If the heart rate cannot be reduced to this level, a beta-adrenoceptor blocking drug or verapamil may be added.

Restoration of sinus rhythm. When atrial fibrillation has been present for many years, and there is associated and untreatable severe heart disease, there is little to be gained by trying to restore normal rhythm because this is not likely to be maintained. Even if it is, the atrial muscle has usually atrophied and is functionally ineffective. When the arrhythmia is of relatively recent onset, and particularly when the heart disease has been alleviated or some complicating condition such as thyrotoxicosis or pulmonary infection corrected, the patient is likely to benefit from its termination.

In some patients sinus rhythm can be restored by pharmacological means. Amiodarone is frequently used for this purpose. Class I antiarrhythmic drugs, such as flecainide, have also been used successfully, but should be used with caution because of the risk of pro-arrhythmia.

Electric shock therapy is the most reliable means of restoring sinus rhythm and is effective in most instances, at least initially. However, there is a considerable relapse rate within the succeeding months.

The maintenance of sinus rhythm presents a difficult problem, particularly in patients with paroxysmal atrial fibrillation. Both amiodarone and class I antiarrhythmic agents are of proven value. However amiodarone may give rise to serious side-effects and there are serious concerns regarding the potential pro-arrhythmic effects associated with the long-term use of class I antiarrhythmic drugs. Their use should be confined to individuals with no underlying heart disease. Other agents, such as the beta-blocker sotalol, have less troublesome side-effects, but are also less effective. Drug selection must therefore be tailored to the severity of the problem posed by recurrent episodes of atrial fibrillation. Digoxin is of no value in preventing recurrences of atrial fibrillation.

Anticoagulation. Patients with atrial fibrillation complicating rheumatic heart disease should be anticoagulated. Recent evidence has shown that patients with non-rheumatic atrial fibrillation, but with demonstrable underlying heart disease, also benefit from anticoagulation. In patients with lone atrial fibrillation the risks of thromboembolism are low and the benefits of anticoagulation remain uncertain. In this group aspirin may be considered as an alternative.

In patients undergoing cardioversion, anticoagulation for a period of 1 month before and 1 month after cardioversion is indicated. This may be omitted if the arrhythmia is of very recent onset (less than 24 h). In patients in whom formal anticoagulation is contraindicated, transoesophageal echocardiography (see p. 74) can be used to exclude the presence of atrial thrombus, prior to cardioversion.

THE CAROTID SINUS AND ARRHYTHMIAS

The carotid sinus is situated at the bifurcation of the common carotid artery and is sensitive to changes in arterial pressure. Impulses arising from the stretch receptors in the carotid sinus pass to the medulla and reflexly slow the heart by stimulating the motor nucleus of the vagus nerve and by inhibiting cardiac sympathetic action. Usually, external pressure on the carotid sinus leads to a slight slowing of the heart rate by reducing the activity of the sinus node. In some individuals in whom the carotid sinus is hypersensitive, external pressure leads to extreme bradycardia and hypotension with resulting syncope.

Carotid sinus pressure plays an important part in the recognition and management of cardiac arrhythmias. It is best to locate the carotid artery on one side first and then to stroke it gently, but firmly. If this is ineffective, the manoeuvre should be repeated on the other side.

- *sinus tachycardia.* Carotid sinus massage causes only slight slowing of the ventricular rate in patients with sinus tachycardia;
- *atrial fibrillation.* Carotid sinus massage causes slight slowing of the ventricular response;
- *paroxysmal supraventricular tachycardia.* Carotid sinus massage causes an abrupt termination of the arrhythmia, if it has any effect at all;
- *atrial flutter.* Carotid sinus massage produces an increase in atrio-

ventricular block, temporarily decreasing the ventricular rate which rises again when the massage is discontinued (Fig. 11.14);

● *ventricular tachycardia.* Carotid sinus massage has no effect;
● *carotid sinus hypersensitivity.* Carotid sinus massage causes a profound bradycardia or asystole, frequently dizziness or syncope.

It is best to carry out carotid sinus massage with ECG control, as excessive bradycardia and even ventricular arrhythmias may result from this procedure. Other dangers include reflex hypotension and cerebrovascular insufficiency. In patients with peripheral arterial disease there is a small risk of precipitating a transient ischaemic attack or stroke.

Ventricular arrhythmias

Ventricular ectopic beats (extrasystoles, premature beats)

An ectopic focus in the ventricles may arise because of ventricular escape, enhanced automatic activity, or re-entry. Ventricular ectopic beats are not uncommon in normal individuals but are encountered frequently in organic heart disease, especially in myocardial infarction. If they occur every second beat (bigeminy or 'coupling') they are frequently due to digitalis therapy.

Patients are seldom aware of ventricular ectopic beats, but may complain of the heart seeming to stop briefly, or of an occasional heavy beat. The diagnosis may be suspected from an irregularity of the pulse interrupting an otherwise regular rhythm, but cannot be made without an ECG, in which there are bizarre and broadened QRS complexes followed by T waves pointing in the direction opposite to that of the main QRS component (Fig. 11.15). The QRS complexes are not preceded by

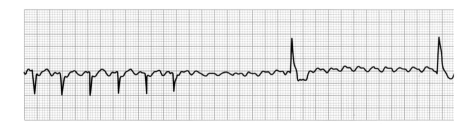

Fig. 11.14   Carotid sinus massage in atrial flutter. The initial tracing shows atrial flutter with 2:1 atrioventricular block. Carotid sinus massage causes a high degree of atrioventricular block, enabling the individual flutter waves to be clearly distinguished. The subsequent QRS complexes are ventricular escape beats.

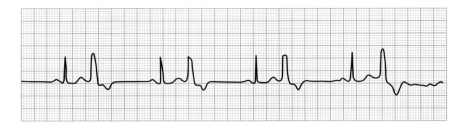

Fig. 11.15 Ventricular ectopic beats. Each sinus beat is followed by a broad complex ventricular ectopic beat. The constant coupling in this example is termed ventricular bigeminy.

a P wave and are usually succeeded by a long period (the compensatory pause) before the next sinus-activated beat appears.

The importance of ventricular ectopic beats depends upon their context. In normal individuals they are virtually of no consequence. Such individuals should undergo clinical examination, echocardiography and exercise testing, as appropriate, to rule out structural heart disease or coronary disease. Ventricular ectopic beats are associated with an impaired prognosis in ischaemic heart disease. But there is no evidence that suppression of ventricular ectopics with antiarrhythmic drugs improves prognosis. On the contrary, the class I antiarrhythmic drugs flecainide and encainide have been shown to increase mortality in patients with ventricular ectopic beats following myocardial infarction, despite reducing the frequency of ectopic beats.

Ventricular tachycardia (Fig. 11.16)

In this condition a tachycardia arises in the ventricles at a rate of 120–220/min; the atria usually remain under the control of the sinus node. It may be a consequence of either re-entry or enhanced automaticity of ventricular pacemaker cells. It is nearly always a complica-

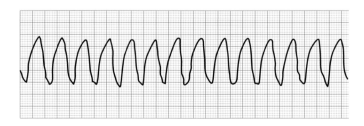

Fig. 11.16 Ventricular tachycardia. Regular wide QRS tachycardia at a rate of 170/min.

tion of serious heart disease, although occasionally seen in an otherwise normal individual. The attacks are liable to occur in paroxysms lasting for seconds or minutes, but may continue for several hours. Ventricular tachycardia is a frequent complication in patients with severe heart failure (see p. 159).

As with supraventricular tachycardia, the first symptom may be that of rapid and regular palpitations, but because of the more serious effects on the circulation, acute breathlessness and ischaemic chest pain tend to be more severe. On examination there is a rapid, regular but small pulse. The independent atrial activity may be responsible for dissociated 'a' waves in the venous pulse and a variation in the intensity of the first heart sound, but these physical signs are difficult to elicit. The ECG shows rapidly occurring broad QRS complexes resembling those of bundle branch block (see Fig. 11.15). P waves may be identified at a rate different from that of the ventricles (Fig. 11.18). The RR intervals are usually equal, but may vary by up to 0.03 s from one another. The lack of response to carotid pressure assists in the differentiation from atrial tachycardia with bundle brach block (see also pp. 195 and 200).

Treatment.   In the patient with good underlying heart function, urgent treatment may not be necessary. Most instances of ventricular tachycardia, however, call for immediate action, particularly in the context of acute myocardial infarction. Lignocaine, 100 mg, may be given intravenously and repeated if necessary. Alternative therapy includes flecainide and amiodarone. If these drugs fail to control the arrhythmia, electric shock may be used.

The drugs mentioned above may be used to prevent recurrences but should not be used empirically. The efficacy of drug therapy should be assessed by electrophysiological testing (see p. 87) to ensure that the arrhythmia is successfully controlled and to guard against the possibility of pro-arrhythmic effects.

In patients with ventricular tachycardia which fails to respond to drug therapy, alternative means of treatment should be considered. These include surgery to identify and remove or destroy the area of diseased muscle giving rise to the arrhythmia. An implantable cardioverter defibrillator (p. 214), to terminate automatically episodes of tachycardia represents another option. These devices detect the onset of tachycardia and pace or shock the heart back to its normal rhythm via implanted electrodes.

Benign ventricular tachycardias

Ventricular tachycardia can occasionally arise in patients with no underlying cardiac pathology. The commonest form is right ventricular outflow tachycardia. This shows a characteristic ECG morphology with left bundle branch block, and an axis directed inferiorly (leads II, III

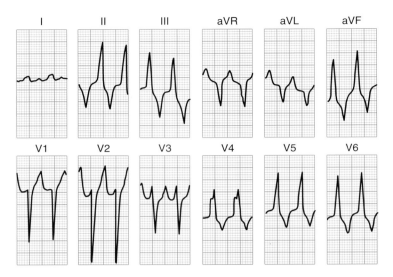

Fig. 11.17 A case of ventricular tachycardia arising from the right ventricular outflow tract. The characteristic features of left bundle branch block and an inferior axis in the frontal plane are evident.

and AVF positive) (Fig. 11.17). Characteristically episodes of tachycardia are provoked by adrenergic stress and exercise. Accordingly the best means of treatment is beta-blockade. In patients with refractory symptoms, radiofrequency ablation is an alternative to drug therapy.

Less commonly, a further form of benign ventricular tachycardia arises within the left ventricle, characteristically within the posterior fascicle of the left bundle. The resultant arrhythmia consequently shows a right bundle branch block morphology accompanying left axis deviation. The arrhythmia is once again amenable to radiofrequency ablation.

Torsades de pointes (Fig. 11.18)

This distinctive type of ventricular tachycardia is associated with a long QT interval, and may be idiopathic, due to hypokalaemia, or the result of the toxic action of such drugs as tricyclic antidepressants and type Ia antiarrhythmics. Its characteristic ECG feature is 'twisting of the points' of the QRS complexes. It usually occurs in repetitive bursts lasting a few seconds; it may progress to ventricular fibrillation. The underlying cause should, if possible, be corrected. Treatment of the arrhythmia with antiarrhythmic drugs should be avoided. Episodes causing haemodynamic compromise should be terminated by d.c. shock. Recurrences can generally be prevented by atrial or ventricular

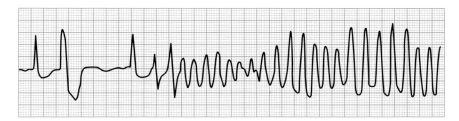

Fig. 11.18   Torsades de pointes. This is a form of polymorphic ventricular tachycardia in which the QRS axis undergoes progressive change. As a result the amplitude of the QRS complexes waxes and wanes.

pacing at 90–100/min. If pacing is not available, an infusion of isoprenaline to increase ventricular rate is an alternative.

Ventricular fibrillation (Fig. 11.19)

In this condition there is a chaotic electrical disturbance of the ventricles, with impulses occurring irregularly at a rate of 300–500/min. Ventricular contraction is uncoordinated and ventricular filling and emptying cease. The cardiac output falls precipitously to zero.

Ventricular fibrillation is the commonest cause of sudden death. It may occur as a primary arrhythmia or as a complication of acute myocardial infarction.

It may also result from drowning, electrocution and overdosage of drugs including digitalis, adrenaline and isoprenaline. Self-terminating episodes are rare but may complicate complete heart block.

Because of its catastrophic effects, ventricular fibrillation gives rise to the clinical features of cardiac arrest, with sudden disappearance of arterial pulses, cessation of respiration, loss of consciousness and dilatation of the pupils. Although it cannot be diagnosed clinically, it is to be suspected in any patient dying with apparent suddenness, particularly in the context of acute myocardial infarction. On the electrocardiogram, there is a chaotic rhythm with ventricular complexes of varying amplitude and rate (Fig. 11.19). Eventually asystole ensues.

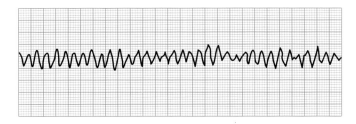

Fig. 11.19   Ventricular fibrillation.

Ventricular fibrillation is almost invariably fatal, and immediate treatment is necessary if death is to be prevented. As with other forms of cardiac arrest, an effective circulation and ventilation must be obtained with 4 min if irreversible brain damage is not to occur. Sinus rhythm can usually only be restored by electric shock, which should be administered as soon as possible. If an electrical defibrillator is not immediately available, the standard treatment of cardiac arrest should be started with closed chest cardiac compression and artificial ventilation (see Chapter 22).

Recurrences of ventricular fibrillation should be prevented in the same way as ventricular tachycardia.

THE DIFFERENTIATION OF SUPRAVENTRICULAR FROM VENTRICULAR TACHYCARDIA

The rapid rate associated with some supraventricular tachycardias may result in bundle branch block, causing a broad QRS complex tachycardia which is difficult to distinguish from ventricular tachycardia. It is occasionally possible to distinguish between the two on clinical grounds. In ventricular tachycardia atrial activity is usually dissociated from that of the ventricles. There may be irregular cannon waves in the jugular veins (see p. 46) and variation in the intensity of the first heart sound. In junctional tachycardia, cannon waves may occur with every beat.

The response to carotid sinus massage is sometimes diagnostic (see p. 194), as this manoeuvre frequently abolishes supraventricular tachycardia but leaves ventricular tachycardia unaffected. However, one should delay applying this test if possible until a 12-lead ECG is available, as one may otherwise miss the opportunity of verifying the nature of the arrhythmia by obtaining a graphic record.

Commonly, a clinical diagnosis is not possible. A 12-lead ECG may provide additional formation. ECG evidence of atrial dissociation

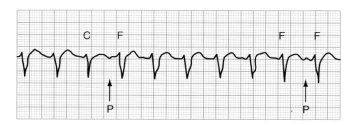

Fig. 11.20 Features of ventricular tachycardia. The ECG shows a slow ventricular tachycardia at a rate of 120/min. Several diagnostic features of ventricular tachycardia are evident: dissociated P waves (P), narrow complex 'capture' beats, and intermediate morphology 'fusion' (F) beats.

confirms a diagnosis of ventricular tachycardia (Fig. 11.20). The following findings are diagnostic:

- dissociated P waves;
- capture beats – the dissociated atrial activity 'captures' the ventricle over the normal conduction pathway, giving a single beat with narrow QRS morphology;
- fusion beats – the dissociated atrial activity is conducted into the ventricles fusing with the tachycardia beats and giving a QRS morphology intermediate between a supraventricular morphology and the tachycardia morphology.

However, these classical diagnostic features are frequently absent and their absence should not be used to infer a supraventricular origin. There are a number of other ECG features which may be helpful in reaching a diagnosis (Fig. 11.21):

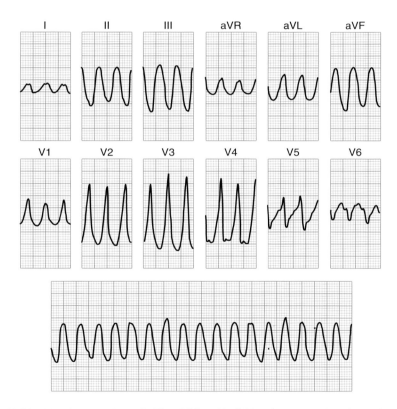

Fig. 11.21 Ventricular tachycardia. The QRS width (200 ms) suggests that the tachycardia is ventricular in origin. For further discussion see text.

- *QRS width.* A tachycardia with a QRS width greater than 140 ms (3.5 small squares) is very likely to be ventricular;
- *QRS axis.* A tachycardia demonstrating left axis deviation is similarly likely to be ventricular.

If doubt remains it is important to remember that ventricular tachycardia is much more common than supraventricular tachycardia with bundle branch block. When in doubt a tachycardia is best treated as ventricular. Intravenous adenosine may also prove of value in distinguishing supraventricular tachycardia with aberration from ventricular tachycardia (see p. 399).

DISORDERS OF CONDUCTION

Sinu-atrial block and sinus arrest

In sinu-atrial block, an impulse from the sinus node fails to activate the atria. This results in a dropped beat; on the electrocardiogram a complete PQRST complex is absent, but the next sinus beat comes in at the predicted time (Fig. 11.22). It is of little clinical importance except that it may be a manifestation of intoxication by digoxin or other antiarrhythmic drugs. It may be a component of the sick sinus syndrome (see p. 181). If it is prolonged, syncope occurs. In sinus arrest, the sinus node fails to initiate an impulse; after a pause, junctional or ventricular escape occurs. Its significance is similar to that of sinu-atrial block.

Atrioventricular (heart) block

The term atrioventricular (AV) block implies that there is some defect in conduction of the impulse from the atria to the ventricles. In first-degree AV block, all the impulses reach the ventricles but they are

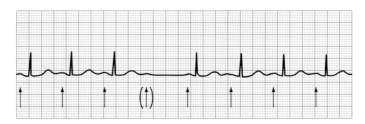

Fig. 11.22 Sinu-atrial exit block. The P waves are regular (arrowed). One P wave is absent (bracketed arrow), but the P wave rhythm is maintained without change in cycle length. The sinus discharge rate has therefore been maintained, although the impulse has failed to exit the sinus node.

delayed in their passage and the PR interval exceeds 0.20 s. In second-degree block, some impulses reach the ventricles while others fail to do so. In complete heart block, no impulses reach the ventricles from the atria, and the ventricles are under the control of a lower pacemaker situated in the junctional tissue, bundle of His, the bundle of branches or Purkinje tissue. In bundle branch block, AV conduction is maintained through one branch, the other being blocked.

First-degree AV block (Fig. 11.23).   First-degree AV block occurs occasionally in normal individuals; it is a characteristic feature of the carditis of acute rheumatic fever and of digitalis overdosage. It cannot be diagnosed clinically and its recognition depends on observing a PR interval of greater than 0.20 s in the ECG. Its only importance is as an index of digitalis intoxication and as a precursor of the more advanced degrees of AV block.

Second-degree AV block.   There are two types of second degree heart block. In the first type (sometimes referred to as *Mobitz type 1* or *Wenckebach block*) the PR interval becomes progressively more prolonged from beat to beat until one P wave is not succeeded by a QRS complex (Fig. 11.24). The next atrial complex is followed at a normal or near normal interval by a QRS complex and the cycle of events recurs.

The pulse is correspondingly irregular. The Wenckebach phenomenon is frequently the result of digitalis intoxication, but both this and the other varieties of second-degree heart block are often due to ischaemic heart disease, particularly myocardial infarction, and to many other types of cardiac disease.

In the second type (*Mobitz type 2*), block occurs without progressive prolongation of the PR interval (Fig. 11.25). This is much rarer than Wenckebach block. Whereas Wenckebach block is indicative of diseased conduction in the AV node, sudden dropped beats, without progressive PR prolongation, suggest disease lower in the His–Purkinje system. In 2:1 block there is no opportunity to observe progressive PR prolongation and consequently it is difficult to categorize the site of conduction disturbance.

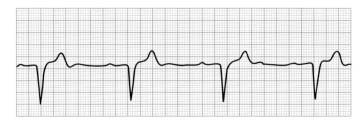

Fig. 11.23   First-degree AV block. The PR interval is prolonged at 320 ms. In this example, bradycardia (rate 40) and QRS widening (130 ms) are also evident.

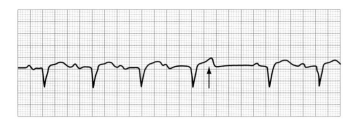

Fig. 11.24 Second-degree AV block: Wenckebach. Progressive PR prolongation is evident, culminating in a P wave (arrowed) which fails to conduct to the ventricle.

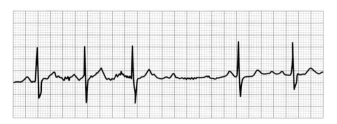

Fig. 11.25 Second-degree AV block: Mobitz 2. A P wave fails to conduct to the ventricles, without any progressive PR prolongation beforehand. The tracing is taken from a Holter recording and high frequency artefact is apparent.

The main significance of second-degree heart block lies in the liability of the patient to develop complete heart block and the Adams–Stokes syndrome. However, if the ventricular rate in second-degree heart block is sufficiently slow, cardiac failure or hypotension may be precipitated. The more distal the site of block in the conduction system, the less reliable becomes the escape pacemaker if complete heart block develops. For this reason the two types of second degree AV block are of differing significance:

- *sudden dropped beats (Mobitz 2)* indicate disease low in the conduction system and a risk of a poor escape rhythm, should complete heart block develop. They are therefore an indication for pacing;
- *progressive PR prolongation (Mobitz 1)*, on the other hand, indicate AV node disease, is more likely to be succeeded by a satisfactory ventricular escape rhythm, should complete block occur. Pacing, therefore, generally is unnecessary.

Occasionally, the slow heart rate accompanying second-degree AV block is responsible for clinical deterioration and the heart must be accelerated. This may be achieved by administering atropine or by artificial pacing.

Complete AV (heart) block (Fig. 11.26)

The ventricular rate is slow (25–50/min). There are cannon waves in the venous pulse (see p. 46) and a varying first heart sound (see p. 51).

Acute complete heart block is most commonly a complication of myocardial infarction, but may also result from cardiac surgery and myocarditis. In myocardial infarction, it usually follows occlusion of the right coronary artery which is responsible for the blood supply of the junctional tissue and bundle of His (see also p. 140). The severely damaged heart may not be able to compensate adequately for the bradycardia by increasing its stroke volume; heart failure and hypotension may ensue. There is also a considerable risk of ventricular asystole. The bradycardia may be temporarily controlled by infusing isoprenaline in a dose of 2–5 mg in 500 ml of 5% dextrose, but insertion of an artificial pacemaker is preferable (see p. 405). If the patient survives, normal AV conduction is usually restored within a week.

In most cases of chronic complete heart block there is fibrosis of both bundle branches of unknown cause. This variety is most commonly seen in the elderly. A congenital form occurs either as an isolated finding or in association with other congenital heart defects. Heart block can also complicate rheumatic or ischaemic heart disease, or follow trauma to the conducting tissue at surgery. A proportion of patients with chronic complete heart block survive for years with no symptoms, but once heart failure or syncopal attacks of the Adams–Stokes variety develop, the expectation of life, if left untreated, is usually only a few months. For this reason, an artificial pacemaker is indicated when symptoms arise.

The Adams–Stokes attack. In an Adams–Stokes attack the patient loses consciousness for a period of some seconds because of transient cardiac arrest. It usually occurs in patients with second-degree or complete heart block who develop sudden loss of ventricular activity. It is particularly common during the progression from second-degree to complete heart block because the ventricular pacemaker necessary for

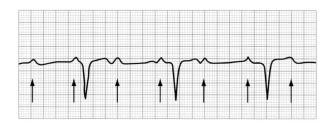

Fig. 11.26   Complete heart block. P waves (arrowed) are completely dissociated from the QRS complexes.

survival may not have become firmly established. In some cases, the Adams–Stokes attack is due not to ventricular asystole but to a short burst of ventricular tachycardia or fibrillation.

The presenting symptom is syncope with or without a preceding period of dizziness. The attack usually lasts some 10–30 s and convulsions may occur. During the attack the patient is pulseless, pale or cyanosed. Consciousness returns rapidly with reappearance of the heart beat, the patient then flushing as blood courses through capillaries dilated by the hypoxia of the attack. Attacks of the Adams–Stokes variety may be separated from one another by a number of months, but occasionally a series occurs over a period of minutes or hours. Sooner or later, the patient is likely to die from ventricular asystole or ventricular fibrillation.

The diagnosis should be considered in any patient presenting with syncope, but is unlikely to be the explanation in the absence of bundle branch block, second-degree block, or complete AV block between the episodes.

During an attack a blow over the cardiac apex may restore the heart action, but if it does not do so, the usual therapy for cardiac arrest should be undertaken (p. 392) with closed-chest cardiac compression and artificial ventilation. Adams–Stokes attacks can be prevented by an artificial pacemaker.

Bundle branch block

In this condition, either the right or the left branch of the bundle of His is not conducting impulses.

Right bundle branch block. Block of the right bundle branch gives rise to a characteristic electrocardiographic appearance (Fig. 11.27). This is often an isolated congenital lesion of no importance but may be associated with other congenital heart defects, particularly atrial septal defect (p. 300); in middle or advanced age, it is usually due to ischaemic heart disease or idiopathic fibrosis. Right bundle branch block may be partial, with QRS width of less than 0.12 s, or complete, in which case the QRS is of 0.12 s duration or more. It may be suspected clinically because the block leads to a delayed activation, and therefore contraction, of the right ventricle. This results in late closure of the pulmonary valve which can be recognized by a wide splitting of the second heart sound (p. 51). Right bundle branch block is of minor clinical significance, except as an indicator of possible heart disease, and as a precursor of complete heart block (especially if associated with left or right axis deviation indicating block in one of the fascicles of the left bundle (see p. 141)).

Left bundle branch block. Left bundle branch block is rare in the otherwise normal individual and is most commonly seen in ischaemic heart disease. It is difficult to recognize clinically, although there may be reversed splitting of the second heart sound (p. 51); it is readily identified on the ECG (Fig. 11.28). Because it is associated with severe ventricular disease (usually ischaemic) it carries a more serious

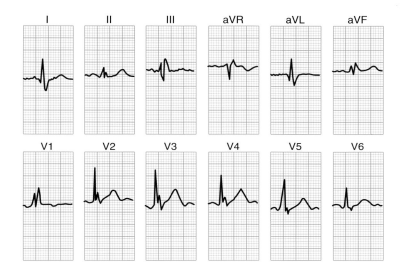

Fig. 11.27   Right bundle branch block and RsR' pattern is evident in lead V1. There is a late S wave in lead V6.

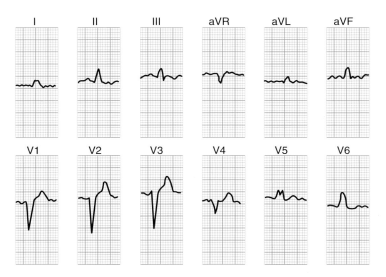

Fig. 11.28   Left bundle branch block.

prognosis than right bundle branch block, but patients with this lesion may survive for many years.

Neither form of bundle branch block requires treatment.

Pre-excitation (Wolff–Parkinson–White syndrome)

In this condition, an anomalous conduction pathway bypasses the AV node. This permits the abnormally early activation of part of one ventricle, the remaining ventricular muscle receiving its impulse normally. This leads to a short PR interval (less than 0.12 s) and a slurred upstroke and widening of the QRS (Figs 11.2 and 11.11).

INVESTIGATION OF ARRHYTHMIAS

Ambulatory ECG monitoring

ECG monitoring is of particular value in the diagnosis and investigation of arrhythmias. The technique is described in Chapter 5 (see p. 77). Ambulatory monitoring can also be used to assess the response of arrhythmias to drug therapy.

Invasive electrophysiological studies

Invasive electrophysiological studies play an important role in the diagnosis and therapy of many arrhythmias. They are also an essential accompaniment to radiofrequency ablation. This approach is described in more detail in Chapter 6 (see p. 90).

MANAGEMENT OF ARRHYTHMIAS

Electrical therapy

CARDIAC PACING

Control over the electrical activity of the heart may be obtained by the use of an artificial pacemaker (Fig. 11.29). A pacemaking system consists of a pulse generator (containing batteries and electronic circuitry) and one or more electrodes. If pacing is to be maintained for only a short period of time, an external power source is used; if long-term pacing is necessary, the pulse generator is implanted.

Electrical pacemaking is potentially hazardous. If the electrical impulse is of sufficient magnitude and falls during the period of ven-

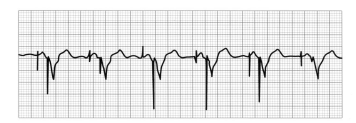

Fig. 11.29   Paced ECG. A dual chamber pacemaker is present, pacing both atrium and ventricle. The first pacing spike is followed by a P wave and the second by a QRS complex.

tricular repolarization, i.e. on the T wave of the ECG, ventricular fibrillation may be induced. This problem is overcome by the use of a 'demand' pacemaker which senses the patient's spontaneous beats and operates only when there is no ventricular complex generated by the patient's own heart. In the absence of a complex, the pacemaker discharges after a selected interval.

Temporary pacing

When pacing is employed in the treatment of heart block in acute myocardial infarction, it is customary to introduce the electrode through a peripheral vein and to position its tip in the apex of the right ventricle. The other end of the electrode is attached to a portable battery-operated demand pacemaker. The electrode is withdrawn when the risks of atrioventricular block have resolved. The procedure for insertion of a temporary pacemaker is described in Chapter 22.

Permanent pacing

In chronic heart block, an electrode is positioned with its tip in the right ventricle, and its proximal end attached to a pacemaker buried under the skin of the axillary region or the anterior chest. The pacing electrode may have a single pole, in which case pacing is between this pole and the can of the pacemaker (unipolar pacing) or two poles in which case pacing is between the two poles (bipolar pacing). Occasionally electrodes may be placed directly on the surface of the myocardium at the time of a thoracotomy or laparotomy and the wires passed subcutaneously to a pacemaker positioned in the abdomen. However, epicardial pacing is less satisfactory than endocardial. Pacemakers should have a life of more than 10 years but regular checking for battery or other failure is necessary.

Numerous types of pacemaker are now available; most are 'programmable', that is the cardiologist can choose the particular type of pacing programme that is most suitable for an individual patient. Programmable functions include:

- *stimulus voltage and duration.* These factors are programmable to provide an adequate safety margin, exceeding the patient's threshold voltage. Excessive voltages should be avoided as these are an unnecessary drain on the generator and may lead to skeletal muscle twitching.
- *sensing threshold.* In patients with an underlying spontaneous rhythm, the threshold voltage for detection of sensed electrograms can be determined. The sensitivity of the pacemaker is then programmed to provide an adequate margin of safety for detection of these electrograms. Problems may, however, arise if the pacemaker unit is made excessively sensitive – musculoskeletal potentials may be detected and misinterpreted as cardiac activity, inhibiting pacing. Most pacemakers have noise detection circuits which switch to fixed rate pacing when electrical noise is detected to guard against this possiblity;
- *pacing rate.* This sets the rate at which the generator unit will discharge impulses. Many units feature, in addition, hysteresis, that is the heart rate must fall to a lower value than the generator's discharge rate, before pacing will be initiated. For example, a rate of 70/min with hysteresis of 20/min would mean that a pacemaker will only start pacing when the spontaneous heart rate falls below 50/min, at which time pacing will commence at 70/min.

Hazards of pacemaking include infection and failure of the components of the pacemaking unit, such as batteries, circuitry and electrodes.

Dual-chamber pacing. Ventricular pacing successfully prevents bradycardias, but it fails to substitute for the heart's normal pacemaker function in two ways. Firstly, the rate of the pacemaker is fixed and cannot adapt to the differing needs of the body, as for example during exercise. Secondly, the normal sequence of atrial and ventricular contraction is lost, which leads to a fall in cardiac output.

In patients who continue to have a normal atrial rhythm, these problems can be prevented by insertion of a dual-chamber pacemaker. Dual chamber pacing involves the use of two intra-cardiac leads, one in the atrium and one in the ventricle. This system ensures the maintenance of normal AV synchrony. The AV interval is a programmable function. The pacemaker may operate in a number of modes. In one it paces both atrium and ventricle. In another, the patient's underlying spontaneous atrial activity is sensed and this is followed, after the AV delay, by a ventricular impulse. This system has the advantage that the rate of discharge of ventricular impulses will be determined by the patient's own intrinsic atrial rate. Heart rate will, therefore, increase appropriately to meet the varying demands of the body.

Dual-chamber pacing improves the exercise tolerance of patients with complete heart block in comparison with single chamber pacing. It also prevents the occurrence of pacemaker syndrome. *Pacemaker syndrome* is a problem which arises in occasional individuals with single chamber ventricular pacemakers. Patients experience transient hypotension and dizziness with the onset of pacing. This is due to loss of AV synchrony and is prevented by dual-chamber pacing.

Rate-responsive pacing. In some patients, particularly those with atrial fibrillation, dual-chamber pacing is not possible. A variety of rate-responsive pacing systems have been developed, to enable heart rate to rise with exercise in a single chamber ventricular pacing system. These pacemakers detect the onset of exercise and increase the ventricular pacing rate. Sensed parameters include the mechanical detection of vibrations, changes in QT interval of the ECG, changes in temperature of the blood returning to the right atrium and changes in respiratory rate. Rate-responsive systems have the advantage of increasing the patient's exercise capacity, in comparison with fixed-rate pacemakers.

Recently, dual-chamber rate-responsive pacemakers have been introduced. These are indicated in patients requiring dual chamber pacing, in whom the response of the sinus node to exercise is reduced. These pacemakers enable the normal sequence of AV synchrony to be maintained, with an accompanying increase in heart rate with exercise.

PACING MODES

The international pacemaker code

A three-letter alphabetic code is used to describe the mode of a pacemaker's operation. Each of the three letters of this code presents specific information:

- the first letter refers to the site of cardiac pacing – **A**trium, **V**entricle or **D**ual (both);
- the second letter refers to the site of sensing – **A**trium, **V**entricle, **D**ual or no sensing (designated O);
- the third letter refers to the response to sensing – **I**nhibited, **T**riggered, **D**ual (both inhibited and triggered) and no response (designated O).

Additional letters can be added to this basic three-letter code to indicate a rate-adaptive pulse generator (R) or to provide information on the type of pacing lead.

Although numerous pacing modes are theoretically possible, in practice relatively few modes are actually used.

VVI mode. This represents single-chamber ventricular-demand pacing. A sensed impulse in the ventricle inhibits the output of the pacemaker. VVI pacing and VVIR (rate-responsive) pacing are the commonest choice of pacemaker worldwide.

AAI mode. This is exactly the same as the VVI mode except that the pacemaker senses and paces the atrium instead of the ventricle. This mode is reserved for patients with sick sinus syndrome with normal AV conduction and hence no need to pace the ventricle.

DDD mode. This represents a dual-chamber pacemaker and is the most sophisticated mode of dual-chamber pacing. The pacemaker can be considered as an AAI pacemaker which paces or senses the atrium with an added AV counter, which emits a ventricular stimulus if no ventricular impulse has been sensed by the end of the AV period. AV synchrony is therefore maintained during atrial pacing while the pacemaker will also 'track' the rate of atrial activity enabling the ventricular rate to respond to physiological changes in sinus rate. This, however, also represents a shortcoming of DDD pacing: the pacemaker will sense atrial arrhythmias and could result in an excessive ventricular tracing rate. To guard against this a maximum tracking rate is programmed to limit ventricular response at high atrial rates. This can be achieved either by imposing a Wenckebach-type block in ventricular response or by programming the pacemaker to switch to VVI mode. In patients with intact VA conduction, a pacemaker-mediated tachycardia can be generated by conduction of a paced ventricular impulse back into the atrium. This is sensed as an atrial event by the pacemaker, leading to ventricular stimulation and completing a tachycardia loop. This complication can generally be avoided by careful programming.

VDD mode. The device senses in the atrium but does not pace. This mode is useful in the management of patients with AV block and normal sinus mode function. This mode has the further advantage that it can be used in combination with a single-lead system in which an atrial cavity electrode is present on a ventricular lead. The cavity electrode senses atrial activity, but is not able to pace the atrium.

Choice of pacemaker and pacing mode

Sinus node disease. In general, dual-chamber pacing is indicated. Single-chamber ventricular pacing is unsatisfactory as intermittent ventricular pacing may cause hypotension and dizziness, termed pacemaker syndrome. In patients in whom AV nodal conduction is not in question, single-chamber atrial pacing is satisfactory.

AV block. Dual-chamber pacing is optimal. In patients with a satisfactory sinus node activity, VDD pacing can be substituted. Single-chamber ventricular pacing is in general suboptimal because of loss of

AV synchrony, but may be acceptable in more elderly or sedentary patients.

Carotid sinus sensitivity. As for sick sinus syndrome, dual-chamber pacing is indicated.

MANAGEMENT OF TACHYARRHYTHMIAS

Direct current (d.c.) shock therapy

The d.c. shock must be timed to avoid the vulnerable period. It is customary to arrange for the defibrillator to discharge 0.02 s after the peak of the R wave. A synchronized discharge of this kind is not possible when there is ventricular fibrillation.

Because the procedure is a painful one, an anaesthetic is usually given, except when there is ventricular fibrillation (because the patient is unconscious). A short-acting barbiturate is often used, but an alternative is to supplement an analgesic such as morphine with diazepam 5–10 mg intravenously. One electrode, smeared with electrode jelly, is placed in the right parasternal region and the other either in the left axilla or posteriorly below the left scapula. The machine is charged to the chosen level and discharged by pressing a button on the electrode. The strength of shock needed varies with the arrhythmia being treated:

- *ventricular tachycardia and ventricular fibrillation.* An initial 200 J shock is appropriate, increased to 360 J for subsequent shocks if the initial shock is ineffective;
- *atrial fibrillation.* The initial amplitude should be 100 J and subsequently increased to 200 and 360 J as necessary;
- *'organized' supraventricular arrhythmias* (atrial flutter, paroxysmal supraventricular tachycardia), a low-amplitude shock is frequently successful; an initial amplitude of 25 J is appropriate.

Apart from slight skin burns, the procedure is usually free from undesirable effects. However, there is a danger of producing serious arrhythmias in the patient with digitalis intoxication, and it is wise to discontinue this drug for 1–2 days prior to electric shock administration if possible.

The indications for electric shock therapy are discussed under the individual arrhythmias, but in general it may be stated that electric shock therapy is almost invariably effective for all types of tachycardia including the supraventricular tachycardias, atrial flutter, atrial fibrillation, ventricular tachycardia and ventricular fibrillation. Some cases of chronic atrial fibrillation are resistant. Electric shock should not be given if it is thought that the arrhythmia is digitalis or quinidine induced.

Anti-tachycardia pacing

Some re-entrant supraventricular tachycardias, particularly AV node re-entry tachycardia, can be terminated by critically timed atrial extrastimuli. Antitachycardia pacemakers have been developed which have the ability to detect the onset of a tachyarrhythmia and deliver critically timed trains of extrastimuli to the right atrium, thereby restoring sinus rhythm. These devices provide an alternative to drug therapy in the management of supraventricular tachycardias, but have largely been superseded by the advent of radiofrequency ablation. They are in general contraindicated in patients susceptible to atrial fibrillation, because of the possibility that a train of atrial extra-stimuli will cause atrial fibrillation rather than restoring sinus rhythm. Because of the special dangers of atrial fibrillation in patients with Wolff–Parkinson–White syndrome they are rarely indicated in this condition.

The implantable defibrillator

Implantable defibrillators have been developed which can deliver a d.c. shock to the heart to terminate episodes of ventricular tachycardia or ventricular fibrillation. Early devices were large and this necessitated implantation in the abdomen. Later devices have decreased in size substantially and are now suitable for prepectoral or subpectoral implantation (Fig. 11.30). While early devices required a thoracotomy for the placement of epicardial patches, defibrillation can now be achieved in the vast majority of patients with an endocardial lead. Much lower energies are required than for external defibrillation. Shocks of 10–20 J are generally sufficient to defibrillate the heart and restore sinus rhythm. In patients with ventricular tachycardia, this can frequently be terminated by anti-tachycardia pacing, without the need to resort to a shock.

Implantable defibrillators are particularly expensive. Their use should be restricted to patients resuscitated from sudden cardiac death and to those with life-threatening ventricular tachyarrhythmias, which are not amenable to other forms of treatment.

Catheter ablation (Fig. 11.31)

Catheter ablation has revolutionized the management of a number of arrhythmias. Radiofrequency current is passed down an electrode catheter positioned in contact with the endocardium, producing a small area of thermal tissue destruction. The technique can be used in the management of a number of arrhythmias:

- accessory pathways, whether overt in patients with Wolff–Parkinson–White syndrome or concealed (only conducting from

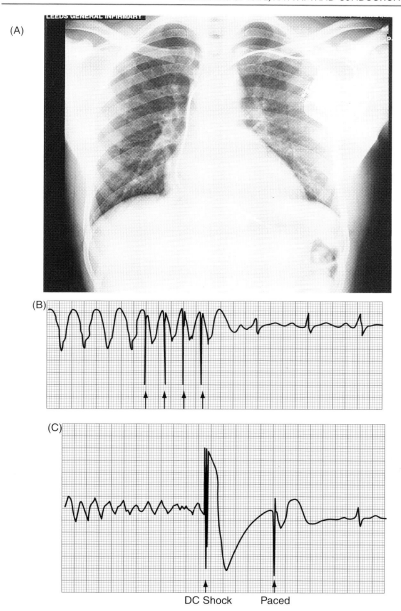

Fig. 11.30 Implanted defibrillator. (A) Chest X-ray in a patient with a prepectoral defibrillator. The shock is delivered between the coil in the right ventricle and the 'active' can of the device. (B) Ventricular tachycardia terminated by a train of four extrastimuli. (C) Ventricular fibrillation terminated by a DC shock delivered by the device (arrowed). The first beat after delivery of the shock is paced.

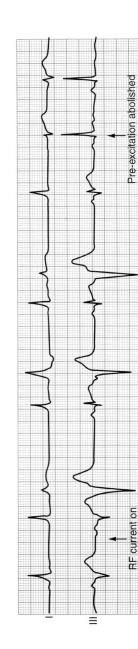

Fig. 11.31 Radiofrequency ablation of an accessory pathway in a patient with Wolff–Parkinson–White syndrome. Six seconds after commencing current application accessory pathway conduction is abolished, with loss of the delta wave and prolongation of the PR interval.

ventricle to atrium and hence not causing pre-excitation, can be successfully destroyed thereby preventing arrhythmia recurrence;
- in patients with AV node re-entrant tachycardia, the re-entry circuit can be interrupted by destroying one of the pathways through the AV node. With this technique there is a small risk of complete destruction of the AV node, resulting in complete heart block and the need for permanent pacing;
- intra-atrial arrhythmias and atrial flutter are also amenable to radiofrequency ablation, but recurrence rates are appreciably higher than for accessory pathway and AV node ablation.
- benign ventricular tachycardias, such as right ventricular outflow tachycardias are readily amenable to ablation. Success has also been reported for the other more common forms of ventricular tachycardia arising as a result of scar formation following myocardial infarction, but these generally involve widespread abnormalities in the ventricles and consequently recurrence rates are high;
- total AV node ablation is an option in patients with refractory atrial fibrillation in whom drugs fail to provide satisfactory rate control. By ablating the bundle of His, complete heart block is produced. The atria continue to fibrillate but the ventricles are protected from the fast rate. Permanent pacing is necessary and dictates the rate of ventricular contraction.

Antiarrhythmic drugs

Before commencing a patient on therapy with an antiarrhythmic drug, it is essential to consider the advantages and disadvantages of drug treatment. As a group, antiarrhythmic drugs have the potential to do harm as well as to do good. It is well established that under some circumstances antiarrhythmic drugs may exacerbate existing arrhythmias or even create new ones. In general, antiarrhythmic drug treatment should only be prescribed when clearly indicated either to treat symptoms or to prevent potentially life-threatening arrhythmias. They are not indicated simply to 'tidy up' the ECG. Although antiarrhythmic agents are highly successful in suppressing ventricular ectopic beats, they may have an adverse effect on more serious ventricular tachyarrhythmias.

Antiarrhythmic therapy is used to:

- Suppress or prevent arrhythmias;
- Slow the ventricular response rate in the case of supraventricular arrhythmias.

Table 11.1   Classification of antiarrhythmic drugs

Class I Membrane-stabilizing drugs		
Subgroup	(A)	Quinidine
		Procainamide
		Disopyramide
	(B)	Lignocaine
		Mexiletine
	(C)	Flecainide
		Propafenone
Class II Anti-sympathetic drugs		
Beta-blockers		
Class III Drugs that prolong action potential duration		
Amiodarone		
Bretylium		
Sotalol		
Class IV Calcium antagonists		
Verapamil		

ANTIARRHYTHMIC DRUG CLASSIFICATION (Table 11.1)

There are four main classes of antiarrhythmic drug action:

- *class I 'membrane-stabilizing'* drugs, which also have a local anaesthetic action, block the inflow of sodium into the cell and, therefore, the rate of depolarization. This has the effect of reducing the automaticity of ectopic pacemaker foci and of slowing conduction, which may abolish a re-entry circuit;
- *class II 'anti-sympathetic' drugs* – notably those that block beta-adrenoceptors;
- *class III drugs that prolong action potential duration*. Amiodarone is the main drug in this category, although sotalol and bretylium also have class III actions;
- *class IV drugs that block the inflow of calcium into the cell*. This affects the activity of certain cells, particularly those of the atrioventricular node, which are dependent more on the calcium inflow than on sodium. Verapamil belongs to this group.

Notes on individual antiarrhythmic drugs

Lignocaine.   Lignocaine is the first-choice drug in the acute management of ventricular tachycardia and ventricular fibrillation. It has virtually no myocardial depressant effect in therapeutic doses and is safer to give intravenously than other class I antiarrhythmic agents. It should not be given in the presence of AV block, which it may aggravate. The drug is used mainly intravenously, and by this route its duration of action is only 10–20 min. Initially, a dose of 50–100 mg (i.e. 5–10 ml of the 1% solution) can be given over a period of 1–2 min and repeated, if necessary, 2 min later. This may be followed by an intravenous infusion of 4 mg/min for 30 min, 3 mg/min for a further 30 min and thereafter 2 mg/min for 24–48 h, if necessary. Serious toxic effects from lignocaine are unusual, but include confusion, convulsions, respiratory depression and coma. The drug is not effective in controlling atrial arrhythmias.

Flecainide. Flecainide is one of the most effective antiarrhythmic drugs, and usually abolishes all ventricular ectopic activity. It is a class Ic antiarrhythmic agent. However, like other drugs in this category it carries a particular risk of pro-arrhythmia. It has been found to be hazardous when given to patients after myocardial infarction, particularly if they have impaired left ventricular function, because it may cause cardiac failure and fatal arrhythmias. Its use in patients with ischaemic heart disease should be restricted to patients with life-threatening ventricular arrhythmias, in whom efficacy has been proven and proarrhythmic effects excluded by invasive electrophysiological investigations. The drug is also of value in the management of some supraventricular arrhythmias (particularly Wolff–Parkinson–White syndrome) in whom the risk of serious pro-arrhythmic effects is extremely low. Oral flecainide is given in a dosage of 100 mg twice daily.

Propafenone. Propafenone is a class Ic drug. It is useful in the management of paroxysmal supraventricular arrhythmias including atrial fibrillation. It is also effective in many cases of ventricular tachycardia but, like other drugs in its class, it is also prone to provoke ventricular arrhythmias. Oral propafenone is given in a dosage of 150–300 mg thrice daily.

Amiodarone. This drug prolongs the action potential and the refractory period; it is therefore of value in blocking re-entrant pathways but the drug is of value in many resistant supraventricular and ventricular arrhythmias. Its toxic effects have precluded its widespread use. It causes corneal deposits, but these appear to be benign and reversible and seldom give rise to symptoms. Other side-effects include a bluish discoloration of the skin following exposure to the sun and thyroid disorders, especially thyrotoxicosis. More rarely, a pneumonitis may occur, which may be fatal. Oral amiodarone may not exert its antiarrhythmic action for up to a week and on stopping the drug may take several weeks for the effects to disappear. The usual dosage is 200 mg thrice daily for a week, gradually reducing thereafter to 200 mg daily. The incidence of side effects is dose related and patients should be reduced to the minimum drug dose compatible with arrhythmia control. In some cases of supraventricular arrhythmias, a 100 mg daily dose may be sufficient to provide arrhythmia control.

Sotalol. Sotalol differs from other beta-blockers in prolonging action potential duration. Its antiarrhythmic effects are weaker than those of amiodarone, but it may none the less prove useful, particularly in the management of supraventricular arrhythmias, when the risks of amiodarone are not thought to be justified. It is given orally in a dose of 80–160 mg twice daily.

Bretylium. Bretylium is an adrenergic blocking agent, which was at one time used in the management of hypertension, but was abandoned because of undesirable side-effects and tachyphylaxis in long-term use. It prolongs action potential without affecting the fast sodium current and is, therefore, categorized as a class III drug. It is relatively ineffective at suppressing ventricular ectopic activity but quite often prevents recurrences of ventricular tachycardia and ventricular fibrillation when other drugs have failed. It is given as 5 mg/kg intramuscularly every 6–8 h, or in the case of an arrhythmia causing serious haemodynamic compromise, as a rapid intravenous injection (initial dose 5 mg/kg).

Verapamil. This calcium antagonist, when used intravenously in a dosage of 5–10 mg is usually effective in abolishing supraventricular tachycardia. It is administered over 30–60 s and should be avoided in those receiving beta-blocking drugs, and given cautiously to patients with compromised ventricular function. Oral verapamil (40–120 mg three times a day) is useful in slowing the ventricular rate in atrial fibrillation.

Digoxin and adenosine

Neither digoxin nor adenosine are included in the traditional classification of antiarrhythmic drug actions. Both act to slow conduction through the AV node and are of use in supraventricular arrhythmias. Digoxin is considered further in Chapter 10 (p. 168).

Adenosine is a selective inhibitor of AV node conduction. The drug is administered intravenously (see Chapter 22, p. 401) and produces a transient AV block lasting a few seconds. It can hence be used to terminate re-entry tachycardias which include the AV node in the re-entry circuit. The drug is also of value in distinguishing broad complex tachycardias, when the diagnosis is in doubt (see p. 399).

General principles of antiarrhythmic drug selection

The above classification of antiarrhythmic drugs is of value in comparing the similarities and differences between the actions of different drugs. However, it is of limited value clinically, when selecting which drug to treat a particular arrhythmia. That is best considered from the

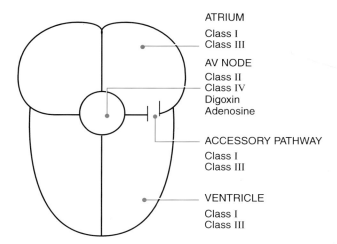

ATRIUM
Class I
Class III

AV NODE
Class II
Class IV
Digoxin
Adenosine

ACCESSORY PATHWAY
Class I
Class III

VENTRICLE
Class I
Class III

Fig. 11.32 Sites of action of antiarrhythmic drugs. Antiarrhythmic drugs can be considered to act at four sites within the heart: the atrium, AV node, accessory pathway and ventricle. For further discussion see text.

anatomical and functional viewpoint of which parts of the conduction system are involved in an arrhythmia. There are four functionally distinct regions, the atrium, the AV node, accessory pathways and the ventricle (Fig. 11.32).

Atrium

The two common examples of intra-atrial arrhythmias are atrial flutter and fibrillation. Either class I or class III drugs may be effective in restoring sinus rhythm. Alternatively, treatment may be selected to limit ventricular response, with drugs limiting AV nodal conduction.

AV node

Digoxin remains the mainstay of treatment to slow AV conduction, and is widely used in the management of atrial fibrillation. Beta-blockers are similarly of value and can be used in combination with digoxin, when digoxin slows the heart rate inadequately. Verapamil is also of value in this context, but should not be given with beta-blockers.

Several re-entrant arrhythmias arise within the AV node or involve the AV node. These commonly present as paroxysmal supraventricular tachycardia. Verapamil is frequently an effective treatment. Class I agents, particularly flecainide, may also be of value.

Accessory pathways

Accessory pathway conduction is slowed by class I agents and once again flecainide is particularly effective. Amiodarone is also of value, increasing the refractory period of the pathway. These drugs are specifically indicated in cases of atrial fibrillation complicating Wolff–Parkinson–White syndrome. They are also of value for re-entrant arrhythmias which involve conduction over an accessory pathway.

Ventricle

Class I drugs are the first line of treatment of ventricular tachyarrhythmias. Amiodarone is particularly effective, but is generally restricted in its use because of potential side-effects. However, if left ventricular function is severely impaired, amiodarone is the treatment of choice. Beta-blockers are of value in patients with exercise or ischaemic-induced arrhythmias.

Although class I drugs are the mainstay of treatment, there is little to guide selection of drugs from within the class. It is not possible to predict from the characteristics of an arrhythmia whether a Ia, Ib or Ic agent is likely to be successful. Choice of treatment is initially empirical, perhaps based on which drug is least likely to cause side-effects. However, treatment should then be validated by electro-physiological testing or 24 hour ECG monitoring, to assess drug efficacy and reduce the possibility of pro-arrhythmic effects.

Further reading

Almendral, J., Ormaetxe, J., Delcan, J. L. (1992) Idiopathic ventricular tachycardia and fibrillation: Incidence, prognosis and therapy. PACE **15**: 627.

Bernstein, A. D., Camm, A. J., Fletcher, R. D. et al. (1987) The NASPE/BPEG generic pacemaker code for antibradyarrhythmia and adaptive-rate pacing and antitachyarrhythmia devices. PACE **10**: 794.

Bloomfield, P. & Miller, H. C. (1987) Permanent pacing. British Medical Journal **295**: 741.

Camm, A. J. (1986) Asystole and electromechanical dissociation. British Medical Journal **292**: 1123.

Griffith, M. J., Garratt, C. J., Mounsey, P. et al. (1994) Ventricular tachycardia as default diagnosis in broad complex tachycardia. Lancet **343(8894)**: 386.

Jackman, W. M., Beckham, K. J., McClelland, J. H. et al. (1992) Treatment of supraventricular tachycardia due to atriventricular nodal re-entry by radiofrequency catheter ablation of the slow-pathway conduction. New England Journal of Medicine **327**: 313.

Kuck, K. H. & Schluter, M. (1993) Junctional tachycardia and the role of catheter ablation. Lancet **341**: 1386.

Mason, J. W. (1987) Amiodarone. New England Journal of Medicine **314**: 455.

Mitrani, R. D., Klein, L. S., Rardon, D. P. et al. (1994) Current trends in the implantable cardioverter defibrillator. In: Zipes, D. P., Jalife, J. (Eds). Cardiac Electrophysiology: From Cell to Bedside. Philadelphia: Saunders, p. 1393.

Opie, L. (1984) The Heart. London: Grune & Stratton.

Shenasa, M. et al. (1993) Arrhythmia Octet. Ventricular tachycardia. Lancet **341**: 1512.

Yee, R., Klein, G. J., Guiraudon, G. M. (1994) The Wolff–Parkinson–White syndrome. In: Zipes, D. P., Jalife, J. (Eds). Cardiac Electrophysiology: From Cell to Bedside. Philadelphia: Saunders, p. 1199.

Diseases of the Pericardium and Myocardium

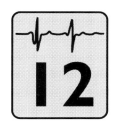

THE PERICARDIUM

The pericardium has several functions: it helps to fix the heart and prevent excessive movement, it acts as a barrier against the spread of infection and malignancy from adjacent organs, and it reduces friction between the heart and its neighbouring tissues. It also limits acute cardiac dilatation and plays a part in the distribution and equalization of hydrostatic forces on the heart, being responsible for 'diastolic coupling', such that the diastolic pressures in the two ventricles are closely correlated when the pericardium is intact, but not when it is absent.

Pericardial disease, which may be acute or chronic, is usually associated either with a generalized disorder or with pulmonary disease.

Pathology

Pericarditis may be fibrinous, purulent or constrictive. In acute fibrinous pericarditis, the serous pericardium is inflamed and covered with an adherent layer of fibrin. There may be an accompanying effusion. In purulent pericarditis, there is usually a thick fibrinous exudate containing polymorphonuclear cells and organisms. In pericardial constriction, the pericardium is a dense mass of fibrous tissue which is often heavily calcified. Sometimes a mixed picture of effusion and constriction is seen ('effusive–constrictive pericarditis').

Acute pericarditis

Aetiology

The causes of acute pericarditis are diverse (Table 12.1). Frequently no cause is identified. It seems probable that most idiopathic cases are due either to an unrecognized viral infection or to allergy or autoimmunity.

Table 12.1   Causes of pericarditis

Infective
  Viral – Coxsackie B, influenza, measles, mumps, chickenpox, human immunodeficiency virus
  Pyogenic
  Fungal
  Tuberculous

Connective tissue disorder
  Rheumatic fever (p. 245)
  Rheumatoid arthritis (p. 366)
  Systemic lupus erythematosus (p. 366)
  Polyarteritis (p. 367)
  Scleroderma (p. 367)
  Sarcoid (p. 367)

Acute myocardial infarction

Autoimmune
  Post-myocardial infarction (Dressler) syndrome
  Post-pericardiotomy syndrome

Neoplastic invasion

Metabolic and endocrine
  Uraemia
  Gout

Trauma

The viruses most frequently identified have been of the Coxsackie B group, but influenza, measles, mumps, chickenpox and human immunodeficiency virus (HIV) may also be responsible. Purulent pericarditis usually results from the spread of infection from adjacent lung. Tuberculous pericarditis is preceded by infection in contiguous mediastinal lymph nodes.

Clinical features and diagnosis

Chest pain is the commonest symptom but is not invariable. Its distribution simulates that of acute myocardial infarction, being central and sometimes radiating to the shoulder and upper arm. The pain may be most severe in the xiphisternal or epigastric regions. It is often sharp and severe, but may be aching or oppressive. Unlike ischaemic cardiac pain, it is accentuated by inspiration, by movement and by lying flat.

  The most definitive sign of pericarditis is a pericardial rub, although this is not always present. A to-and-fro scratchy or grating noise may be heard in systole, mid-diastole and presystole, or in only one of these phases. It is often localized to a small area but varies in position from time to time. It is usually accentuated if the patient leans forward, with the breath held in expiration, but is sometimes heard better towards the end of inspiration. Although the rub may disappear with the development of the pericardial effusion, it does not necessarily do so. Other signs may include those of pericardial effusion and, occasionally, of pericardial tamponade.

Investigations. In the early stages, the ECG usually shows widespread ST elevation with the ST segment concave upwards (Fig. 12.1). After a few days the ST segment returns to the iso-electric line and the T wave becomes inverted. The ECG may simulate that of myocardial infarction, but Q waves are not seen and the ST segment elevation is of a different configuration (see Fig. 2.12).

The chest radiograph is not helpful unles there is a large pericardial effusion or there is concomitant pulmonary or pleural disease. Echocardiography is of value in the detection of pericardial effusion.

Differential diagnosis. Acute pericarditis is most likely to be confused with acute myocardial infarction, spontaneous pneumothorax and pleurisy. In differentiating it from acute myocardial infarction, the following points are of importance:

- *history.* The character of the pain, the absence of pre-existing angina, and the history of an upper respiratory infection or of pyrexia preceding the onset of chest pain;

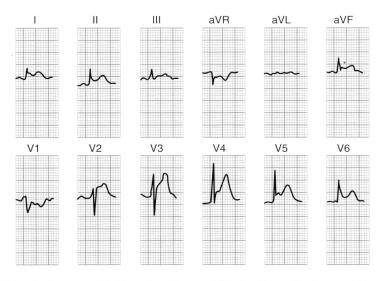

Fig. 12.1   Acute pericarditis. There is widespread ST elevation, with characteristic upward concavity of the ST segments.

- *the absence of Q waves* and of the characteristic infarction type of ST elevation on the ECG;
- *the absence of serum enzyme changes.*

In spontaneous pneumothorax, the diagnosis can usually be made without difficulty by the detection of hyper-resonance and absent breath sounds over the affected lung or by the radiological demonstration of air in the pleural space. There is sometimes a coexistent pneumo-mediastinum which can cause a crunching or crackling sound with each heart beat. Pleurisy can be distinguished by the location and character of the pain, the presence of a pleural rub and, sometimes, by the clinical and radiological evidence of pleural effusion. Pleurisy and pericarditis commonly coexist.

Aetiological diagnosis

Viral pericarditis should be suspected if there is a history of an upper respiratory infection and fever preceding the chest pain, and can be confirmed by the demonstration of changing titres of viral antibodies in the blood, or the culture of viruses from the stools.

Tuberculous pericarditis may be difficult to diagnose, because there is often no evidence of either pulmonary or miliary infection. Usually, however, there is a history of malaise and weight loss for some weeks prior to the pericarditis. Tuberculosis is unlikely if tuberculin skin tests are negative. If necessary the diagnosis may be confirmed by pericardial aspiration or biopsy.

In pericarditis due to staphylococci, streptococci or pneumococci, there is usually infection in the lungs or elsewhere in the body. In rheumatic fever, there is accompanying evidence of the rheumatic process as well as of myocarditis and endocarditis. In pericarditis due to hypersensitivity or autoimmunity, there is no preceding respiratory infection but there is often a history of similar episodes in the past.

Acute pericarditis may also occur in patients with acquired immune deficiency syndrome (AIDS). Some cases are idiopathic, while others are related to specific viral pathogens, particularly cytomegalovirus. Tuberculous pericarditis may also occur in patients with AIDS.

Treatment

This consists of the symptomatic relief of pain with anti-inflammatory analgesics such as indomethacin or ibuprofen, the removal of fluid when this is causing pericardial tamponade (see p. 229), and the treatment of the underlying cause when this is possible. No specific therapy is usually necessary for viral or allergic pericarditis, although corticosteroids may be used to abbreviate their course if this is protracted. Tuberculous pericarditis requires prolonged treatment with antituberculous drugs and corticosteroids. Pericardial resection may be necessary even during the acute phase if pericardial constriction develops. Bacterial pericarditis should be treated with the appropriate antibiotics; surgical removal of pericardial pus may be necessary.

Pericardial effusion

Pericardial effusion may result from:

- transudation (in cardiac failure);
- exudation of serous fluid or pus (in pericarditis);
- blood (from trauma or malignant disease).

It is also a feature of myxoedema. The hydropericardium of cardiac failure causes few, if any, symptoms, although it may cause compression of the lungs and reduce the vital capacity. Pericardial effusion due to other causes may produce pain and pericardial tamponade.

Large effusions may be detected by percussion. With the patient lying flat, increased dullness may be noted in the second left interspace, as well as in the fourth and fifth right interspaces, and to the left of the apex beat.

Auscultation may reveal pericardial friction and heart sounds which are often, but not always, soft.

Investigations. The chest radiograph is valuable in diagnosis, particularly if several films are taken over a period of days – a sudden increase in the cardiothoracic ratio being very suggestive of pericardial effusion. When there is a considerable effusion, the cardiac silhouette is enlarged and the normal demarcation between the chambers is obliterated (Fig. 12.2). Similar abnormalities may be seen in some cases of cardiac failure, but the presence of a very large heart shadow in the absence of pulmonary vascular congestion makes the diagnosis of pericardial effusion likely.

Pericardial effusion produces low-voltage ECG complexes which may vary considerably in amplitude from cycle to cycle ('electrical alternans'), reflecting changes in the position of the heart within the pericardial effusion.

Echocardiography is the most useful diagnostic method. When fluid separates the contracting and relaxing posterior wall of the heart from the stationary posterior pericardium, an echo-free space is produced (Fig. 12.3). Similarly, the anterior wall of the heart is separated from the chest wall.

Paracentesis may occasionally be required for diagnostic purposes, e.g. to identify a causative organism. No specific treatment is required for a pericardial effusion unless there is tamponade.

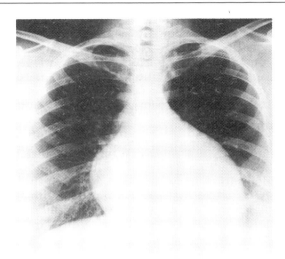

Fig. 12.2 Chest X-ray of pericardial effusion. The cardiac contour is markedly enlarged with a rounded appearance.

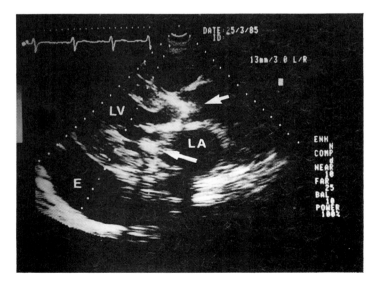

Fig. 12.3 Cross-sectional echocardiogram in the long axis parasternal view of a patient with a large pericardial effusion. An echo-free space is seen behind the posterior left ventricular wall. No effusion is seen. LV = left ventricle. E = pericardial effusion. The arrows point to a thickened aortic valve and a calcified mitral valve.

Pericardial tamponade

The pericardium does not normally impede ventricular distension during diastole. An accumulation of pericardial fluid, or pericardial fibrosis or calcification may prevent adequate filling. This may develop acutely, as when the pericardium fills with fluid, or slowly, as in chronic pericardial constriction. Probably the commonest causes are neoplasm and idiopathic or viral pericarditis, but it may develop in such conditions as uraemia, myocardial infarction, and after a traumatic cardiac catheterization, perforation by a pacing wire, cardiac surgery and chest injury.

The inability of the ventricles to fill during diastole leads to raised diastolic pressures in right and left ventricles, an increase in systemic and pulmonary venous pressures, and a fall in cardiac output.

Clinical features

Clinical features include:

- sinus tachycardia;
- elevation of jugular venous pulse. A further rise may occur during inspiration – Kussmaul's sign;
- fall in systemic blood pressure and shock in severe cases;
- variation in systemic blood pressure in relation to the respiratory cycle – pulsus paradoxus.

Investigations. Echocardiography is the most important investigation in pericardial tamponade. Echocardiographic findings include:

- right and left atrial diastolic collapse;
- right ventricular diastolic collapse;
- inspiratory increase in tricuspid flow;
- inspiratory increase in right ventricular dimensions and decrease in left ventricular dimensions.

Treatment

The management of cardiac tamponade depends on the extent of haemodynamic compromise. Severe cases may be rapidly fatal, and relief by emergency pericardial aspiration may be required (see p. 404). In less critical cases, particularly if the underlying cause of tamponade is likely to recur, formal surgical drainage is preferable, with formation of a drainage window to prevent reaccumulation of pericardial fluid. The same objective can also be achieved percutaneously, by balloon inflation to create a tear in the pericardium.

Pericardial constriction ('constrictive pericarditis')

Constriction of the heart by a fibrosed or calcified pericardium is relatively uncommon. In most patients, no identifiable cause can be found, although in some communities a tuberculous infection is responsible for the majority of cases. Constriction can also be a late complication of other types of infection, neoplastic invasion and intrapericardial haemorrhage.

Adequate filling of the ventricles during diastole is prevented by thick, fibrous and, often, calcified pericardium. Although extension of the disease process may affect the superficial areas of the myocardium, the rest of the heart is usually normal.

Clinical features and diagnosis

The inability of the ventricles to distend during diastole leads to an increase in diastolic pressure and to a consequent rise in pressure in the left and right atria and in both pulmonary and systemic veins. The stroke volume is low and there is a compensatory tachycardia.

The onset may be subacute or chronic. Symptoms resemble those of right-sided cardiac failure. The presenting complaint is often that of abdominal swelling due to ascites, but dyspnoea and ankle swelling are also common.

- *The pulse* is of small volume and may exhibit paradox. Sinus tachycardia is usually present, but atrial fibrillation develops in the advanced case.
- *The neck veins* are grossly engorged and show two characteristic features; a rapid 'y' descent (Fig. 4.4, p. 46) and an increase in pressure on inspiration.
- *The first and second heart sounds* are soft, and there is nearly always an early diastolic sound heard best at the lower end of the sternum. This is an unusually early third heart sound associated with rapid but abbreviated ventricular filling.
- *The liver* is enlarged and often tender, although it may be difficult to feel because of gross ascites. In contrast with the severity of the ascites, peripheral oedema is comparatively slight.

Investigations. One of the most characteristic features of pericardial constriction is a shell-like rim of calcified pericardium, which is particularly well seen in lateral radiographs of the heart (Fig. 12.4). However, calcification is not invariable, nor does its presence necessarily imply constriction. The heart is usually small or of normal size, but is occasionally large. Computed tomography (CT) and magnetic resonance imaging (MRI) are of value, demonstrating thickening of the pericardium in almost all cases.

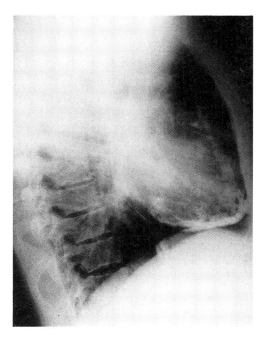

Fig. 12.4 Lateral chest X-ray showing a rim of calcification over the inferior aspect of the ventricles.

The ECG is not diagnostic, but usually shows low-voltage QRS complexes associated with flattened or slightly inverted T waves. If atrial fibrillation is not present, the P waves are often broad and bifid. Cardiac catheterization reveals:

- raised left ventricular diastolic, left atrial, pulmonary arterial, right ventricular diastolic and right atrial pressures. Characteristically, the diastolic pressures are identical in all four cardiac chambers;
- the right ventricular pressure pulse shows an early diastolic dip followed by a plateau (Fig. 12.5). This appearance is not specific to pericardial constriction and may be seen in restrictive cardiomyopathy.

Differential diagnosis. Pericardial constriction is suggested by a small and paradoxical pulse, a high venous pressure, a quiet heart with an early third heart sound and pericardial calcification, although not all these features are necessarily present. An important clue to the diagnosis is the combination of advanced right-sided failure with a normal-sized heart.

Pericardial constriction is most likely to be confused with cirrhosis of the liver, but the characteristic arterial and venous pulses in pericardial constriction should permit differentiation. In other forms of right-sided heart failure, cardiac valve lesions or pulmonary disease are usually evident.

Differentiation of pericardial constriction from restrictive cardiomyopathy may be difficult. In restrictive cardiomyopathy:

- the heart is generally enlarged;
- the left ventricular end-diastolic pressure generally exceeds the right ventricular end-diastolic pressure;
- there is no pericardial thickening.

Treatment

The medical treatment of the failure associated with pericardial constriction is seldom successful, although some improvement may follow the use of diuretics. Digoxin is of value only if atrial fibrillation supervenes.

The only effective treatment is surgical removal of the thickened pericardium. However, pericardial constriction sometimes occurs during the acute or subacute phase of tuberculous pericarditis, and preliminary treatment should then be undertaken with antituberculous drugs and corticosteroids. In some patients the pericardium may be densely calcified and adherent to the underlying heart muscle. In such cases, ultrasonic debridement can provide a useful surgical adjunct.

Progress following pericardiectomy is usually satisfactory but may not be so if there has been extensive myocardial involvement or severe liver damage. In such patients, a low output syndrome may ensue, resulting in a high operative mortality rate. Pericardiectomy should probably not be attempted routinely in such patients.

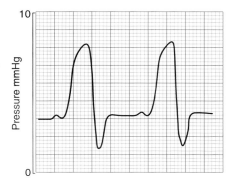

Fig. 12.5 Characteristic right ventricular pressure pulse in pericardial constriction. Note early diastolic dip, followed by a plateau.

CARDIOMYOPATHY AND MYOCARDITIS

Myocardial disease

The myocardium is involved in most types of heart disease. The terms *myocarditis* and *cardiomyopathy* are reserved for those relatively uncommon types of myocardial disease which cannot be attributed to coronary atherosclerosis, congenital or valvar heart disease or hypertension.

Myocarditis is used to describe inflammatory disorders of the myocardium due to infection and toxins. *Cardiomyopathy* is used for chronic disorders of heart muscle; the term may be restricted to those disorders whose cause is unknown, and the term 'specific heart muscle disease' for those of identified aetiology.

MYOCARDITIS

Myocarditis usually forms part of a generalized infection (particularly viral) but can also be due to physical and chemical agents (see Table 12.2). It is often associated with pericarditis. Occasionally, septicaemia may lead to focal suppurative lesions. Myocarditis is an important component of acute rheumatic fever (see Chapter 13).

Mild forms of myocarditis occur in a large number of infectious diseases but often cause only sinus tachycardia and non-specific ECG changes. They may, however, give rise to arrhythmias such as atrial

Table 12.2 Causes of myocarditis

Infective
Viruses – Coxsackie B, cytomegalovirus, infectious mononucleosis, human immunodeficiency virus
Mycoplasma
Bacteria
Spirochaetes
Rickettsiae
Fungi
Parasites and protozoa
Radiation
Drugs – Sulphonamides, doxorubicin, lithium, emetine, cyclophosphamide
Heavy metals
Hypersensitivity states
Insect stings

fibrillation or supraventricular tachycardia without producing other overt cardiac effects.

Clinical features

There are three basic ways by which an infectious agent can lead to myocardial damage:

- direct invasion of the myocardium;
- toxin production, e.g. diphtheria;
- immunologically mediated damage.

In the case of viral myocarditis, immune mechanisms are predominantly responsible for myocardial damage, rather than direct damage caused by the virus itself.

In severe cases, tachycardia may be marked, or, particularly in diphtheria, there may be a bradycardia due to heart block. The symptoms and signs of left and right cardiac failure may develop, with dyspnoea, gallop rhythm, cardiac enlargement and murmurs due to dilatation of the ventricles. Chest pain is common, but usually attributable to associated pericarditis. There is a risk of acute circulatory failure (shock) and of serious ventricular arrhythmias and sudden death. Minor ECG abnormalities are common, but such changes may occur in infections even in the absence of myocarditis. Occasionally, there is ST elevation (due to pericarditis) or depression, or inversion of T waves, or disturbances of conduction and rhythm. There may be enzyme evidence of myocardial necrosis. Echocardiography and radionuclide imaging may be useful in demonstrating ventricular dysfunction.

Viral myocarditis

The diagnosis may be supported by the isolation of a virus from tissue or fluid specimens, or by increases in the titre of virus-neutralizing, complement-fixing or haemagglutination-inhibiting antibodies. Endomyocardial biopsy is of some limited value in confirming the diagnosis. In Europe and North America most cases of myocarditis are thought to be viral in origin. In South America, Chagas' disease (caused by *Trypanosoma cruzi*) is the commonest cause of myocarditis.

There is a spectrum of clinical expression of myocarditis, ranging from mild local inflammation which may only be inferred from ST-segment changes in the ECG, to fulminant congestive cardiac failure. The outcome after viral myocarditis is similarly variable. In most cases, the myocarditis is self-limiting and recovery is complete. However, in a small minority of patients, myocarditis may culminate in dilated cardiomyopathy as a consequence of virally mediated immunological damage.

There is no specific treatment. Therapy is primarily supportive, treating the complications of heart failure and arrhythmias if they occur. Bed rest is advisable, followed by a period of restricted activity for approximately 6 months.

The role of corticosteroids remains controversial. Corticosteroids are frequently administered to patients with progressive disease who have evidence of an inflammatory cell infiltrate on endomyocardial biopsy, although the benefits of such treatment are not proven. Nonsteroidal anti-inflammatory agents are contraindicated during the acute phase because they increase myocardial damage.

A large number of viruses may cause viral myocarditis. Coxsackie B is a particularly common cause, but other possibilities include cytomegalovirus, infectious mononucleosis, influenza and HIV. Myocarditis characteristically develops several weeks after the original viral infection, suggesting that damage is immunologically mediated.

Human immunodeficiency virus (HIV). Clinically apparent cardiac involvement occurs in about 10% of patients with AIDS. Manifestations include myocarditis, pericarditis, endocarditis, dilated cardiomyopathy and metastatic involvement from Kaposi's sarcoma. Most cases of myocarditis are thought to be related to the HIV itself, although myocarditis secondary to opportunistic pathogens may also occur.

Clinical features of viral myocarditis. Congestive heart failure is the commonest clinical manifestation. Conventional drug treatment with diuretics and angiotensin-converting enzyme (ACE) inhibitors provides effective short-term treatment of the failure, but is unlikely to alter the course of the underlying myocarditis.

Cardiomyopathy related to specific heart muscle diseases

Aetiologically, cardiomyopathies fall into two groups: those in which the heart disease is the major or only abnormal feature, and those in which the myocardial disease is a complication of a generalized disorder. Systemic diseases associated with cardiomyopathy are listed in Table 12.3.

Table 12.3 Systemic disorders causing cardiomyopathy

Connective tissue disorders (systemic lupus erythematosus, scleroderma and polyarteritis)
Amyloidosis
Sarcoidosis
Neuromuscular diseases (Friedreich's ataxia, progressive muscular dystrophy and myotonic
   dystrophy)
Haemochromatosis
Glycogen storage diseases

There are three distinctive clinical patterns of cardiomyopathy:

- dilated;
- hypertrophic;
- restrictive.

DILATED CARDIOMYOPATHY

Dilated (congestive) cardiomyopathy is the commonest type of heart muscle disease. In many patients no aetiological agent can be identified, but it is likely that a substantial proportion follow a viral myocarditis. Alcohol abuse is an important factor in many cases. Other causes of dilated cardiomyopathy are listed in Table 12.4. In occasional cases dilated cardiomyopathy can be familial.

Dilated cardiomyopathy is not a single specific disease entity, but a final common pathway which is the end result of myocardial damage produced by a variety of different mechanisms.

The major physiological defect is the decreased contractile force of the left ventricle, with slow and inadequate systolic emptying. The ventricle dilates and the pressure rises in the left atrium. Subsequently, pulmonary hypertension and right ventricular failure occur.

Clinical features

Patients usually present with dyspnoea and oedema whose onset may be abrupt or insidious. Tachycardia is common as are ventricular ectopic beats and atrial fibrillation. The venous pressure is raised and there may be systolic venous pulsation from tricuspid regurgitation. Cardiac enlargement affects both left and right ventricles. Third and

Table 12.4 Some causes of dilated cardiomyopathy

Infection
   Viral myocarditis
   Human immunodeficiency virus

Toxins and drugs
   Ethanol
   Anthracyclines (e.g. doxorubicin, daunorubicin)
   5-Fluorouracil

Nutritional and related deficiencies
   Thiamine deficiency
   Hypocalcaemia
   Hypophospataemia

Pregnancy

---

fourth heart sounds are common. There may be the pansystolic murmurs of mitral or tricuspid regurgitation.

Investigation. The ECG frequently demonstrates arrhythmias, as well as abnormalities of the ST segment and T waves. The absence of Q waves (suggesting previous myocardial infarction) is an important negative finding. The chest radiograph confirms cardiac enlargement affecting all chambers. Echocardiography and radionuclide imaging reveal dilated, poorly contracting ventricles. Contractile impairment is global, in contrast to the regional impairment which occurs following myocardial infarction. Cardiac catheterization and angiocardiography are of little value in diagnosis as they merely demonstrate evidence of ventricular failure and, occasionally, tricuspid and mitral regurgitation.

Differential diagnosis. The diagnosis requires the exclusion of coronary artery disease, thyrotoxicosis, hypertension, rheumatic heart disease and congenital heart disease as aetiological factors; it is supported by evidence of one of the generalized disorders associated with cardiomyopathy. Endomyocardial biopsy is occasionally of value in confirming an underlying aetiology, but most often simply shows an end-stage fibrotic process, without providing clues as to the pathogenesis.

Treatment

As the cause of idiopathic dilated cardiomyopathy is unknown, there is no specific treatment for the underlying disease process and treatment is instead directed at the consequences of the disease, most particularly the management of failure. Treatment depends on the stage of disease. Alcohol should be forbidden. Bed rest may be necessary in severe cases.

Drug management is substantially similar to that of other causes of heart failure. Drug therapies that may be considered include:

- *diuretics* control the symptoms of both right and left heart failure;
- *ACE inhibitors* are of value to control symptoms and to improve prognosis;
- *beta-blockers* are surprisingly well tolerated. They improve symptoms and may also improve prognosis. They should be excluded only in patients with the most severe degrees of failure;
- *dihydropyridine calcium antagonists* such as amlodipine may have a particular role in the management of dilated cardiomyopathy. Improvement of prognosis has been shown in one study;
- *antiarrhythmic drugs.* There is no generalized indication for antiarrhythmic drug therapy. In patients requiring treatment because of symptomatic arrhythmias, amiodarone is the agent of choice because of lower negative inotropic effects and a lower

potential for pro-arrhythmia than other antiarrhythmic agents. Digoxin is indicated in patients with atrial fibrillation;

- *anticoagulants* should be considered in all patients with dilated cardiomyopathy and are particularly indicated in the presence of atrial fibrillation.

Cardiac transplantation is indicated if disability is severe and life expectancy short (p. 173). Patients with life-threatening ventricular arrhythmias should be considered for an implantable cardioverter defibrillator (p. 214).

Prognosis

The prognosis of patients with dilated cardiomyopathy is extremely variable. Many patients have minimal or no symptoms and have a reasonable long-term prognosis. In those with more severe or progressive symptoms, deterioration can be rapid. Amongst newly diagnosed patients referred to major centres the 1-year mortality rate is 25% and the 5-year mortality rate 50%. Greater ventricular enlargement and more severe impairment of function correlate with poor prognosis.

Alcoholic cardiomyopathy

Excessive alcohol consumption is one of the commonest causes of dilated cardiomyopathy in the Western world. Myocardial damage may arise by three basic mechanisms:

- direct toxic effects of alcohol;
- nutritional deficiencies, particularly thiamine deficiency;
- toxic effects of additives (e.g. cobalt) in alcoholic beverages.

Identification of the aetiological role of alcohol is of particular importance because, in contrast to other causes of dilated cardiomyopathy, ceasing alcohol consumption can halt the progression of the disease and may lead to an improvement in ventricular function. In patients with associated thiamine deficiency, thiamine administration may improve ventricular function.

HYPERTROPHIC CARDIOMYOPATHY

In this condition there is massive hypertrophy of the ventricles. The rigid non-compliant chambers impede diastolic filling. The ventricular septum is often the site of the most conspicuous hypertrophy, which may obstruct the left ventricular outflow tract (obstructive cardiomyopathy). The obstruction increases as systole progresses, and the more vigorously the ventricle contracts the more severe is the obstruction.

Pathogenesis

The characteristic macroscopic feature of hypertrophic cardiomyopathy is disproportionate hypertrophy of the interventricular septum and anterolateral wall of the left ventricle compared with the posterolateral free wall. Other patterns of hypertrophy seen more rarely are symmetrical hypertrophy with uniform thickening of the septum and free wall, and hypertrophy confined to the apex.

Histological features demonstrated on microscopy include disorganization of the myofibrillar architecture. This finding is present in almost all patients with hypertrophic cardiomyopathy. Considerable progress has been made in understanding the genetic disorders underlying this myofibrillator disarray. The disorder is not due to a single gene. At least five different genes on four different chromosomes are involved. The first gene identified was localized to the long arm of chromosome 14, and subsequently recognized as coding for the beta cardiac myosin heavy chain (*CMH1* gene).

In about 50% of cases autosomal dominant Mendelian inheritance is present and a family history of heart disease or sudden death can be recognized in relatives. Consequently family screening is an important part of the assessment of any patient with hypertrophic cardiomyopathy. In the case of the *CMH1* gene, this can be detected in DNA extracted from blood lymphocytes, enabling mutations of this gene to be detected in childhood, even before the disease becomes clinically evident. However, the fact that a number of different gene mutations can result in the phenotypic expression of hypertrophic cardiomyopathy means that there is no single genetic marker that enables the diagnosis to be excluded.

Pathophysiological consequences

Hypertrophic *obstructive* cardiomyopathy is characterized by a pressure gradient in the outflow from the left ventricle. Two factors contribute to this gradient, a muscular sphincter action in the outflow and the abutment of the anterior leaflet of the mitral valve against the hypertrophied septum in systole. Outflow gradients in hypertrophic cardiomyopathy are characteristically dynamic, increasing under conditions of adrenergic stimulation.

Only a minority (about a quarter) of patients with hypertrophic cardiomyopathy demonstrate an outflow gradient. By contrast, abnormalities of diastolic function are very common, leading to impaired relaxation and increased filling pressures.

Clinical features

The clinical features in patients with hypertrophic cardiomyopathy vary widely. Many are asymptomatic or minimally symptomatic, and may only be identified during screening of a relative with the disease. In more severely affected individuals, symptoms are often similar to those that occur in aortic stenosis, including dyspnoea, angina and syncope. Arrhythmias are common and there is a high risk of sudden death.

Physical signs include:

- steep pulse upstroke due to the rapid ejection of blood by the hypertrophied ventricle during early systole;
- the venous pulse may show a large 'a' wave, and there may be evidence of both left and right ventricular hypertrophy;
- left ventricular outflow obstruction causes the systolic murmur and thrill of subaortic stenosis, maximal at the lower left sternal edge or apex;
- there may be a double impulse on apical palpation, reflecting forceful atrial systole, or even a triple impulse, with the third component due to late systolic bulging of the left ventricle;
- the pansystolic murmur of mitral regurgitation is frequent; less often there may be the signs of tricuspid regurgitation or of pulmonary stenosis;
- a fourth heart sound.

The 'a' wave, fourth heart sound and presystolic apical impulse are due to forceful atrial contraction against the non-compliant hypertrophied ventricle.

Investigations. The ECG shows left ventricular hypertrophy and, sometimes, conduction defects.

The echocardiogram is of great value. Characteristic features are:

- asymmetrical hypertrophy of the septum (ASH);
- systolic anterior movement of the mitral valve (SAM) (Fig. 12.6);
- mid-systolic closure of the aortic valve;
- cross-sectional echocardiography demonstrates the asymmetrical hypertrophy and the obliteration of the ventricular cavity during systole.

The chest radiograph may show left ventricular hypertrophy.

On cardiac catheterization, a systolic pressure difference can frequently be demonstrated between the body and the outflow tract of the left ventricle if there is obstruction. This difference is increased by drugs such as isoprenaline, which increase myocardial contractility, and may be abolished by drugs such as propranolol, which decrease myocardial contractility. Angiocardiography demonstrates a small left ventricular cavity with narrowing of the outflow tract and, often, mitral regurgitation.

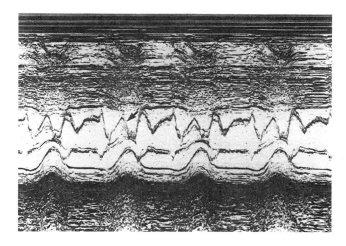

Fig. 12.6   M-mode echocardiogram in hypertrophic cardiomyopathy. The arrow indicates a systolic anterior movement of the mitral valve (SAM). The interventricular septum is grossly thickened.

Differential diagnosis. Obstructive cardiomyopathy has usually to be differentiated from other types of aortic stenosis. In valvar aortic stenosis, the pulse is usually small and flat and there is either an early systolic click or calcification of the aortic valve. In congenital subaortic stenosis, the pulse is small and flat and there is frequently aortic regurgitation, which is not a feature of obstructive cardiomyopathy. The systolic murmur of hypertrophic cardiomyopathy characteristically increases during a Valsalva manoeuvre, in contradistinction to the murmur of aortic stenosis which decreases in intensity.

It is also important to distinguish hypertrophic cardiomyopathy from the 'physiological' hypertrophy of trained athletes. Factors favouring hypertrophic cardiomyopathy over athlete's heart include:

- unusual and unequal distribution of hypertrophy (e.g. septal hypertrophy);
- decreased left ventricular cavity size;
- left atrial enlargement;
- abnormal ECG;
- family history of hypertrophic cardiomyopathy;
- the maintenance of hypertrophy on detraining.

Natural history and prognosis

The clinical course of hypertrophic cardiomyopathy is extremely variable. Clinical deterioration is usually slow. About 10% of patients develop left ventricular dilatation and progress to a dilated cardiomyopathy.

The greatest threat is sudden death. Identification of patients at particular risk of sudden death is extremely difficult; risk factors include:

- young age;
- family history of sudden death;
- history of recurrent syncope;
- sustained ventricular or supraventricular arrhythmias;
- non-sustained ventricular tachycardia on Holter monitoring.

Management

Beta-blockers and calcium antagonists are both helpful in relieving symptoms of chest pain and shortness of breath (especially the combination of beta-blocker and nifedipine). In patients with frequent ventricular arrhythmias, on 24-h ECG recording, amiodarone is indicated, as there is some evidence that amiodarone treatment can prevent sudden death. Amiodarone is also indicated for the maintenance of sinus rhythm in patients developing atrial fibrillation.

In patients with frefractory symptoms, surgical resection of part of the intraventricular septum is occasionally indicated. Alternatively some patients benefit from dual-chamber pacing. This can be thought of as changing the ventricular activation sequence, such that the body of the ventricle is activated earlier than the septal region responsible for outflow obstruction. A short AV delay is required to minimize activation over the His–Purkinje system, while maintaining normal AV synchrony.

Patients should be advised to refrain from vigorous competitive sports to minimize the risk of sudden death.

RESTRICTIVE AND INFILTRATIVE CARDIOMYOPATHIES

Restrictive cardiomyopathy is the least common of the three major functional categories of cardiomyopathy (dilated, hypertrophic and restrictive). In restrictive cardiomyopathy the ventricles are abnormally stiff and impede ventricular filling, with the result that there is abnormal diastolic function. Systolic function, by contrast, may remain normal.

Restrictive cardiomyopathy may arise due to a variety of pathological processes (Table 12.5). These may involve infiltration of the myocardium or endomyocardial scarring.

The haemodynamic presentation and clinical features closely resemble constrictive pericarditis (p. 230). Differentiation from cases of constrictive pericarditis may be extremely difficult. There is frequently cardiac enlargement in patients with restrictive cardiomyopathy,

Table 12.5   Causes of restrictive cardiomyopathy

Infiltrative
  Amyloid
  Sarcoid

Storage diseases
  Haemochromatosis
  Glycogen storage diseases

Endomyocardial
  Endomyocardial fibrosis
  Hypereosinophilic syndrome
  Carcinoid

whereas it is unusual for the heart to be enlarged in constrictive pericarditis. Conversely, CT or MRI scan generally shows pericardial thickening in constrictive pericarditis and a normal pericardium in restrictive cardiomyopathy.

Clinical features

Shortness of breath is the commonest presenting symptom. Other patients may present with signs of right heart failure. Features on clinical examination include:

- tachycardia. Because of compromised ventricular filling, heart rate increases to maintain cardiac output;
- elevated jugular venous pulse, with a further increase on inspiration (Kussmaul's sign);
- enlarged liver, ascites and peripheral oedema;
- S3, S4 or both.

Conduction disturbances and arrhythmias may occur if the disease process involves the conduction system. Sudden death is common.

Management

There is no specific therapy. Treatment is seldom effective and disease is commonly progressive. Use of low doses of diuretics and vasodilators may provide symptomatic benefit. Caution is necessary as decreased ventricular filling pressures may reduce cardiac output and cause excessive hypotension. In patients with eosinophilia, steroids and cytotoxic drugs may be helpful.

ARRHYTHMOGENIC RIGHT VENTRICULAR DYSPLASIA

This is a rare form of cardiomyopathy involving predominantly the right ventricle. The aetiology is unknown, although some cases are familial. The disease differs from other forms of cardiomyopathy in that arrhythmias are the commonest presenting feature. Patients commonly present with features of palpitations, dizziness or syncope, although features of heart failure may also occur. In some cases there may also be left ventricular involvement.

The diagnosis should be considered in patients with ventricular tachycardia with a left bundle branch block morphology, suggesting a right ventricular origin. Echocardiography generally shows right ventricular dilatation. The diagnosis can be confirmed using myocardial biopsy to demonstrate characteristic fatty infiltration of the myocardium. MRI also plays an increasing role in diagnosis, revealing abnormal infiltration, wall thinning and abnormal contraction patterns.

Management in general involves the control of any arrhythmias. Beta-blockers, particularly sotalol, are useful, although class I antiarrhythmics or other class III antiarrhythmics may be necessary. In occasional patients with localized disease, this may be amenable to radiofrequency ablation. The disease may result in sudden death, and in patients with refractory arrhythmias causing haemodynamic compromise an implantable defibrillator should be considered.

Further reading

Abelmann, W. H. & Lovell, B. H. (1989) The challenge of cardiomyopathy. *Journal of the American College of Cardiology* **13**: 1219.

Dec, G. W., Fuster, V. (1994) Medical progress: Idiopathic dilated cardiomyopathy. *New England Journal of Medicine* **331**: 1564.

Fontaine, G., Fontaliran, F., Lascault, G. *et al.* (1994) Arrhythmogenic right ventricular dysplasia. In Zipes, D. P., Jalife, J. (Eds). *Cardiac Electrophysiology: From Cell to Bedside*. Philadelphia: Saunders.

Goodwin, J. F. (Ed.) (1985) *Heart Muscle Disease*. Lancaster: MTP Press.

Louie, E. F., Edwards, L. C. (1994) Hypertrophic cardiomyopathy. *Progress in Cardiovascular Diseases* **36**: 275.

Olsen, E., Goodwin, J. (1993) *Cardiomyopathies*. Berlin: Springer-Verlag.

Shabetai, R. (1978) The pericardium: an essay on some recent developments. *American Journal of Cardiology* **42**: 1036.

Spyrou, N., Foale, R. (1994) Restrictive cardiomyopathies. *Current Opinion in Cardiology* **9**: 344.

Rheumatic Fever and its Sequelae

Acute rheumatic fever is a disease which follows infection by group A haemolytic streptococci and produces manifestations in many tissues and organs. Arthritis is often the most conspicuous feature, but cardiac involvement is of much greater importance. The duration of rheumatic activity is very variable; it may cease in 2 weeks or persist for many months. Recurrences are common. Death is rare in the acute phase but chronic rheumatic heart disease is responsible for a considerable morbidity and mortality.

Aetiology

Rheumatic fever seems to occur only after a group A streptococcal infection. It is a complication of less than 1% of episodes of streptococcal pharyngitis, developing some 10–20 days after the onset of the sore throat. No history of sore throat, however, can be obtained in some 30–50% of cases; none the less virtually all patients with acute rheumatic fever have a streptococcal antibody response.

It is probable that rheumatic fever is a result of a hyperimmune reaction either to bacterial allergy or to autoimmunity.

Over the last 50 years, rheumatic fever has been becoming progressively less frequent and is now rare in many countries, including the UK, the United States and Scandinavia. However, in the rapidly expanding cities of Asia, Africa and South America, rheumatic heart disease is the commonest cause of cardiac death. The decline of rheumatic fever in Western countries is not solely the result of the use of antibiotics for it preceded their discovery. It may be attributed both to a change in the virulence of streptococci and to improving social conditions. Rheumatic fever most commonly occurs between the ages of 5 and 15 years, with the peak about the age of 8 years. It is rare under the age of 4 and becomes progressively less common after the age of 15, although occasional cases are seen even after the age of 30.

Microscopic evidence of acute rheumatic fever is widespread, but particularly affects tissues lined by endothelium such as blood vessels,

245

the endocardium, the pericardium and synovial membranes. The earliest lesion is one of swelling in and around collagen fibres, accompanied by oedema and lymphocytic infiltration. Later, and more specifically, granulomatous Aschoff nodules appear. These are formed by collections of round cells, fibroblasts and multinucleated giant cells, and are usually surrounded by an area of polymorphonuclear cells, lymphocytes and plasma cells.

The lesions of rheumatic fever are most obvious in relation to the heart valves and the pericardium. The valve cusps become thickened by oedema and by the infiltration of capillaries. Grey or yellow warty vegetations ('verrucae') form along the lines of closure. These are common on the mitral and aortic valve cusps, and seldom affect the tricuspid or pulmonary valves.

Chronic rheumatic heart disease is a sequel to acute rheumatic carditis, and many of its features are the result of fibrosis occurring during the healing of the acute lesion. Its pathology will be discussed in more detail later in this chapter.

Clinical features

In most cases, some 2–3 weeks after the onset of acute pharyngitis, the child begins to feel unwell, loses his or her appetite and complains of pains in the limbs. Fever is present, but it is not usually high. The major clinical features are carditis, polyarthritis, subcutaneous nodules, erythema marginatum and chorea.

Carditis.   The heart is involved in about half of the first attacks of rheumatic fever.

Endocarditis, with valvar involvement, is suggested by the appearance of cardiac murmurs. An apical pansystolic murmur indicates either mitral valve damage or functional mitral regurgitation associated with myocarditis. Rheumatic involvement of the mitral valve is also strongly suggested by the appearance of a low-pitched and short mid-diastolic apical murmur (Carey Coombs). This murmur is usually transient, but may persist for months or years until the characteristic features of mitral stenosis develop. Mid-systolic murmurs in the aortic or pulmonary area are less certain evidence of cardiac involvement, as they are common in febrile children without heart disease and usually disappear as recovery takes place. The diastolic murmur of aortic regurgitation is not uncommon, and usually persists after the acute rheumatic process has subsided.

Myocarditis is a common feature of acute rheumatic fever, but is difficult to diagnose with confidence. It is suggested by a tachycardia and by cardiac enlargement. More diagnostic is the appearance of left-sided or right-sided heart failure when this cannot be attributed to valve damage. The symptoms include dyspnoea, orthopnoea and oedema. A gallop rhythm is frequent.

When clinical evidence of *pericarditis* is present, the carditis is usually severe and involves the myocardium and endocardium as well (pancarditis). Retrosternal pain and pericardial friction occur and there may be a pericardial effusion.

When rheumatic activity has subsided, there are often residual signs of valve damage.

Polyarthritis. Characteristically, the joints become swollen, painful and hot, but in the younger child there may be only vague aches. The arthritis usually affects one joint after another, giving the impression of 'flitting'. The knees, ankles, shoulders, wrists and elbows are most commonly involved. The inflammation in each joint usually develops within a few hours and may take up to a week to subside. Even in the absence of treatment, the polyarthritis usually disappears within 3 weeks and leaves no residual abnormality.

Subcutaneous nodules. These seldom give rise to symptoms but are of diagnostic importance. They are firm painless structures which are attached to tendon sheaths, joint capsules and fascia, and the skin is movable over them. They occur mainly over the extensor surfaces of the wrists, elbows, knuckles, knees and Achilles tendons and also over the scalp. They usually last about a week.

Erythema marginatum. This consists of lesions which develop rapidly from small macules or papules into large circles with pink, slightly raised, sharply circumscribed edges and pale centres. As these circles intersect, a pattern of segments develops. These appear and disappear within a period of hours. Erythema marginatum affects the trunk and limbs, but never involves the face.

Chorea (St Vitus' dance). This is a neurological manifestation of the acute rheumatic process. It often occurs without the other features, but cardiac involvement is common. The onset is usually insidious with the development of an apparent clumsiness in an otherwise healthy child. Jerky and non-repetitive movements occur and muscle tone is reduced.

Laboratory investigations

In most cases there is a moderate leucocytosis of 12 000–15 000 white blood cells/mm^3, an increased erythrocyte sedimentation rate (ESR) and a raised level of C-reactive protein.

In only about one-quarter of patients can a group A streptococcus be grown from the throat. The presence of a raised or rising anti-streptolysin 'O' (ASO) titre provides good evidence of recent infection, particularly if it rises and falls. Other antibody tests, such as those for anti-DNase B and anti-streptozyme (ASTZ), are also of value.

A number of electrocardiographic abnormalities occur in acute rheumatic fever. Amongst these are a prolonged PR interval and, more rarely, more advanced degrees of atrioventricular block. Non-specific T wave changes are common and the ST and T wave changes characteristic of pericarditis may be seen.

The diagnosis of rheumatic fever

There is no certain way of establishing the presence of rheumatic fever, but the combination of certain clinical features and laboratory findings is highly suggestive. It may be diagnosed with some confidence if evidence of a recent streptococcal infection is present together with two or more of the following:

● carditis;
● polyarthritis;
● chorea;
● erythema marginatum;
● subcutaneous nodules.

The diagnosis is also probable if evidence of streptococcal infection is combined with one of the clinical features mentioned together with two or more of the following:

● arthralgia;
● fever;
● raised ESR or C-reactive protein level;
● prolonged PR interval.

(Revised Jones Criteria, American Heart Association, 1992.)

The absence of microbiological or serological evidence of group A streptococcal infection makes the diagnosis of acute rheumatic fever extremely unlikely.

Patients with a previous history of rheumatic fever are at increased risk of recurrent episodes. This should lead to an increased index of suspicion in considering possible recurrences.

Differential diagnosis

The diagnosis of rheumatic fever is often difficult because the complete picture is seldom present. Furthermore, although the criteria described are valuable, they depend upon accurate observation and the correct timing and performance of laboratory tests. A history of sore throat may be misleading, as this is often due to organisms other than streptococci. Likewise, polyarthritis may be wrongly diagnosed when only the vague limb pains so common in childhood have occurred. Cardiac signs can also be deceptive, as functional systolic murmurs often come and go in the child with pyrexia from any cause. Another problem is posed by the patient with chronic rheumatic heart disease who develops a sore throat. Nevertheless, if the above-mentioned criteria are adhered to, the correct diagnosis will usually be made.

Diseases which are particularly important to differentiate from rheumatic fever are bacterial arthritis, rheumatoid arthritis and sub-acute infective endocarditis. In most cases of acute septic arthritis, the disease process is confined to a single joint and the inflammation is liable to extend into adjacent soft tissue. The diagnosis can be confirmed by bacteriological examination of fluid from the joint. Staphylo-coccal and meningococcal septicaemias can be diagnosed from blood cultures. Rheumatoid arthritis tends to involve smaller joints than rheumatic fever, but observation over a long period may be necessary in order to be certain of the diagnosis. Subacute infective endocarditis may be difficult to differentiate from rheumatic fever if blood cultures are negative, but a polyarthritis is rare, and some of the characteristic features such as microscopic haematuria and anaemia, which are seldom found in rheumatic fever, are usually present.

Course and prognosis

The course of rheumatic fever is variable and unpredictable. In some apparently severely ill patients, complete recovery takes place within a few days, whereas in others the disease drags on for months.

The first attack is seldom fatal, but recurrences may lead to increasing cardiac damage and heart failure. More than two-thirds of patients who have experienced rheumatic fever eventually develop chronic rheumatic valve disease.

There can be no doubt that many cases of rheumatic fever escape diagnosis because about half of the patients with proven chronic rheumatic disease give no history of an acute episode.

Treatment

During the acute phase of the disease the subject wants and needs bed rest. When the temperature, pulse rate and ESR have returned to normal and the evidence of acute arthritis and carditis has disappeared, the patient may be gradually mobilized and rehabilitated. Active carditis requires complete rest, and this may have to be continued for several weeks. Subsequent increases in activity must depend upon the individual response, and a full resumption of normal physical activity usually has to be delayed to 6 months from the time when the last signs of active carditis have resolved.

Both salicylates and corticosteroids have a dramatic effect on the fever and polyarthritis of rheumatic fever. Although controversy continues as to the relative merits of the two forms of drug therapy, it is now common practice to use salicylates for rheumatic fever without carditis, and to add or substitute corticosteroids if there is undoubted evidence of cardiac involvement. However, it does not seem that any drug prevents the development of chronic valve damage. It is important not to give large doses of salicylate which can lead to salicylate intoxication; it is particularly undesirable to administer large doses of sodium salicylate as the sodium may precipitate cardiac failure. For children, 50 mg of acetylsalicylic acid per kilogram body weight may be given daily, and the dose subsequently adjusted to control symptoms. For adults, 4–8 g a day may be appropriate, in divided doses, given every 4 h. Salicylates should be continued until signs of rheumatic activity have ceased. There is great variation in the dosage of corticosteroids necessary to control activity. An initial dose of 40 mg of prednisone daily may be given and subsequently reduced to 20 mg daily, continued for 6 weeks and gradually withdrawn. Some patients have a rebound of rheumatic activity subsequently, and it is best to try to control this with salicylates.

The manifestations of cardiac failure are often suppressed by corticosteroids but diuretics and digitalis should be administered if necessary.

Prevention of rheumatic fever

Rheumatic fever may be prevented by the prophylaxis and treatment of acute streptococcal infections.

Acute streptococcal infections are probably most effectively treated by a single injection of 0.6–1.2 mega-units of benzathine penicillin, but this is painful. Alternatively, oral phenoxymethylpenicillin may be given for 10 days.

All patients who have experienced acute rheumatic fever should receive long-term prophylactic therapy. For this purpose, benzathine penicillin may be injected monthly in a dosage of 0.6–1.2 mega-units, or oral therapy given as 125 mg phenoxymethylpenicillin twice daily or sulphadiazine 0.5 g twice daily. It is not known how long prophylaxis should be continued, but it is common practice to recommend this up to the age of 25 years.

The healing of rheumatic carditis and the development of chronic rheumatic heart disease

Chronic rheumatic heart disease is the result of damage produced by recurrent attacks of acute rheumatic carditis and the subsequent healing process. These changes are largely confined to the valve structures, although in some instances myocardial damage may also be severe. Because valve damage predominates in patients with chronic rheumatic heart disease, this condition will be considered in detail under the individual valve lesions. Nevertheless it is important to recognize that myocardial damage coexists and that correction of a valve abnormality will not necessarily restore normal cardiac function.

The pathological processes that cause valve deformity include thickening and distortion of the cusps at the time of rheumatic fever, contracture of the valve structures, fusion of the commissures, shortening of the chordae tendineae and, finally, calcification during the phase of healing. The nature of the valve lesion depends upon the relative importance of these factors in the individual case. Stenosis occurs if fusion of the cusps predominates; regurgitation is produced by shortening of the chordae tendineae and contracture of the valve leaflets.

The valve deformities may take many years to develop and, in particular, narrowing is not critical until the affected orifice is reduced to less than a quarter of its normal size. Regurgitation may be important from the time of the attack of acute rheumatic fever but its appearance as a symptomatic disorder, also, is likely to be delayed. Therefore, although the signs of mitral and aortic regurgitation may be present in childhood or early adult life, symptoms due to these lesions seldom develop until the third or fourth decade. The same is true for mitral stenosis; in aortic stenosis symptoms are often postponed even longer.

Further reading

American Medical Association (1992) Guidelines for the diagnosis of rheumatic fever. Jones Criteria 1992 update. *Journal of the American Medical Association* **268**: 2069.
Mitha, A. S. (1994) Acute rheumatic fever. In Julian, D. G., Camm, A. J., Fox, K. M., Hall, R. J. C., & Poole-Wilson, P. A. (Eds) *Disease of the Heart*, 2nd edn. London: Saunders.

Disorders of the Cardiac Valves

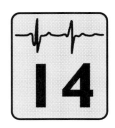

Disorders of the cardiac valves may be secondary to a number of inflammatory, degenerative or infective processes. As a result of disease, a valve may become stenotic (when it fails to open normally) or regurgitant (when it fails to close normally). The causes and consequences of stenosis and regurgitation of each of the four heart valves are discussed below. This is followed by a description of infective endocarditis which may involve any of the heart valves.

MITRAL VALVE DISEASE

The normal mitral valve (Fig. 14.1) consists of the valve ring, two unequal cusps (leaflets), chórdae tendineae and papillary muscles. The larger antero-medial (or aortic) cusp is interposed between the mitral and aortic orifices, and forms part of the outflow tract of the left ventricle (Fig. 14.2). The circumference of the valve is approximately

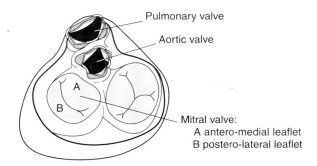

Fig. 14.1 Appearances of the heart valves during systole, with the atria and great vessels removed. The heart is viewed from behind, with the left ventricle and mitral valve on the left.

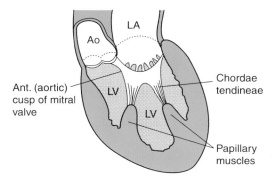

Fig. 14.2 Diagrammatic representation of relationships of left atrium (LA), left ventricle (LV) and aorta (Ao). Note the aortic cusp of the mitral valve separates the mitral valve orifice from the outflow tract of the left ventricle.

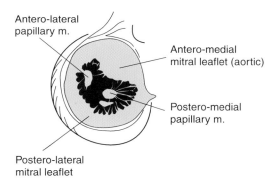

Fig. 14.3 Open mitral valve viewed from the left atrium. Note that the papillary muscles arise opposite the commissures and are attached to the cusps on either side of the commissures by the chordae tendineae.

10 cm and the length of the commissure (where the two leaflets are in contact with each other) is approximately 4 cm. The papillary muscles arise from the ventricular wall opposite the commissures and are attached to the cusps on either side of the commissures by the chordae tendineae (Fig. 14.3). The chordae are collagenous strands, which, when tensed by the contracting papillary muscles, prevent the cusps from prolapsing into the left atrium during ventricular systole.

Chronic mitral valve disease may take the form of mitral stenosis with or without some degree of regurgitation, in which case it is virtually always the consequence of rheumatic endocarditis. Pure mitral regurgitation in Western countries is seldom rheumatic in origin; mitral valve prolapse is the common abnormality. Regurgitation may also be due to ruptured or defective chordae tendineae, papillary muscles or valve cusps, or to dilatation of the valve ring following left ventricular enlargement from a variety of causes.

Mitral stenosis

Pathology

Mitral stenosis is usually the result of recurrent rheumatic inflammation followed by healing. The leaflets adhere at their commissures, leaving a central orifice. In some instances the valve cusps remain pliant and mobile; in others fibrosis and calcification make them rigid. In about 10% of cases severe shortening of the chordae tendineae produces a funnel-shaped orifice.

Pathophysiology

Serious haemodynamic consequences develop only when the mitral valve orifice is reduced from the normal size of approximately 5 cm^2 to about 1 cm^2. In severe mitral stenosis, the orifice is a slit less than 1 cm long and 0.5 cm across.

In the normal heart there is little pressure difference across the mitral valve between its opening in early ventricular diastole and its closure. In mitral stenosis, a pressure difference develops which depends upon the area of the mitral valve orifice and the volume of blood flowing through it (Fig. 14.4).

When the stenosis is relatively mild, the mean pressure in the left atrium may be normal at rest (i.e. less than 12 mmHg) but increases on exercise as the cardiac output rises. In more severe stenosis, the pressure is raised even at rest, and in the most severe grades is persistently elevated to 25 mmHg or more. The left ventricular pressure is normal, provided there is no disease affecting this chamber.

When the stenosis is slight, the cardiac output may be normal, but as the narrowing increases, the cardiac output diminishes to about half the normal value, and may not rise in response to exercise.

The pressure in the pulmonary veins and capillaries parallels that in the left atrium. If the pulmonary capillary pressure rises rapidly to 30 mmHg, pulmonary oedema develops as the hydrostatic pressure exceeds plasma osmotic pressure. If the process takes place slowly, fluid exudes into the alveolar wall and a physical barrier eventually develops between capillaries and alveoli consisting of a thickened capillary basement membrane, increased collagen and oedema. These changes increase the tissue tension of the alveolar wall and limit the exudation of fluid. As a consequence, patients with mitral stenosis can sometimes tolerate high pulmonary capillary pressures without developing severe pulmonary oedema. Because of the increased fluid in the interstitial tissues, the lymphatics become engorged.

As the pulmonary capillary pressure increases, there is a concomitant rise in pulmonary arterial pressure. However, in many cases of tight mitral stenosis, pulmonary arterial hypertension is much more severe than can be accounted for by this passive rise. The dispropor-

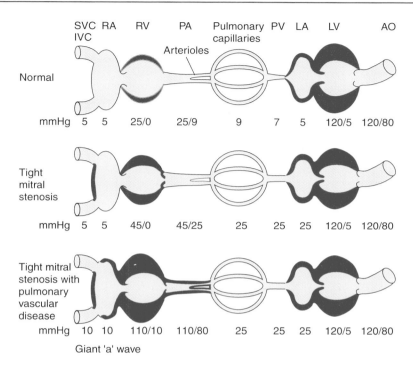

	SVC IVC	RA	RV	PA	Pulmonary capillaries	PV	LA	LV	AO
Normal				Arterioles					
mmHg	5	5	25/0	25/9	9	7	5	120/5	120/80
Tight mitral stenosis									
mmHg	5	5	45/0	45/25	25	25	25	120/5	120/80
Tight mitral stenosis with pulmonary vascular disease									
mmHg	10	10	110/10	110/80	25	25	25	120/5	120/80

Giant 'a' wave

Fig. 14.4 The haemodynamic effects of mitral stenosis. In the normal heart, the pressure in the left atrium is similar to that of the left ventricle during ventricular diastole. With the development of mitral stenosis, the pressure in the left atrium rises, and this rise is transmitted to the pulmonary veins, capillaries and arteries. When pulmonary vascular disease develops, there is a narrowing of the pulmonary arterioles which leads to a disproportionate rise in the pulmonary arterial and right ventricular systolic pressures. With right ventricular failure, both the right ventricular end-diastolic pressure and the mean atrial pressure may rise to 10 mmHg.

tionate elevation of pulmonary arterial pressure is largely due to an increase in tone in the small pulmonary arteries. Severe pulmonary arterial hypertension is disadvantageous in that it leads to right ventricular hypertrophy and failure. However, the increased resistance of the pulmonary arterial vessels prevents an abrupt rise in right ventricular output on exercise and therefore protects the lungs from a sudden increase in pulmonary capillary pressure.

The pulmonary vascular congestion typical of mitral stenosis leads to increased rigidity (decreased compliance) in the lungs. As a consequence, patients with severe mitral stenosis may have to double or treble the work of breathing.

Complications

- Atrial fibrillation develops sooner or later in most cases of mitral stenosis. At first this may be paroxysmal, but it is usual for it to become permanent. At its onset the ventricular rate is often more than 140/min and the patient may be rapidly precipitated into acute pulmonary oedema. It is an important complication, both because it contributes to the development of cardiac failure and because it is responsible for atrial stasis and the consequent risk of thrombosis and embolism.
- Pulmonary embolism and infarction frequently occur, especially when the disease is far advanced, as thrombosis is encouraged by atrial fibrillation, cardiac failure and bed rest.
- Systemic embolism is common and often follows the onset of atrial fibrillation. The embolism is cerebral in a high proportion of cases but may involve the mesenteric, renal or other arteries.
- The congested respiratory tract makes the patient liable to attacks of acute bronchitis and to the development of chronic bronchitis.
- Infective endocarditis is rare in pure mitral stenosis but is commoner as a complication of mixed mitral stenosis and regurgitation.

Symptoms

The patient with mitral stenosis, who is often symptom-free for many years, eventually develops features of left-sided cardiac failure and, later, those of right-sided failure. Various factors, such as pregnancy and the onset of atrial fibrillation, may suddenly precipitate the patient from one of these stages into the next.

The major symptom of mitral stenosis is shortness of breath. This occurs at first only on strenuous exercise, but as time passes less and less exertion is required to evoke it. Eventually, orthopnoea develops and the patient is liable to attacks of paroxysmal dyspnoea and acute pulmonary oedema. Acute pulmonary oedema is less likely when severe pulmonary arterial hypertension has developed.

Haemoptysis occurs in some 10–20% of patients with mitral stenosis but is seldom severe. In some cases, the sputum is frothy and pink due to acute pulmonary oedema, but frankly bloody sputum may be expectorated by a patient who is almost free of breathlessness. This is probably due to the rupture of dilated pulmonary or bronchial veins. Another important cause of haemoptysis is pulmonary infarction.

Patients may also complain of palpitation, cough and angina pectoris. Severe breathlessness and orthopnoea have usually been present for years before right-sided heart failure develops. The earliest symptom of this is oedema of the legs, but abdominal discomfort due to engorgement of the liver or to ascites also occurs.

Physical signs

Patients with long-standing mitral stenosis often have a characteristic facies – a dusky malar discoloration. This may be attributed to peripheral cyanosis associated with a low cardiac output and vasoconstriction.

The arterial pulse is usually normal in volume but may be small, and is often irregular due to atrial fibrillation. In the earlier stages, the venous pressure is normal, but rises with the onset of right-sided heart failure. When there is severe pulmonary hypertension, there may be a large venous 'a' wave due to forceful right atrial contraction against the hypertrophied non-compliant right ventricle.

The apex beat is usually in the normal place but may be deviated to the left by right ventricular hypertrophy. It often has a tapping quality, which is associated with the characteristic loud first heart sound. In more advanced cases, right ventricular hypertrophy produces a heaving impulse to the left of the lower sternum. Mid-diastolic and presystolic thrills may be present at, or internal to, the apex beat.

There are four cardinal auscultatory features of mitral stenosis (Fig. 14.5):

- a loud first sound;
- an opening snap;
- a mid-diastolic murmur;
- a presystolic murmur.

The first sound is accentuated and the opening snap loud when the cusps are mobile; these signs may disappear with the development of rigidity and calcification of the valves. A mid-diastolic murmur is usually present, and its length, but not its intensity, gives an indication of

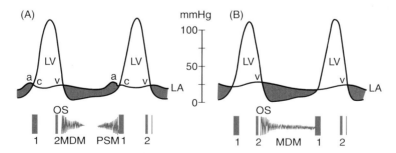

Fig. 14.5 (A) The pressure pulses in left ventricle and left atrium and the phonocardiographic appearances in mitral stenosis. A pressure difference is present throughout diastole (shaded area), and is accentuated by atrial contraction ('a' wave). Mid-diastolic and presystolic murmurs result. (B) Atrial fibrillation has developed with loss of the 'a' wave and of the presystolic accentuation of the murmur.

the severity of the lesion. The presystolic murmur is often an early sign but may not be heard unless the patient is exercised and then turned into the left lateral position. A mitral systolic murmur signifies concomitant mitral regurgitation.

The second sound splits normally, but the pulmonary component is often accentuated because of pulmonary hypertension. An apical third heart sound is impossible in significant mitral stenosis because the rapid filling of the left ventricle necessary for its production cannot occur.

The ECG

If sinus rhythm is present, there is usually P mitrale (Fig. 14.6). Atrial fibrillation is common; other atrial and ventricular arrhythmias occur occasionally. Evidence of right ventricular hypertrophy develops in cases with severe pulmonary hypertension.

Radiological appearances

The most characteristic radiological feature of mitral stenosis is the selective enlargement of the left atrium, which, in the posteroanterior view, produces a bulge below the pulmonary artery on the left border of the heart, and a rounded dense shadow within or outside the middle part of the right border of the heart (see Fig. 5.4). Left atrial enlargement can be confirmed by observing the displacement of the barium-filled oesophagus in the lateral view. Other radiological features may include calcification of the mitral valve, a normal or small left ventricle, and a normal or small aorta. The upper pulmonary veins are usually prominent. When the pulmonary capillary pressure is high, horizontal septal lines (Kerley's B lines) appear in the costophrenic angles, and the radiological features of pulmonary oedema may be seen. Haemosiderosis may produce mottling of the lungs. Pulmonary artery, right ventricular and, occasionally, right atrial enlargement may also be present when there is pulmonary arterial hypertension (Fig. 14.7).

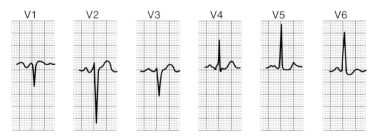

Fig. 14.6 P mitrale. There is a biphasic P wave in lead V1, with deep inversion of the terminal segment. In the left-sided leads the P wave is bifid, most clearly seen in leads V4 and V5 in this example.

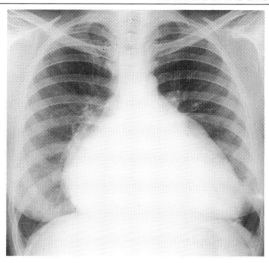

Fig. 14.7 Mixed mitral valve disease. Gross cardiac enlargement in a severe case of mixed mitral valve disease.

Echocardiography

Echocardiography is the investigation most commonly used to confirm the diagnosis of mitral stenosis and to assess its severity. Two-dimensional echocardiography will demonstrate thickened mitral valve leaflets with restricted opening (Fig. 14.8). The left atrium is usually enlarged and there may be a 'swirling' appearance in the left atrium which has been termed 'spontaneous contrast'. This appearance is caused by a red cell aggregation in the slow moving blood. If present, this appearance indicates severe mitral stenosis, although it is not specific for mitral valve disease and can occur in other conditions of low cardiac output. In some patients with severe mitral stenosis, left atrial thrombosis may be visible on two-dimensional echocardiography (Fig. 14.9). Analysis of the mitral leaflet motion with the M-mode cursor shows three characteristic abnormalities in mitral stenosis:

- a reduction in the diastolic closure rate of the anterior mitral valve leaflet (Fig. 14.10);
- increased echogenicity of both leaflets;
- the anterior and posterior leaflets appear to move in the same direction (anteriorly) during diastole.

Doppler examination allows assessment of the functional severity of the stenosis. In a normal heart, the opening of the mitral valve at the onset of diastole is followed by a period of rapid ventricular filling as blood flows through the open mitral valve into a compliant left ventricle. This results in rapid equalization of the pressures in the left atrium

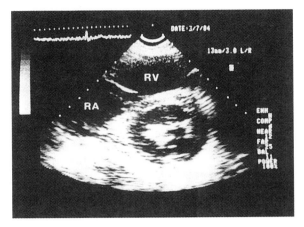

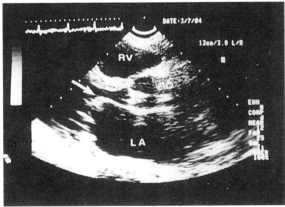

Fig. 14.8   Cross-sectional echocardiogram in mitral stenosis. The upper panel shows a short axis parasternal view. The mitral valve orifice is small and there is considerable thickening particularly on the left hand side of the orifice. The lower panel shows the long axis parasternal view with the hammocking appearance of the anterior cusp as it comes to the end of its opening movement (arrowed).

and left ventricle. In mitral stenosis, antegrade flow through the stenotic mitral valve is impeded; in mild mitral stenosis, the left atrial and left ventricular pressures will take longer to equilibrate, whereas in severe mitral stenosis the pressures will not equilibrate during diastole and a gradient will still be present at the end of diastole. Using pulsed-wave Doppler examination, blood velocity through the mitral valve can be measured and the rate of decay of blood velocity (and thus driving pressure) throughout diastole can be estimated (Fig. 14.11). A measurement in common usage is the mitral valve pressure half-time,

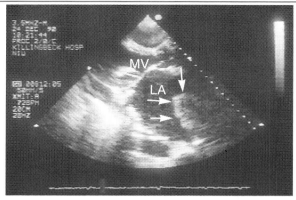

Fig. 14.9 Left atrial thrombus (arrowed) in a patient with severe mitral stenosis. Note the thickened mitral valve (MV) and dilated left atrium (LA).

which is the time taken for the pressure gradient between the left atrium and left ventricle at the onset of diastole to decay to half of its initial value. In a normal mitral valve, the pressure half-time is no greater than 60 ms. The longer the pressure half-time, the more severe the mitral stenosis (see Table 14.1). A mitral pressure half-time of 220 ms is equivalent to a mitral valve area of 1 cm^2.

Cardiac catheterization

This investigation is seldom required for diagnostic purposes, but may be helpful in assessing the severity of the stenosis. This is most accurately done by simultaneously measuring the pressure on either side of the mitral valve and estimating the cardiac output. Angiocardiography is mainly of value in assessing the severity of any associated mitral or aortic regurgitation.

Combined valve disease

Mitral stenosis is frequently complicated by disease of the other cardiac valves. The combination of rheumatic aortic regurgitation with

Table 14.1 Mitral valve pressure half-time and stenosis

Pressure half-time (ms)	Stenosis
< 60	Normal
60–100	Mild
100–200	Moderate
> 200	Severe

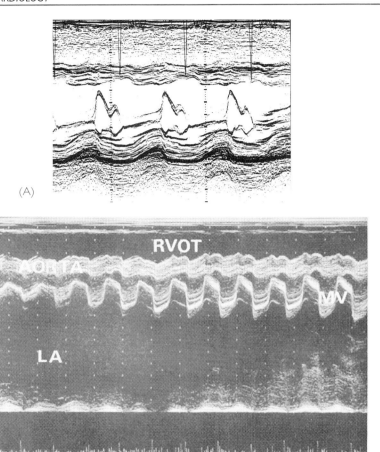

Fig. 14.10 M-mode echocardiogram of (A) a normal and (B) a stenotic mitral valve. In the normal valve, note the characteristic 'm' shape of movement of the anterior leaflet. The first upstroke is caused by passive filling of the left ventricle; this is followed by partial closure of the mitral valve as the pressures equilibrate. The second upstroke is caused by atrial contraction. In the stenotic valve, the diastolic closure rate is reduced (i.e. the slope becomes flatter) because the left ventricular and left atrial pressures do not equilibrate. The stenotic leaflets also show increased echogenicity.

mitral stenosis is a common one; in most cases the aortic regurgitation is the less important defect. The severity of the aortic regurgitation can be judged with reasonable assurance by the pulse volume, and by the diastolic pressure, which in severe cases is usually less than 60 mmHg.

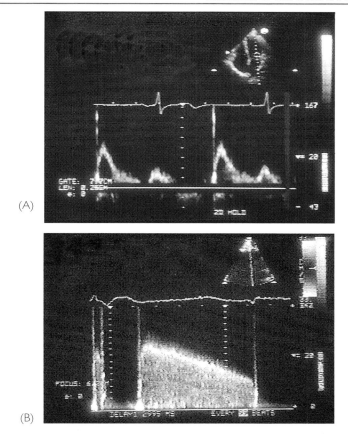

Fig. 14.11 Doppler examination of flow in diastole through (A) a normal and (B) a stenotic mitral valve. The 'flatter' the slope of decline in velocity, the more severe is the stenosis (see text for details).

The combination of severe mitral stenosis and aortic stenosis is unusual but important, because one may mask the presence of the other.

Severe tricuspid stenosis complicates about 3% of cases of mitral stenosis and often obscures its signs.

Tricuspid regurgitation is common in advanced mitral stenosis because the tricuspid valve ring dilates with right ventricular enlargement. The associated pansystolic murmur may be heard not only at the left sternal edge but as far out as the apex. This may lead to the erroneous diagnosis of mitral regurgitation. Systolic venous pulsation in the neck, the increase in the murmur on inspiration, and the lack of transmission of the murmur to the axilla serve to identify its tricuspid origin.

Diagnosis

The presence of mitral stenosis can often be suspected from a history of rheumatic fever combined with progressive dyspnoea, a small and irregular pulse, and a mitral facies. In the milder case, these features may be absent, and palpation and auscultation first reveal the diagnosis. A high proportion of patients have a tapping apex beat, right ventricular heave, loud first sound, opening snap, and mid-diastolic and presystolic murmurs. The experienced auscultator is usually first struck by the loud first sound and the opening snap rather than by the diastolic murmurs, which may be audible only if they are specifically sought with the patient lying in the left lateral position. The diagnosis is supported by P mitrale in the ECG, by the demonstration of left atrial enlargement in the radiograph and by the characteristic echocardiographic and catheterization features.

Probably the commonest cause for the mistaken diagnosis of mitral stenosis if the misinterpretation of normal splitting of the first sound for a presystolic murmur (a presystolic murmur is seldom the only auscultatory abnormality in mitral stenosis). A third heart sound may be wrongly interpreted as being an opening snap or a mid-diastolic murmur, and differentiation may be impossible without a phonocardiogram. One should hesitate to diagnose mitral stenosis on the basis of either a presystolic murmur or a short 'mid-diastolic murmur' alone without collateral evidence.

When an apical pansystolic murmur complicates the physical signs in mitral stenosis, it may be difficult to establish whether there is a significant degree of mitral regurgitation. This is unlikely if there is a loud first sound and an opening snap, or if there is evidence of advanced pulmonary hypertension. Important mitral regurgitation is probable if the systolic murmur is loud and radiates to the axilla, or if there is left ventricular hypertrophy, a soft first heart sound or a third sound rather than an opening snap. Doppler ultrasonography and angiography are valuable in the diagnosis and assessment of regurgitation.

Mitral stenosis may be simulated by the mid-diastolic murmurs encountered in conditions leading to high flow through the mitral valve, such as ventricular septal defect and persistent ductus arteriosus, and by the Austin Flint murmur associated with severe aortic regurgitation as well as by the mid-diastolic murmur of left atrial myxoma. The possibility that a mid-diastolic murmur is not due to mitral stenosis should be considered particularly if there is neither a loud first sound nor an opening snap. In left atrial myxoma, the signs may entirely mimic those of mitral stenosis, but tend to vary from time to time. Echocardiography is partciularly valuable in differentiating the mid-diastolic murmur of mitral stenosis from that due to other causes.

Course and prognosis

The characteristic physical signs of mitral stenosis, which can be present within a year of acute rheumatic fever, may precede the development of symptoms by 10–20 years. Breathlessness, usually the first complaint, is most likely to start between the ages of 20 and 30 years, but may be delayed much longer. In those in whom complications do not develop, the course is slowly but steadily downhill over a number of years. However, in Western countries, patients with signs of rheumatic mitral valve disease are now mainly seen in middle or old age, whereas in parts of Asia and Africa it is predominantly found in adolescents and young adults.

Sooner or later, some complication usually arises which leads to temporary or permanent deterioration. In young women, pregnancy is often responsible for the onset or aggravation of breathlessness; in the patient with severe stenosis, parturition may lead to pulmonary oedema and death. Once right-sided heart failure has developed, the prognosis without direct intervention on the valve is poor.

Medical treatment

Surgery or balloon valvuloplasty are eventually required in most cases, but it is usually necessary to prepare the patient for these procedures by appropriate medical therapy. Even after relief of the stenosis, treatment is often needed for the control of arrhythmias and the prevention of emboli.

Patients with mitral stenosis should be encouraged to live reasonably normal lives, but to avoid excessive exertion. They should be advised against being overweight, and discouraged from smoking. Infections must be treated promptly with appropriate antibiotics. Anticoagulants should be used in all patients with atrial fibrillation unless there are exceptional circumstances. Even patients in sinus rhythm who have mitral stenosis are at risk of embolic events including stroke, and anticoagulation should be considered in these patients. Careful supervision is required during pregnancy.

Digitalis is required for atrial fibrillation, but is of no value in pure stenosis in sinus rhythm. Cardiac failure is otherwise treated by the usual means (see Chapter 10). An attempt to restore sinus rhythm should be made after mitral valve surgery in patients with atrial fibrillation, particularly if this is known to be of recent onset.

Surgical treatment and balloon valvuloplasty

Pure mitral stenosis can be treated by balloon valvuloplasty or by surgery. In the past, patients with pliant valves could be treated by a closed valvotomy (i.e. without direct vision of the valve and without cardiopulmonary bypass), but this procedure is largely being replaced

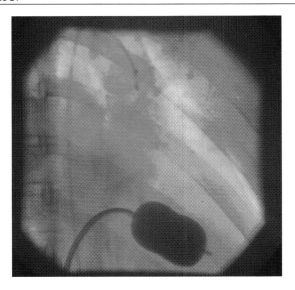

Fig. 14.12 Left ventricular angiogram after successful balloon dilatation of the mitral valve showing no mitral regurgitation. The valvuloplasty balloon is introduced from the femoral vein and is then advanced across the inter-atrial septum into the left atrium.

by balloon valvuloplasty in which a balloon is passed through the artrial septum into the left atrium using the trans-septal technique, and the balloon dilated within the valve (Fig. 14.12). Transoesophageal echocardiography is useful in assessing whether or not balloon valvuloplasty is likely to be successful.

If the valve leaflets are pliant and mobile, valvuloplasty is usually effective in relieving symptoms for a period of several years, but restenosis of the valve frequently takes place after 5–10 years. Successful valvuloplasty is effective in reducing symptoms, but signs of residual stenosis usually persist. The loud first heart sound and opening snap remain, but the diastolic murmurs are shortened or abolished. If the valve leaflets are rigid or calcified, or there is significant pre-existing mitral regurgitation, then valvuloplasty is unlikely to be successful and the patient should be considered for mitral valve replacement under cardiopulmonary bypass.

The mortality of mitral valve surgery depends on the severity of the disease and the presence of complications. If the patient is in reasonably good health before the operation, and free of severe pulmonary hypertension and mitral regurgitation, the mortality rate should be less than 5% and, in the most favourable cases, less than 1%. Where there is advanced pulmonary hypertension or right-sided failure, the mortality rate may rise to 10% or more.

Operation should be avoided in the presence of rheumatic activity. Surgery should also be deferred until cardiac failure has been brought under control or when there has been recent pulmonary or systemic embolism. 'Prophylactic' intervention (either by valvuloplasty or by surgery) should be considered in young women with moderate or severe symptoms to avoid operation during pregnancy.

Mitral regurgitation

A number of different conditions may lead to mitral regurgitation by different mechanisms:

- *rheumatic endocarditis* is the major cause in areas where rheumatic fever is prevalent, and is often accompanied by mitral stenosis. The valve cusps are usually rigid and deformed and the chordae tendineae fused and shortened. Calcification is common. Regurgitation may develop at the time of rheumatic fever, especially if this is severe, but does not usually produce major haemodynamic effects for several years because the progression of valve damage is slow;
- *mitral valve prolapse.* Prolapse of the mitral valve is a common condition which may be associated with rheumatic and ischaemic heart disease and with the Marfan syndrome. Usually, however, there is no other disease process; in such cases, there is a myxomatous change of the valve leaflets, which are voluminous and redundant. This most commonly involves the posterior mitral valve leaflet but may include the anterior or both leaflets. It is important to distinguish between billowing and prolapsing leaflets. Leaflets may billow into the left atrium but the line of co-aption between the two leaflets may still be in the normal position and there may be no mitral regurgitation. Prolapse implies displacement towards the left atrium of the commissural surfaces of a leaflet and is usually accompanied by regurgitation. The usual auscultatory finding is a mid-systolic click and/or a late apical systolic murmur, but the click and murmur may occur at other times during systole. In any individual, the auscultatory features may vary considerably from time to time, and can be made to do so by standing, sitting and straining in the Valsalva manoeuvre. Most patients are asymptomatic, but some complain of left-sided chest pain or palpitation. The ECG may show minor ST abnormalities. Echocardiography, which has demonstrated this abnormality in some 5% of normal young people, characteristically reveals a mid-systolic 'buckling' of one or both leaflets into the left atrium. Most of these patients have trivial mitral regurgitation which will not progress. Some, however, will develop haemodynamically significant mitral regurgitation and will require mitral

valve surgery. All patients with mitral valve prolapse should receive antibiotic prophylaxis against infective endocarditis.

- *infective endocarditis* may produce destruction or perforation of the cusps, or rupture of chordae tendineae;
- *congenital mitral regurgitation* occurs with or without other congenital abnormalities;
- *papillary muscle malfunction* or rupture may result from myocardial infarction;
- *mitral valvotomy* may produce tearing of cusps;
- *left ventricular dilatation* from any cause, such as hypertension, coronary artery disease and aortic valve disease, may lead to dilatation of the valve ring. The mitral regurgitation so produced leads to further enlargement of the left ventricle, and therefore further dilatation of the valve ring, with the development of a vicious circle;
- *spontaneous rupture of chordae tendineae* of unknown aetiology may occur.

Pathophysiology

The severity of mitral regurgitation depends on a number of factors:

- the size of the mitral valve orifice during ventricular systole. Although this can be of fixed size, as it is when the valve is calcified, it may be variable, depending on the degree of left ventricular dilatation;
- the pressure relationships between the left ventricle, aorta and left atrium;
- the left ventricular output.

Any factor which augments left ventricular output or raises aortic impedance increases mitral regurgitation. The degree of mitral regurgitation is limited by the distensibility of the left atrium and pulmonary veins. However, the pressure in the left atrium is much lower than that in the aorta; with a large valve orifice, therefore, as much blood may regurgitate into the left atrium during systole as is ejected into the aorta. A feature of chronic severe mitral regurgitation is that the left atrium is much larger than is usual in mitral stenosis.

During systole, the pressure in the left atrium may rise to a high 'v' peak, but will not do so if the regurgitated blood is readily accommodated in a voluminous left atrium. When mitral regurgitation develops abruptly, as with the rupture of papillary muscles or chordae tendineae, the left atrium is often small and the 'v' wave tall (see Fig. 6.1).

In diastole, there is a large flow from left atrium to left ventricle, consisting of the blood received from the pulmonary circulation combined with that which regurgitated during the preceding systole. At this time the pressure in the left atrium falls rapidly to the ventricular level.

Therefore, although there may be a high 'v' wave, the mean left atrial pressure is often not greatly raised, and the pulmonary capillary pressure is seldom as high as that encountered in mitral stenosis. Eventually, however, with the development of left ventricular failure, the pulmonary capillary pressure rises and, with it, the pulmonary arterial pressure. Severe pulmonary hypertension and right-sided cardiac failure are unusual unless there is also an appreciable degree of mitral stenosis.

Complications

The complications are similar to those of mitral stenosis. Atrial fibrillation is frequent when mitral regurgitation is of rheumatic origin but less so when other disease processes are responsible. Infective endocarditis is not uncommon when the regurgitation is rheumatic or due to prolapse.

Symptoms

In cases of rheumatic origin, the physical signs precede symptoms by many years. When symptoms do occur, they usually increase slowly. Fatigue, perhaps attributable to the low cardiac output, may be the first complaint, but eventually dyspnoea on exertion, orthopnoea and, rarely, paroxysmal nocturnal dyspnoea develop.

When mitral regurgitation is due to perforation of a cusp, or to rupture of chordae tendineae or papillary muscles, the onset of symptoms is abrupt; the patient may present with acute pulmonary oedema.

Physical signs

The pulse is usually of normal volume; irregularity due to atrial fibrillation is common. The venous pressure is normal except when there is right-sided cardiac failure. The apex beat, which may be displaced downwards and outwards, often has the vigorous thrusting character of left ventricular hypertrophy and dilatation, and there is sometimes a systolic thrill.

The first sound is usually soft and introduces an apical pansystolic murmur which radiates to the axilla. The murmur may be of the same intensity throughout systole, but often increases towards the end of this period. When the regurgitation is due to papillary muscle malfunction or ballooning of a mitral cusp, the murmur may be exclusively in late systole. Rarely, it may radiate to the left sternal edge rather than to the axilla and may be mistaken for aortic stenosis. The intensity of the murmur bears some relation to the severity of the regurgitation, but is not a reliable guide. In most severe cases there is a third heart sound, followed by a short mid-diastolic murmur due to rapid filling of the left ventricle.

The ECG

The ECG may be normal but P mitrale is often present if atrial fibrillation has not supervened. Left ventricular hypertrophy occurs in severe mitral regurgitation, but if there is significant stenosis there may be evidence of biventricular hypertrophy or no abnormality.

Radiography

Radiologically, the most conspicuous feature is the marked enlargement of the left atrium, but there may also be left ventricular enlargement. Calcification of the mitral valve is often visible in rheumatic cases. Evidence of pulmonary dilatation and pulmonary oedema develops when there is left ventricular failure.

When mitral regurgitation is of acute onset due to malfunction or rupture of valve cusps, papillary muscles or chordae tendineae, there may be little left atrial or left ventricular enlargement in spite of high left atrial pressure and pulmonary oedema.

Echocardiography

Two-dimensional echocardiography allows examination of the mitral valve leaflets and may reveal thickening in rheumatic disease or prolapse of the anterior (Fig. 14.13) or posterior (Fig. 14.14) leaflets, or of both leaflets together. Echocardiography may also demonstrate the flail leaflet caused by ruptured chordae or papillary muscles. If the degree of regurgitation is haemodynamically significant, the left atrium will be dilated. Doppler examination and colour flow mapping are very sensitive techniques for detecting mitral regurgitation. Indeed, colour flow mapping will often demonstrate a small jet of mitral regurgitation in normal valves. Assessing the severity of mitral regurgitation by echo is more difficult but it is usually possible to differentiate mild, moderate and severe mitral regurgitation, particularly if the transoesophageal approach is used. Transoesophageal echocardiography is also useful in analysing the mechanism of mitral regurgitation. This may demonstrate such diverse causes of regurgitation as prolapse of a leaflet, tethering of a leaflet, perforation of a leaflet (usually a consequence of endocarditis) or structurally normal leaflets which fail to meet at the commissure because of dilatation of the mitral valve ring. This information is particularly useful to the surgeon if mitral valve repair is being considered.

Cardiac catheterization and angiography

These procedures are seldom used for diagnosis, but quantitation can be obtained by injecting radio-opaque contrast medium into the left ventricle. Left ventriculography is of particular value in assessing the

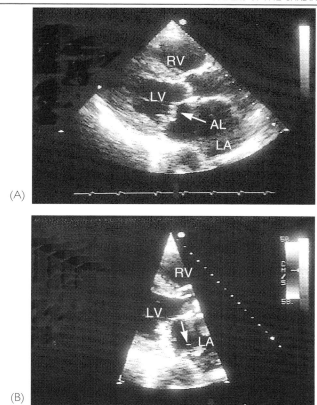

Fig. 14.13   (A) Mitral valve demonstrating prolapse of the anterior leaflet (AL). (B) The regurgitant jet is directed behind the posterior leaflet towards the free wall of the left atrium (LA).

severity of mitral regurgitation complicating mitral stenosis. The presence of left ventricular failure may be confirmed by finding a high left ventricular end-diastolic pressure. A tall 'v' wave in the left atrial or pulmonary arterial wedge pressure tracing is suggestive of, but not diagnostic of, mitral regurgitation. In patients being considered for mitral valve surgery, it is normal practice to carry out coronary angiography in areas where the prevalence of coronary artery disease is high, because unsuspected coronary artery disease might lead to serious complications at the time of cardiac surgery.

Diagnosis

The diagnosis is usually based on the finding of an apical pansystolic murmur radiating to the axilla. The pansystolic murmur of tricuspid

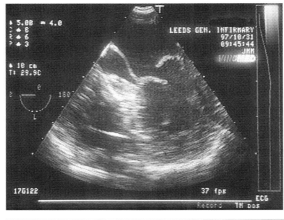

(A)

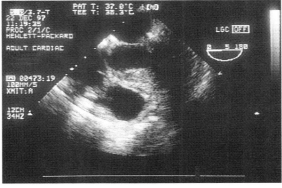

(B)

Fig. 14.14 (A) Prolapse of the posterior leaflet of the mitral valve. This results in severe mitral regurgitation. (B) Following mitral valve repair and insertion of a mitral valve ring, there is no longer any prolapse of the posterior leaflet and the mitral regurgitation has been abolished.

regurgitation may reach the apex, but does not radiate further and is usually increased on inspiration. The systolic murmur of aortic stenosis may be heard best at the apex, but is mid-systolic and does not radiate to the axilla. The murmur of ventricular septal defect is heard best at the lower left sternal edge.

It may be difficult to differentiate mitral regurgitation from a benign systolic murmur, but benign murmurs are never pansystolic, are seldom of grade 3 or greater intensity and tend to vary with posture and respiration.

Suggestive evidence of mitral regurgitation is provided by left atrial and left ventricular enlargement on the chest radiograph, and by P mitrale and left ventricular hypertrophy on the ECG. The definitive diagnosis is usually made by echocardiography or by ventriculography.

In mitral regurgitation of non-rheumatic origin, the diagnosis may be suggested by the sudden appearance of a loud apical systolic murmur accompanied by left ventricular failure.

Course and prognosis

The course of patients with mitral regurgitation is very variable. Those with mild regurgitation and without cardiomegaly may live a normal life span, although exposed to the risk of infective endocarditis. In rheumatic mitral regurgitation of moderate severity, the course is one of slow deterioration over 10–20 years with gradually increasing heart size until left ventricular failure develops. Unless this has been precipitated by a complication that can be corrected, the prognosis is then poor and death is likely to occur within a few years. When mitral regurgitation has been due to ruptured chordae tendineae, papillary muscles or cusps, the prognosis is generally poor, although the regurgitation is occasionally slight and well tolerated.

Medical treatment

Patients with mitral regurgitation should be advised to have antibiotic prophylaxis to cover surgical and major dental procedures. If the degree of regurgitation is mild, then no other medication is required. If the patient is symptomatic, or if there is left ventricular dilatation, then patients should be treated with a loop diuretic and an angiotensin-converting enzyme (ACE) inhibitor. The patient should be anticoagulated when atrial fibrillation supervenes.

Surgical treatment

The most commonly performed operation for patients with severe mitral regurgitation is mitral valve replacement (see Chapter 21). However, surgeons are increasingly attempting to preserve and repair the mitral valve if at all possible. This requires precise knowledge of the mechanism of regurgitation, which is usually gained from transoesophageal echocardiography. Surgical repair techniques may include insertion of a ring to prevent annular dilatation, partial resection of a prolapsing leaflet, transposition of chordae from one leaflet to another, or the insertion of prosthetic chordae.

Timing of surgical treatment. In the past, mitral valve surgery was carried out only when patients had severe symptoms. As the risks of surgical treatment have fallen, so there has been a tendency to operate earlier in the disease process. Serial echocardiography is a useful investigation to detect progressive left ventricular dilatation, which may be an indication for surgery even when symptoms are mild or absent.

AORTIC VALVE DISEASE

The normal aortic valve consists of three semi-lunar cusps attached to a fibrous valve ring. Immediately above the insertion of the valve cusps are the sinuses of Valsalva, from two of which the coronary arteries arise. In about 1% of individuals the aortic valve has only two cusps.

The aortic valve and adjacent structures may be involved in congenital, rheumatic, bacterial, syphilitic and atherosclerotic changes. Both stenosis and regurgitation may occur as isolated lesions but are often combined. Calcification of the cusps is an important factor in the development of aortic valve disease and is often responsible for the stenosis that occurs in those with congenitally bicuspid valves.

Aortic stenosis

Aortic stenosis is most commonly the result of disease of the aortic valve cusps, but may also be due to narrowing in the outflow tract of the left ventricle below the cusps (subvalvar) and, very rarely, a constriction in the first part of the aorta (supravalvar stenosis).

Aetiology and pathology

Aortic valve stenosis may be congenital, rheumatic or sclerotic. Most instances of aortic stenosis occur in middle-aged or elderly patients, in whom there is no evidence of involvement of other valves. Calcification of the valve is usually severe and largely responsible for the stenosis. Even at necropsy it is seldom possible to determine the aetiology, but many have congenitally bicuspid valves. Rheumatic aortic stenosis results from adherence of adjacent cusps with thickening, fibrosis and subsequent calcification.

Subvalvar aortic stenosis may result from a congenital membrane or from fibrous tissue situated in the outflow tract of the left ventricle. This may be combined with valve stenosis, and thus form a tunnel in the outflow tract. A distinctive form of subvalvar stenosis is caused by hypertrophy of the muscle of the outflow tract of the left ventricle, particularly affecting the interventricular septum. This disorder has received a large variety of names including 'idiopathic hypertrophic subvalvular aortic stenosis' and 'hypertrophic obstructive cardiomyopathy' (see also p. 238).

Supravalvar aortic stenosis is congenital and may be associated with a distinctive facial appearance and mental disability.

Aortic stenosis is commonly associated with regurgitation. This is especially so in rheumatic and congenital valve stenosis and in congenital subvalvar stenosis. It is seldom severe in the calcific stenosis of the elderly and almost unknown in hypertrophic subaortic stenosis.

Mitral valve disease usually predominates over aortic stenosis in rheumatic valve disease.

The left ventricle hypertrophies in response to the pressure load imposed upon it. The weight of the heart is often doubled in severe cases. There is usually little ventricular dilatation unless there is associated aortic regurgitation. Coronary artery disease may coexist with aortic stenosis, but commonly the coronary arteries are larger than normal. In aortic valve stenosis, there is a dilatation of the ascending aorta (an effect of the jet of blood which is propelled through the valve).

Pathophysiology

A minor degree of stenosis has little or no effect upon the function of the heart; only when the area of the valve orifice is reduced to a quarter of the normal are there serious consequences. The left ventricle responds to the pressure load by contracting more forcibly, and the left ventricular systolic pressure increases (see Fig. 14.15). A systolic pressure difference develops between the left ventricle and aorta (Fig. 14.16). The magnitude of this difference in pressure depends on the size of the orifice and the flow of blood through it. The obstruction delays emptying of the left ventricle, so that the phase of ejection becomes prolonged. The cardiac output is usually maintained within the normal range but at the expense of a considerable increase in left ventricular work. In consequence, left ventricular hypertrophy

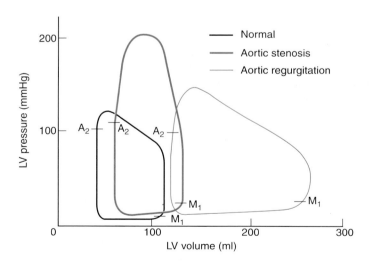

Fig 14.15 Relationships between left ventricular volume and pressure in the normal heart, in aortic stenosis and in aortic regurgitation. M_1 = mitral valve closure. A_2 = aortic valve closure. Note high pressure generated in aortic stenosis and large end-diastolic volume (at M_1), with increased stroke volume in aortic regurgitation.

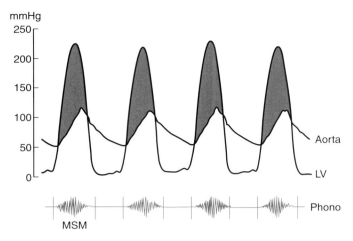

Fig. 14.16 Simultaneous pressure recordings and phonocardiographic appearances in aortic stenosis. Note the systolic pressure difference ('gradient') between the left ventricle and aorta, and the corresponding midsystolic murmur (MSM).

increases progressively as the valve orifice narrows. Although the hypertrophy is a compensatory phenomenon, it eventually contributes to the burden on the heart. The thickened ventricle is less compliant and is therefore less easily filled during diastole; atrial contraction contributes more and more to the filling process. The hypertrophied muscle increasingly outstrips the ability of the coronary arteries to supply it with blood.

Symptoms

There is a characteristic triad of symptoms:

- breathlessness;
- syncope on exertion;
- angina pectoris.

To these may be added the liability to sudden death.

Breathlessness is the earliest symptom in most cases. Later orthopnoea and paroxysmal nocturnal dyspnoea may occur. Eventually, right-sided heart failure with peripheral oedema may develop.

Syncope is much commoner in aortic stenosis than in other types of valvar heart disease and its relationship to exertion is of diagnostic value. Its mechanism is uncertain, but it may be due to the inability of the heart to increase its output sufficiently, or to reflex vasodilatation, or to arrhythmias.

Like syncope, anginal pain is much commoner in aortic stenosis than in other valve lesions. It does not differ in character from that seen in coronary artery disease.

Death is often sudden and may not be preceded by any symptoms. However, it is particularly likely to occur in those who have experienced syncope or angina pectoris. It is believed that ventricular fibrillation is usually responsible.

Physical signs

An aortic systolic murmur is the first abnormality to appear and may be present for decades before evidence of severe stenosis develops.

The pulse is abnormal in most severe cases (Fig. 14.17). Characteristically it is small in volume, rises slowly to its peak, and takes an unusually long time to pass the finger. The pulse pressure is correspondingly small. When there is an appreciable degree of aortic regurgitation as well, the pulse pressure may be normal or large, and the pulse may take on a 'bisferiens' quality in which a double pulse is felt.

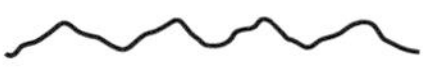

Fig. 14.17   Small, flat pulse in aortic stenosis.

The apex beat may be in the normal position or displaced downwards and to the left. It has a slow heaving quality. A systolic thrill can often be felt in the second right intercostal space, and also in the carotid arteries and along the left edge of the sternum.

There is a mid-systolic murmur, which is usually loud and harsh. This may be best heard in the second right interspace, along the left sternal edge, or even at the apex. It is often audible over the carotid arteries. It is accompanied by an early systolic ('ejection') click in those cases in which there is aortic valve stenosis without heavy calcification. This sign is probably due to sudden tension of the valve cusps at the time of opening. Other signs may include a fourth (atrial) heart sound over the left ventricle and reversed splitting of the second heart sound. This latter sign is due to delay in left ventricular emptying and aortic valve closure. The aortic component of the second heart sound may not be audible if there is calcification.

ECG, chest radiography and echocardiography

The ECG usually shows left ventricular hypertrophy, the extent of which roughly parallels the severity of the stenosis. Other abnormalities which sometimes occur include asymmetrical inversion of T waves and left bundle branch block. The chest radiograph may be normal, but the ascending aorta is usually dilated in aortic valve stenosis. Left ventricular enlargement may be evident (Fig. 14.18).

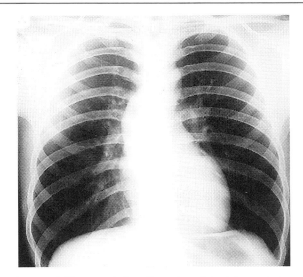

Fig. 14.18 Aortic stenosis. The rounded configuration of the left ventricular outline suggests left ventricular hypertrophy. The ascending aorta shows post-stenotic dilatation.

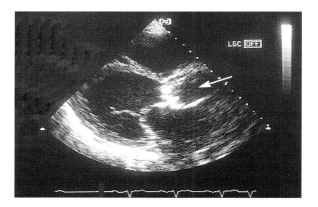

Fig. 14.19 Thickened and stenotic aortic valve producing dense echoes (arrowed).

Two-dimensional echocardiography will demonstrate the thickened aortic valve leaflets with restricted opening (Fig. 14.19). The left ventricular cavity is usually small with marked hypertrophy of the walls. Doppler examination can be used to estimate the severity of aortic stenosis. Using the Bernoulli equation (p. 73), the blood velocity through the stenotic aortic valve can be measured and the aortic valve gradient estimated (Fig. 14.20). This requires considerable patience and skill. In heavily disorganized valves, the aortic jet is often eccentric;

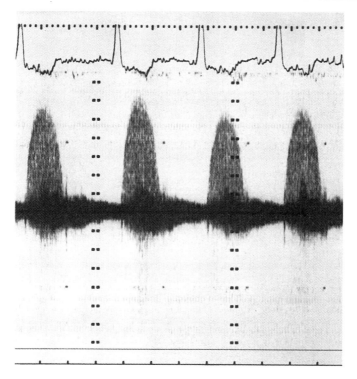

Fig. 14.20 Continuous wave Doppler recording in a patient with aortic stenosis and atrial fibrillation. The height of the signal varies with the velocity of the jet and in this case varies from cycle to cycle depending on the preceding cycle length. The maximum velocity is 6 metres per second which calculates out at a gradient of 144 mmHg.

multiple transducer positions will be required to align the Doppler signal with the aortic jet and so record the maximum gradient. Failure to do so may result in a serious underestimation of the aortic valve gradient. The advent of Doppler examination has, in many cases, obviated the need for cardiac catheterization to establish a diagnosis of aortic stenosis.

Cardiac catheterization

The systolic pressure difference across the stenosis is measured with catheters in the left ventricle and aorta or by the withdrawal of a catheter from left ventricle to aorta (Fig. 14.21). If the stenosis is severe, the left ventricular systolic pressure exceeds that in the aorta by more than 50 mmHg. For technical reasons, the gradient recorded at catheterization is usually lower than that recorded at echocardiography. In advanced cases of aortic stenosis with left ventricular

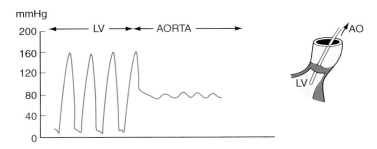

Fig. 14.21   Pressure tracing recorded as catheter is withdrawn from left ventricle to aorta in aortic valve stenosis. Note sudden fall in systolic pressure as the catheter tip enters the aorta.

dysfunction, the gradient, both at catheterization and by echo, may be low despite the presence of severe stenosis. A reported gradient of 30–40 mmHg should be interpreted with caution, therefore, if the left ventricular function is poor.

Complications

The most frequent cause of death is cardiac failure, but there is considerable risk of sudden death. Infective endocarditis may occur and, by eroding the cusps, cause severe aortic regurgitation.

Diagnosis and differential diagnosis

The diagnosis is often suggested by the triad of symptoms (dyspnoea, angina, syncope on exertion), or by the finding of the typical murmur associated with a thrill and a small pulse. Hypertrophic subaortic stenosis can be differentiated from other varieties by the pulse, which rises rapidly rather than slowly, and by the absence of an ejection click, valve calcification and aortic regurgitation; the diagnosis is established by echocardiography.

Prognosis

Cases of mild aortic stenosis have a good prognosis; if there is no appreciable degree of left ventricular hypertrophy, the patient is likely to survive for many years. Once the symptoms of breathlessness, angina or syncope have developed, death is likely to occur suddenly at any time, or within 5 years from heart failure.

Treatment

Little or no benefit can be expected from medical treatment. When symptoms have developed, strenuous activity should be avoided and the conventional treatment of heart failure and angina pectoris employed. Surgery is indicated in nearly all patients and usually takes the form of aortic valve replacement. The mortality rate associated with aortic valve replacement varies greatly from centre to centre, but averages about 2%. Mortality, however, is higher if the patient also requires coronary bypass surgery. This risk must be weighed against the grave prognosis in those with advanced symptoms. Balloon valvuloplasty of the aortic valve has been attempted but probably has no place in current practice.

Aortic regurgitation (synonyms: aortic incompetence, insufficiency)

Aetiology

Aortic regurgitation is commonly due to rheumatic heart disease. It can also be of congenital origin, in which case it is usually of less importance than the lesions which accompany it, such as aortic and subaortic stenosis and ventricular septal defect. Other causes include bicuspid valves, hypertension, infective endocarditis, the Marfan syndrome, dissecting aneurysm, syphilitic aortitis, ankylosing spondylitis and Reiter's disease. In a substantial proportion of cases no cause can be found, i.e. they are 'idiopathic'.

Pathology

Aortic regurgitation can result either from damage to the cusps or from dilatation of the aorta and the valve ring. In rheumatic heart disease, the cusps are thickened and shortened and there may be some fusion of commissures. Varying degrees of stenosis and regurgitation occur. Calcification of the valve, which is usually severe in aortic stenosis, is seldom of importance in pure aortic regurgitation.

Syphilitic aortitis leads to aortic regurgitation as a result of dilatation of the aorta and the valve ring; stenosis is not a feature.

Infective endocarditis can cause erosion or perforation of the cusps, which have usually had some pre-existing abnormality.

Pathophysiology

In aortic regurgitation, a large volume of blood is regurgitated into the left ventricle in each diastole. The left ventricular output may be more than doubled. The increased stroke volume necessary to achieve this is associated with dilatation of the left ventricle. The regurgitant flow is greatest in early diastole when the difference in pressure between the aorta and left ventricle is maximal. The amount of blood that regurgitates is largely determined by the severity of the aortic valve disease but is also influenced by the compliance of the left ventricle and the systemic vascular resistance.

The dilated left ventricle contracts more powerfully in accordance with Starling's law, but there is an increased tension in the myocardium and increased oxygen consumption. The initial dilatation thus leads eventually to hypertrophy.

The diastolic pressure in the aorta is abnormally low, partly due to the leak and partly to peripheral vasodilatation. The left ventricular end-diastolic pressure is normal in the milder case but rises when cardiac failure supervenes.

Clinical features

Rheumatic aortic regurgitation usually develops at the time of acute rheumatic carditis and persists subsequently. Many years elapse between the appearance of the murmur and the onset of symptoms.

Almost invariably the first complaint is that of dyspnoea on exertion, although fatigue is also frequent. Other minor symptoms include dizziness and an awareness of the vigorous heart action.

The dyspnoea progresses slowly; eventually orthopnoea and paroxysmal dyspnoea may develop. Typical angina pectoris is infrequent except when the regurgitation is severe. In the advanced case, signs of right-sided failure complicate those of left-sided failure.

The arterial pulse in aortic regurgitation, often called 'collapsing' or 'water-hammer', rises rapidly and falls abruptly. This is most easily appreciated by placing the palm of one's hand on the anterior aspect of the patient's forearm (the arm being held vertically upright) because by this means one may accentuate the backflow of blood during diastole. Sometimes the pulse is of bisferiens type, i.e. is felt to have two equally prominent waves, particularly if the regurgitation is accompanied by stenosis. The cardiac rhythm is usually normal unless there is associated mitral valve disease. The systolic pressure is often abnormally high and the diastolic low. In a severe case the systolic pressure may be 250–300 mmHg and the diastolic 30–50 mmHg. Vigorous arterial pulsation is often visible in the neck.

If the regurgitation is substantial, the apex beat is displaced outwards and downwards and is overactive and heaving. The essential feature on auscultation is an early diastolic murmur, usually best heard over the midsternal region or at the lower left sternal edge. In some cases, particularly in syphilitic aortitis, it is loudest in the second right intercostal space. There is often an accompanying systolic murmur; this does not necessarily indicate coexistent aortic stenosis but may be due to the increased stroke volume. The early (or 'immediate') diastolic murmur is often difficult to hear, and is frequently overlooked by the inexperienced. It must be specifically sought, with the stethoscope diaphragm placed at the lower left sternal edge, with the patient sitting up, the breath held in expiration.

In some patients with advanced aortic regurgitation, a mid-diastolic murmur may be heard even in the absence of mitral stenosis. This murmur (known as the Austin Flint murmur) has been attributed to the effect of the regurgitant jet on the aortic leaflet of the mitral valve which is interposed between the mitral and aortic valve orifices (see Fig. 14.2). One should hesitate to diagnose an Austin Flint murmur in rheumatic heart disease because concomitant mitral stenosis is likely, particularly if there is a loud first sound or opening snap.

ECG, chest radiography and echocardiography

The ECG shows increasing evidence of left ventricular hypertrophy as the disease process advances. On the chest radiograph, there is usually left ventricular enlargement, with an elongated heart shadow and dilatation of the ascending aorta. Two-dimensional echocardiography may show a thickened aortic valve leaflet although the leaflets can appear normal even in severe regurgitation. If the regurgitation is haemodynamically significant, the left ventricle will be dilated and there may be early closure of the mitral valve. Before the advent of colour flow mapping, the fine oscillation of the anterior mitral valve leaflet was an important echocardiographic sign of aortic regurgitation. This movement was caused by the regurgitant jet striking the anterior leaflet. With the advent of colour flow mapping, the regurgitant jet or jets can now be seen easily (Fig. 14.22). Factors such as the width of the regurgitant jet and the distance into which it penetrates the left ventricle can provide a semi-quantitative estimate of severity.

Cardiac catheterization

Gross aortic regurgitation is so readily recognized clinically and by non-invasive methods that cardiac catheterization is seldom required for diagnostic purposes. This investigation is, however, necessary when the degree of severity is in doubt; it is of particular value in evaluating the significance of an aortic diastolic murmur in a patient needing surgery for concomitant mitral valve disease. The cineangiographic demonstration of the regurgitation of contrast medium injected into the aorta provides a good estimate of severity.

Differential diagnosis

The clinical diagnosis of aortic regurgitation is usually not difficult if it is moderate or severe. A large pulse pressure is also observed in other

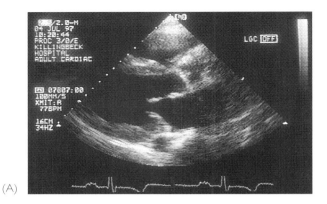

(A)

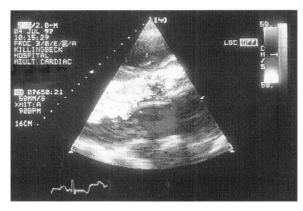

(B)

Fig 14.22 (A) Grossly thickened aortic valve (arrowed). (B) Colour flow doppler examination demonstrates severe regurgitation through the valve and into the left ventricular cavity.

conditions, such as persistent ductus arteriosus, arteriovenous fistulae, pregnancy, anaemia and thyrotoxicosis. The early diastolic murmur may be confused with that of pulmonary regurgitation, but this rare lesion is seldom found in the absence of severe pulmonary hypertension.

In determining the aetiology of aortic regurgitation, it is important to look for other valve lesions and for evidence of disease in other systems. The signs of mitral stenosis or regurgitation suggest a rheumatic origin. Syphilis should be suspected particularly when there is aneurysmal dilatation of the aorta or calcification of the ascending aorta. Congenital aortic regurgitation is usually overshadowed by aortic or subaortic stenosis.

Clinical course and prognosis

Minor degrees of aortic regurgitation are compatible with freedom from symptoms and a normal life span although the risk of infective endocarditis is ever present. In the moderate to severe case, symptoms and signs develop slowly, and it is usually not until the fourth or fifth decade that disability sets in. The severity of aortic regurgitation can be judged, to a large extent, by the pulse pressure and the size of the left ventricle. Increasing dyspnoea and an enlarging heart are signs that the patient is unlikely to survive for more than a few years. Sudden death is unusual in asymptomatic patients but may occur when an advanced stage has been reached.

Treatment

In less severe cases, considerable symptomatic improvement can be obtained by conventional treatment of cardiac failure such as the restriction of activity, and the use of diuretics and ACE inhibitors. When symptoms or heart size are increasing in spite of medical measures, surgery should be considered. In good hands the results of aortic valve replacement, either by artificial valves or bioprostheses, are reasonably satisfactory, but there is an operative mortality rate of about 2%. Artificial prostheses necessitate anticoagulant therapy; bioprostheses do not but are less durable and may require replacement within 5–10 years. Successful surgery is accompanied by a diminution in heart size, although not necessarily to normal. Symptoms are relieved, but medical measures may still be required.

Combined aortic stenosis and regurgitation

Aortic stenosis and regurgitation are often combined. When the lesion is congenital, atherosclerotic or calcific, the stenosis is usually the more important. In rheumatic heart disease, all gradations between the two can occur. In deciding which is dominant, the character of the pulse and the pulse pressure are of great value. A collapsing pulse is incompatible with severe stenosis; a small pulse makes major regurgitation unlikely. The murmurs can be deceptive as loud aortic systolic murmurs are not uncommon in aortic regurgitation even when stenosis is slight or absent. Likewise, the intensity of an aortic diastolic murmur is an unreliable guide to the severity of regurgitation. Echocardiography and, if necessary, cardiac catheterization and angiography permit adequate assessment of the relative contribution of each lesion. Doppler ultrasonography, supplemented, if necessary, by cardiac catheterization and angiocardiography, permits adequate assessment of the relative contribution of each lesion.

TRICUSPID VALVE DISEASE

The structure of the tricuspid valve is similar to that of the mitral valve, except for the presence of three cusps. It may be affected by either stenosis or regurgitation. Tricuspid stenosis is nearly always rheumatic in origin and is rarely the dominant cardiac lesion. Some degree of tricuspid stenosis occurs in about 10% of cases of rheumatic heart disease, but is of significance in only about 3%. Organic tricuspid regurgitation, which is uncommon, is usually due to rheumatic heart disease. Functional tricuspid regurgitation is a frequent complication of right ventricular failure whatever the cause.

When tricuspid valve lesions are due to rheumatic heart disease, the pathological appearances are similar to those seen in the mitral valve. The valve cusps are thickened and the chordae may be adherent and shortened. Dilatation of the tricuspid valve ring is a major factor in regurgitation and occurs as a result of either dilatation of the right ventricle or the rheumatic process.

Tricuspid stenosis

The narrowed valve obstructs flow from the right atrium to the right ventricle during ventricular diastole. As a consequence, right atrial pressure rises, cardiac output falls, and the right atrium and venae cavae dilate. Atrial contraction becomes increasingly forceful and produces large 'a' waves in the venous pulse if sinus rhythm is preserved, as it usually is. Hepatic engorgement follows and ascites and peripheral oedema eventually develop.

In most cases of tricuspid stenosis, mitral stenosis is also present and dominates the clinical picture. For this reason, breathlessness is the commonest symptom, but because tricuspid stenosis restricts right ventricular throughput, pulmonary congestion is often less severe than it is in isolated mitral stenosis. The patient with mitral stenosis may become less breathless as tricuspid stenosis progresses, but at the expense of right-sided cardiac failure.

Large flicking venous 'a' waves may be seen even in early cases. When the lesion is more advanced the venous pressure as a whole is elevated. The 'a' wave disappears when atrial fibrillation develops. The flow of blood from the atrium into the ventricle during diastole is slow and the 'y' descent of the venous pulse is therefore prolonged. The liver is enlarged and may exhibit presystolic pulsation corresponding with the large 'a' waves. On auscultation, mid-diastolic and presystolic murmurs may be heard at the lower left sternal edge which are similar in timing to those of mitral stenosis but of a rather more scratchy quality. The murmurs are accentuated by inspiration, because of increased venous return to the right atrium at this time. The signs of mitral stenosis may be masked.

On the ECG the only characteristic feature is the presence of the tall P waves of right atrial enlargement. The chest radiograph shows enlargement of the right atrium and superior vena cava; the features of mitral stenosis are also usually present. The lung fields are often relatively clear. Echocardiography may demonstrate thickening and reduced movement of the tricuspid valve leaflet. As in the assessment of mitral stenosis, it is possible to measure a tricuspid pressure half-time which will be prolonged in patients with tricuspid stenosis.

On cardiac catheterization, a diastolic pressure difference can be demonstrated between right atrium and right ventricle, and there is usually a large 'a' wave in the right atrial pulse.

The prognosis of patients with tricuspid stenosis is often relatively good. However, if the lesion is severe, progressive signs of right-sided cardiac failure develop; ascites, jaundice and cachexia are characteristic.

In the majority of patients with tricuspid stenosis, the lesion is insufficiently severe to warrant surgery, which should be undertaken only if the stenosis is responsible for major symptoms. Valvotomy seldom restores normal valve function; replacement by a prosthesis is usually necessary.

Tricuspid regurgitation

Functional tricuspid regurgitation is a common complication of right ventricular failure and pulmonary hypertension. Since most patients with this condition have evidence of rheumatic heart disease, it is often difficult to be certain whether or not there is organic tricuspid disease as well.

The features of tricuspid regurgitation are the consequence of a large volume of blood being regurgitated through the valve from the right ventricle. As a result, the forward flow into the pulmonary circuit is reduced and the right ventricle has to cope with a large volume load. When regurgitation is severe, large systolic ('cv') waves develop in the right atrium, which are transmitted to the peripheral veins and liver. There is a high flow of blood through the tricuspid valve during diastole, as both the regurgitated and the forward flow must be transported at this time. Both diastolic and systolic flow through the valve are increased on inspiration as an increased volume of blood is drawn into the heart.

Coexistent mitral valve disease usually dominates the clinical picture and dyspnoea is the major symptom. Tricuspid regurgitation may reduce the effects of the mitral valve disease on the lungs at the expense of producing right-sided heart failure. As the disease progresses, there is an increase in venous pressure, hepatic enlargement, ascites and peripheral oedema. Large systolic waves are present in the jugular veins; systolic pulsation of the liver may be felt. A systolic murmur is heard at the lower left sternal edge; this is usually increased on inspiration. There may also be a tricuspid diastolic murmur due either to concomitant tricuspid stenosis or to high flow through the orifice during this phase.

There are no specific ECG features of tricuspid regurgitation; the chest radiograph usually shows right atrial enlargement. If the tricuspid regurgitation is secondary to mitral valve disease and pulmonary hypertension, the characteristic radiological features of these lesions will be present. On echocardiography, the right ventricle and right atrium will usually be dilated and colour flow mapping will show a broad jet of tricuspid regurgitation.

At cardiac catheterization, the chief feature is the large systolic venous wave of the right atrial pulse. The finding of severe pulmonary hypertension suggests the regurgitation is functional. A near normal pulmonary artery pressure is an indication that the tricuspid disease is organic.

It is often difficult to differentiate mitral regurgitation from tricuspid regurgitation, or to determine whether there is a combination of the two. Mitral regurgitation is suggested by radiation of the murmur to the axilla and by left ventricular enlargement, tricuspid regurgitation by systolic venous pulsation and by inspiratory accentuation of the murmur. Tricuspid regurgitation is often tolerated for a long time, but sooner or later the features of advanced right-sided cardiac failure become disabling, often with jaundice and cachexia. Severe oedema and ascites develop and are progressively less responsive to treatment.

If the tricuspid regurgitation is functional, there may be striking improvement with digitalis and diuretic therapy. Usually, surgery for associated mitral valve disease is required, and, if successful, leads to the disappearance of the tricuspid leak. Often the surgeon will inspect and repair the tricuspid valve at the time of mitral valve surgery. Occasionally replacement by a prosthesis is necessary.

PULMONARY VALVE DISEASE

Pulmonary valve disease is relatively uncommon. Pulmonary stenosis is usually of congenital origin and is discussed in Chapter 15. Other causes of pulmonary stenosis include rheumatic heart disease and malignant carcinoid. Obstruction of the outflow tract of the right ventricle may occur in hypertrophic cardiomyopathy and mediastinal tumours.

Pulmonary regurgitation is usually secondary to pulmonary hypertension, but occasionally occurs as a consequence of infective endocarditis, as a complication of the surgical relief of pulmonary stenosis, and as a congenital anomaly. It is nearly always overshadowed by the heart disease to which it is secondary. In most cases, there are signs of pulmonary hypertension, and the only feature which suggests the diagnosis is an early diastolic murmur (the Graham Steell murmur) in the second or third left intercostal spaces which becomes louder on inspiration. It is often difficult to decide whether a murmur in this position is due to pulmonary or aortic regurgitation. Pulmonary regurgitation is unlikely in the absence of signs of pulmonary hypertension and right ventricular hypertrophy. Aortic regurgitation is suggested by a collapsing pulse and the signs of left ventricular hypertrophy, although these signs may be absent if the regurgitation is slight. The diagnosis may be confirmed by echocardiography and Doppler examination.

INFECTIVE ENDOCARDITIS

Infective endocarditis may be due to bacteria, fungi, *Coxiella* or *Chlamydia*. Endocarditis has classically been described as subacute or acute, based on the clinical course observed before the advent of antibiotic therapy but the term infective endocarditis is now preferred. Subacute referred to less aggressive organisms which resulted in a much more protracted course of many months and even years.

The commonest variety is bacterial in origin and subacute in its course. Infective subacute endocarditis seldom affects a previously normal heart. The process is most frequently superimposed upon pre-existing disease. Prosthetic valves may also become infected and an increasing number of cases are being seen in intravenous drug abusers. Acute endocarditis (most frequently *Staphylococcus aureus*) may occur on previously normal hearts.

Native valve endocarditis

The majority of patients have a predisposing cardiac lesion. The pattern of underlying cardiac disease has been changing, reflecting the decline in the incidence of rheumatic heart disease. Currently the commonest underlying lesions in decreasing frequency are mitral valve prolapse, degenerative aortic and mitral lesions, and rheumatic heart disease. The most common congenital lesions predisposing to endocarditis in the adult are bicuspid aortic valve, ventricular septal defect, coarction of the aorta and pulmonary stenosis.

Endocarditis in intravenous drug abusers

Endocarditis in the absence of underlying cardiac disease is common amongst intravenous drug abusers. The tricuspid valve is the focus of infection in about 50% of cases, with the mitral and aortic valves each accounting for about 20% of cases. Pulmonary valve endocarditis also occurs but is rare.

The presentation of right-sided endocarditis differs from left-sided. Typically, patients may present with pneumonia or multiple septic pulmonary emboli.

Prosthetic valve endocarditis

Prosthetic valve endocarditis is divided into categories of early and late. By definition endocarditis is early when symptoms occur within 60 days of valve implantation and late if they occur after this time. Early infection is generally due to contamination in the perioperative period, from sources such as intravenous cannulae, central lines or urinary catheters. The majority of cases are due to staphylococcal infection. The bacteriology of late prosthetic valve endocarditis more closely resembles native valve endocarditis.

Pathology

A large number of different organisms may cause bacterial endocarditis. Common organisms include:

- *Streptococcus viridans*. An oral commensal of several varieties, this is the organism most frequently responsible for endocarditis, accounting for some 50–70% of cases. Most are highly sensitive to penicillin;
- *Streptococcus faecalis*. These organisms normally inhabit the gastrointestinal tract. The organisms are generally resistant to penicillin. High doses must be used and an aminoglycoside added to achieve a bactericidal effect;
- *Streptococcus bovis*. This organism is frequently associated with the presence of colonic polyps or colonic malignancy. It is highly sensitive to penicillin;
- *Staphylococcus aureus*. This skin organism accounts for about 25% of cases of native valve endocarditis. It is the commonest cause of endocarditis amongst intravenous drug abusers, in whom it is responsible for some 60% of cases. The majority of organisms are highly resistant to penicillin. Multiple metastatic abscesses are common;
- *Staphylococcus epidermidis*. This organism is a relatively rare cause of native valve endocarditis, but a common cause of prosthetic valve endocarditis. Different strains vary in their sensitivity to penicillin.

Other rare causes of endocarditis include *Neisseria gonorrhoeae*, *Coxiella burnetii* (Q fever) and *Chlamydia psittaci* (psittacosis).

The infection leads to the formation of friable vegetations which have necrotic tissue, platelets, fibrin, white cells and red cells in their base, with superficial layers of fibrin and micro-organisms. Ulceration may lead to erosion or perforation of the valve cusps or of a sinus of Valsalva. The location of the endocarditis depends upon the underlying lesion. In aortic regurgitation, endocarditis affects the ventricular surface of the valve; in mitral regurgitation it involves the atrial surface of the mitral valve. In a ventricular septal defect, the vegetations may form around the defect itself but are often located either on the tricuspid valve or where the jet impinges on the right ventricular wall. Invasion of the adjacent myocardium is common and may proceed to abscess formation, and to pericardial involvement.

Embolization from the vegetations is frequent and is responsible for many of the clinical features of the disease. Large emboli may cause occlusion of the cerebral, renal or splenic arteries. Micro-emboli affect nearly all parts of the body and, in particular, lead to skin lesions and a glomerulonephritis. Pulmonary emboli develop when the right side of the heart is involved, as it is when there is a ventricular septal defect or persistent ductus arteriosus.

Several of the manifestations of the disease, including arthritis and glomerulitis, are thought to be due to immune complex deposition.

Clinical features

A history of dental treatment or infection is present in some patients, and in a small proportion there has been preceding urethral, pelvic or cardiac surgery.

The onset is often insidious with malaise and feverishness being the earliest complaints. The symptoms often mimic those of influenza. If left untreated, a characteristic clinical picture develops which was common in the days before antibiotic therapy. The complete syndrome of fever, anaemia, petachiae in the skin, clubbing, splenomegaly, a cardiac murmur and microscopic haematuria is seldom seen nowadays.

Abnormal clinical features in patients with endocarditis include:

- *heart murmurs.* The appearance of a new murmur or change in character of an existing murmur are particularly suggestive of endocarditis. A murmur may also disappear because of worsening valvar regurgitation;
- *petechiae.* These may develop on any part of the body. They may be embolic or vasculitic. They should be sought particularly in the conjunctivae, in the mouth and in the ocular fundi (Roth's spots are small oval, retinal haemorrhages with a pale centre). Haemorrhagic lesions on the palms and soles are termed Janeway lesions;
- *splinter haemorrhages.* These are small linear streaks in the nailbed of fingers and toes;
- *Osler's nodes.* These are small tender nodules in the tips of the fingers and toes;

- *clubbing*. This arises only if the disease is present for several months;
- *splenomegaly*. This too takes several months to develop and is a feature of long-standing disease;
- *proteinuria and microscopic haematuria;*
- *neurological complications* are common and are due to embolic occlusion of cerebral vessels or to mycotic aneurysms.

Investigations. Most patients with infective endocarditis have a normochromic normocytic anaemia. The C-reactive protein level will be raised, although this is not a specific abnormality for infective endocarditis. Chest radiography and ECG are of little value except in the diagnosis and assessment of the underlying cardiac abnormality. Confirmation of the diagnosis depends on obtaining a positive blood culture, which is possible in some 90% of cases. At least six specimens of blood should be obtained over a period of 1–2 days. The blood should be incubated aerobically and anaerobically, and special cultures should be set up for fungi. If the patient has received penicillin previously, penicillinase should be incorporated in the culture medium. Complement fixation tests must be undertaken for the diagnosis of *Coxiella* and *Chlamydia* infection.

Echocardiography is an important investigation of this disorder, both because of its ability to demonstrate vegetations and because it can help in the assessment of the severity of valvar involvement. Vegetations are seen in only 60% of cases by the cross-sectional technique. The absence of vegetations on echocardiography, therefore, does not exclude endocarditis. Transoesophageal echocardiography can achieve higher success rates, and can identify the presence of vegetations in some 90% of patients with endocarditis.

Prognosis. Recovery from infective endocarditis is rare unless effective and prolonged antiobiotic therapy is given. Death, which may be due to heart failure, emboli or renal failure, often does not occur until several months after the onset. Even if the infection is cured, damage to the valves may be so serious as to lead to intractable heart failure. Even with modern antibiotic treatment, the mortality rate is still in the region of 30%.

Complications. Complications are a common occurrence in patients with endocarditis:

- *congestive heart failure* may occur due to progressive valve destruction;
- *systemic emboli* are a particular concern, and may result in stroke or myocardial infarction;
- *mycotic aneurysm formation* may lead to occlusion of vessels or to haemorrhage. Neurological complications may be due either to emboli or to the presence of a mycotic aneurysm;

- *renal failure.* This may arise due to immune complex deposition causing glomerulonephritis. Aminoglycoside antibiotics may also impair renal function;
- *intracardiac abscess formation.* Aortic root abscess formation is a serious complication and an indication for surgical intervention. It should be suspected in patients with persistent or recurrent pyrexia. Septal extension from an abscess may cause widening of the PR interval and heart block. Abscess cavities can usually be seen on transoesophageal echocardiography.

Treatment

It is important that the responsible organism should be identified without delay, so that the appropriate antibiotics can be given. However, the start of therapy should not be postponed beyond 2–3 days in spite of negative blood cultures. Bactericidal agents should be employed, because bacteriostatic drugs produce only temporary suppression of the infection. Following isolation and identification of an organism, careful discussion with the microbiology department is advisable to guide antibiotic selection. The microbiology department can also undertake back titrations to ensure that adequate antibiotic levels are achieved to kill the organism.

Antibiotic selection

- When the organism is penicillin sensitive (e.g. *Streptococcus viridans* or *Streptococcus bovis*), a penicillin (penicillin G or ampicillin) is given. Administration is usually intravenous, at least for the first 2 weeks, and adequate dosage (e.g. penicillin G, 8 million units/day), preferably confirmed by laboratory testing, is essential. Change to oral therapy may be possible later, given a good response.
- In penicillin-resistant infection (e.g. *Streptococcus faecalis*) a combination of a penicillin (penicillin G or ampicillin) and an aminoglycoside (e.g. gentamicin, vancomycin) will be necessary.
- Penicillin-sensitive staphylococci will respond to penicillin, but the more common penicillin-resistant strains demand large doses of penicillinase-resistant drugs (e.g. flucloxacillin 2 g intravenously every 4 h). An aminoglycoside is commonly added for possible synergistic benefit. Coagulase-negative staphylococci such as *Staphylococcus epidermidis* are frequently methicillin-resistant and resistant to all beta-lactam antibiotics. In cases of methicillin resistance, vancomycin should be substituted for flucloxacillin, with or without the addition of an aminoglycoside. Oral rifampicin is also of value in the management of penicillin-resistant staphylococci.

- Blood culture-negative native valve endocarditis should be treated as for *S. faecalis* infections, infection with *Coxiella* and *Chlamydia* having first been excluded. In cases of culture-negative prosthetic valve endocarditis, vancomycin should be added.

A minimum of 4 weeks' therapy is thought necessary in all cases. Antibiotic therapy is constantly changing as new drugs become available and as organisms become resistant to those in current use. Serial measurements of C-reactive protein levels are useful in monitoring the efficacy of treatment.

The temperature usually falls to normal within 3 days of the start of effective antibiotic therapy. If pyrexia recurs, there are several possible explanations:

- emergence of resistant organisms;
- superinfection with another organism;
- development of a reaction to the antibiotic;
- development of an abscess.

Surgery

In most cases it is appropriate to undertake medical management and first to attempt to control and cure the infection. Surgery is indicated in patients with:

- refractory heart failure due to valvar regurgitation;
- a paravalvar abscess;
- ineffective therapy or repeated relapses;
- multiple embolic episodes.

In patients with prosthetic endocarditis, achieving a cure with antibiotics alone is particularly difficult. For this reason the threshold for surgical intervention should be correspondingly lower.

Anticoagulation. The use of anticoagulants in the management of endocarditis is problematic. On the one hand embolic phenomena are common. On the other, anticoagulation will not necessarily reduce the incidence of emboli and increases the potential risk of bleeding from a mycotic aneurysm. In general, if a patient is already on anticoagulant therapy (e.g. for a mechanical valve prosthesis), this should be continued, but anticoagulants should not be commenced *de novo* unless very clear-cut indications exist.

Antibiotic prophylaxis

Although endocarditis may occur in the absence of any obvious cause and in patients without known heart disease, in other cases the risk can be identified and many cases are preventable. A number of medical or dental procedures may provoke bacteraemia and place predisposed individuals at risk of endocarditis. In practice, the most commonly encountered risk arises with dental treatment. Antibiotic prophylaxis should be considered in any individual at risk of endocarditis undergoing any dental procedure likely to provoke gingival or mucosal bleeding. These include cleaning and scaling, but exclude simple fillings above the gum line. Careful attention to oral hygiene may be as important as antibiotic prophylaxis in safeguarding against orally acquired infection. Antibiotic prophylaxis is also advisable in at-risk individuals for many gastrointestinal, urological, gynaecological or obstetric procedures.

Patients can be divided into groups at relatively high risk, intermediate risk and very low or negligible risk (Table 14.2). Antibiotic prophylaxis is indicated before bacteraemia-producing procedures in individuals at high and intermediate risk, but not in those at low risk. The standard prophylactic regimen for dental procedures is 3 g amoxycillin orally given 1 h before the procedure and 1.5 g 6 h after the procedure. For high-risk patients or high-risk gastrointestinal or genitourinary procedures an aminoglycoside may be added. In patients allergic to penicillin, erythromycin may be substituted in low-risk procedures and vancomycin in high-risk procedures.

Table 14.2   Patients at risk of endocarditis

Relatively high risk
   Previous infective endocarditis
   Prosthetic heart valves
   Cyanotic congenital heart disease
   Patent ductus arteriosus
   Aortic regurgitation or stenosis
   Mitral regurgitation
   Ventricular septal defect
   Aortic coarction
   Surgically repaired congenital heart disease with residual haemodynamic abnormality

Intermediate risk
   Mitral valve prolapse with a mitral regurgitant murmur
   Pure mitral stenosis
   Tricuspid valve disease
   Pulmonary stenosis
   Hypertrophic cardiomyopathy
   Bicuspid or calcified aortic valve
   Surgically repaired intracardiac disease with no haemodynamic abnormality within 6 months
   of surgery

Very low or negligible risk
   Mitral prolapse without a regurgitant murmur
   Trivial valve regurgitation or echo without structural abnormality
   Isolated secundum atrial septal defect
   Cardiac pacemaker or defibrillator

Further reading

Greenberg, B. H. & Murphy, E. (Eds) (1987) *Valvular Heart Disease*. Littleton: PSG.
Hall, R. J. C. & Julian, D. G. (1989) *Diseases of the Cardiac Valves*. Edinburgh: Churchill Livingstone.
Hall, R. J. C. & Kirk, R. (1992) Balloon dilatation of heart valves. *British Medical Journal* **305:** 487.

Congenital Heart Disease

15

A congenital abnormality of the heart is present in nearly one in every hundred babies born. About half of the affected babies die either from their heart disease or from some associated congenital anomaly during the first year of life if untreated. The prognosis of those who survive this period is reasonably good; from 5 years of age until early adult life, the prevalence of congenital heart disease remains at about three per thousand. The less severe types of lesion then begin to take their toll and it is unusual for patients with uncorrected congenital heart disease to survive much beyond the age of 40. Most forms of congenital heart disease are amenable to surgery; in some cases this leads to cure, but in others some residual abnormality is left that may require continuing attention.

Embryology

At an early stage, the heart consists of a simple tube of endocardium surrounded by myocardium and epicardium. As it grows, the tube twists into an S shape and by the fourth week of pregnancy it is divided by constrictions into five segments:

- the sinus venosus, which receives the systemic veins;
- the common atrium;
- the common ventricle;
- the bulbus cordis;
- the truncus arteriosus (Fig. 15.1).

Between the fifth and eighth week, changes of the greatest importance occur; it is at this time that congenital abnormalities are most likely to arise through arrested or faulty development. Septa develop in the atria and in the ventricles to sub-divide each of these chambers into two. Simultaneously, the atria are divided from the ventricles by endocardial cushions from which the mitral and tricuspid valves are formed (Fig. 15.2A). A spiral septum divides the bulbus cordis into the outflow

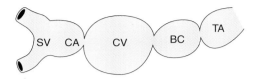

Fig. 15.1 The heart at the fourth week of pregnancy, divided by constrictions into sinus venosus (SV), common atrium (CA), common ventricle (CV), bulbus cordis (BC) and truncus arteriosus (TA).

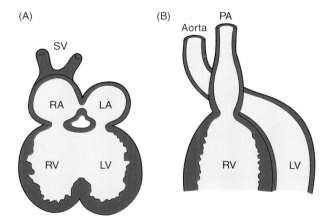

Fig. 15.2 (A) The heart at 8 weeks. The ventricles and atria are each being divided by septa into two chambers. Endocardial cushions develop from which the mitral and tricuspid valves are formed. (B) The spiral septum divides the bulbus cordis into the outflow tracts of the left and right ventricles, and the truncus arteriosus into the aorta and pulmonary arteries.

tracts of the left and right ventricles respectively, and the truncus arteriosus into aorta and pulmonary artery (Fig. 15.2B).

By the end of the eighth week, the heart has largely assumed the features which it retains until birth. The right atrium in the fetal circulation then receives blood from the superior vena cava and from the vitello-umbilical veins which later become the inferior vena cava. A proportion of the venous blood, particularly that from the superior vena cava, flows into the right ventricle, thence into the pulmonary artery and, by way of the ductus arteriosus, into the descending aorta. Only about 5% of the blood flow traverses the pulmonary circulation. Most of the highly oxygenated inferior vena caval blood is directed through the foramen ovale in the atrial septum into the left atrium and thence, by the left ventricle, into the ascending aorta. Within a few hours or, at most, days of birth the ductus arteriosus closes, and the relatively high pressure in the left atrium keeps the valve of the foramen ovale shut.

Aetiology

No aetiological factor can be found in most cases of congenital heart disease. In a minority there is evidence of either a genetic abnormality or an environmental factor affecting the mother during the early stages of pregnancy.

When congenital malformations are multiple, particularly in Down's syndrome (mongolism or trisomy 21), Turner's syndrome and Marfan's syndrome, the heart is often involved. Congenital heart disease rarely affects more than one member of a family. If rubella occurs during the first 3 months of pregnancy, there is a considerable risk of cardiac malformation in the fetus. Other virus infections may occasionally be responsible, as may some drugs, including thalidomide, warfarin and alcohol.

THE VARIETIES OF CONGENITAL HEART DISEASE

The varieties of congenital heart disease can be divided into three types.

Communications between the left (systemic) and right (pulmonary) circulations, e.g. atrial septal defect, ventricular septal defect and persistent ductus arteriosus.

The impedance to flow is normally lower on the right side of the heart and in the pulmonary artery than it is on the left side of the heart and in the aorta. Consequently, the intracardiac pressures are relatively low on the right side. When the two sides of the heart are in communication, provided there is no other abnormality, there is a shunt of blood from left to right through the defect and an increased blood flow through the lungs. In ventricular septal defect and persistent ductus arteriosus, the volume load falls predominantly on the left ventricle, which enlarges accordingly. In atrial septal defect, the load falls on the right ventricle.

The greatly increased pulmonary blood flow frequently leads to a moderate elevation of pulmonary arterial pressure. In most cases, the resistance of the pulmonary arteries is normal but, sometimes, changes take place in the arterial walls which cause a high pulmonary vascular resistance. Severe and irreversible pulmonary hypertension may then ensue and, eventually, lead to reversal of the shunt (Eisenmenger syndrome p. 314).

Obstructive lesions, e.g. coarctation of the aorta, aortic stenosis and pulmonary stenosis.

When these lesions are isolated, they impose a burden on the related ventricle and may eventually cause cardiac failure on this account. They may be combined with abnormal communications, the most important anomaly being that of tetralogy of Fallot, in which there is pulmonary stenosis with a ventricular septal defect.

Displacement or absence of chambers, vessels or valves. These may be associated with abnormal communications or obstructions. Some displacement lesions such as dextrocardia and right-sided aorta may be unimportant. Others, such as transposition of the great arteries, are associated with a high mortality rate.

Abnormal communications

ATRIAL SEPTAL DEFECT (ASD)

The foramen ovale, which is unsealed in some 25% of adults, does not normally permit the flow of blood from the left atrium to the right atrium because of its valvar construction (Fig. 15.3A).

There are three types of abnormality which permit a flow of oxygenated blood into the right atrium:

- The ostium secundum defect, which may be large but does not encroach upon the atrioventricular valves. This is much the commonest variety (Fig. 15.3B).
- The ostium primum defect which is situated close to the atrioventricular valves and is often associated with abnormalities of these valves and, sometimes, with a partial or complete atrioventricular septal defect ('endocardial cushion' defect) (Fig. 15.3D). In the complete form, there is a ventricular septal defect and a common atrioventricular orifice.
- One or more of the pulmonary veins may be attached to the right atrium or great veins instead of the left atrium (Fig. 15.3C). There is usually an atrial septal defect as well. This is termed anomolous pulmonary venous drainage.

The right ventricle is normally thinner and more distensible than the left and, at a given pressure level, more easily filled with blood. Therefore, when both atria are in communication, blood flows preferentially into the right ventricle from both atria and the shunt through the defect is almost exclusively from left to right. The pulmonary blood flow is usually two or three times the aortic blood flow, but the distensibility of pulmonary arterioles is such that they can readily accommodate this with little or no increase in pulmonary arterial pressure. The increase of pulmonary blood flow maintained over many years, however, sometimes leads to changes in the small pulmonary vessels which increase pulmonary vascular resistance and cause severe pulmonary hypertension.

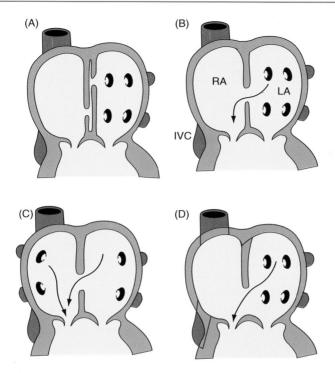

Fig. 15.3   (A) Unsealed foramen ovale. The valvar construction of the foramen ovale prevents shunting from left to right. (B) Atrial septal defect of ostium secundum type. The valve cusps are not affected. (C) Anomalous drainage of the right pulmonary veins into the right atrium, associated with an atrial septal defect of the secundum type. (D) Ostium primum defect, associated with abnormalities of the mitral or tricuspid valves.

The ostium secundum type of defect seldom gives rise to disabling symptoms before the third decade of life, but breathlessness and fatigue are likely to develop before the age of 40. Symptoms are usually progressive and are exacerbated when atrial arrhythmias develop, as they commonly do. By contrast, the complete atrioventricular septal defect often presents in the first year of life with heart failure, respiratory infection, and failure to gain weight.

The arterial pulse is relatively small; the venous pressure is usually normal. The right ventricle is strikingly overactive. Splitting of the second sound is wide, and varies little with respiration ('fixed' splitting of the second sound). This is due to relatively late closure of the pulmonary valve as a consequence of delayed emptying of the overburdened right ventricle. A systolic murmur in the second left interspace due to high flow across the pulmonary valve is almost invariable. Larger defects cause mid-diastolic murmur at the lower left sternal edge, accentuated by inspiration, and produced by increased flow through the tricuspid valve. In the ostium primum type of defect, in which an abnormal mitral valve may permit regurgitation, there may be left ventricular enlargement and an apical systolic murmur.

The ECG nearly always shows the features of partial right bundle branch block ('RSR' complex). In the common ostium secundum type, there is frequently right axis deviation, whilst in the ostium primum type there is usually left axis deviation. This feature is of importance in differentiating the two types of defect (Fig. 15.4).

On the chest radiograph, the heart is usually slightly enlarged, and the pulmonary artery and its branches prominent, as are the right atrium and the right ventricle (see Fig. 5.11). The aorta is abnormally small and may not be visible. Expansile pulsation of the pulmonary arteries ('hilar dance') may be a striking feature on fluoroscopy.

Echocardiography, in ostium secundum defect, demonstrates 'paradoxical' motion of the interventricular septum. As a result of right ventricular overloading, the septum moves towards the right ventricle in systole instead of its usual movement towards the posterior left ventricular wall at this time. In ostium primum defects, abnormalities of the mitral valve are usual.

Cross-sectional echocardiography reliably demonstrates primum and secundum defects and differentiates easily between them. Doppler ultrasonography provides supporting evidence and may permit an assessment of the shunt.

These clinical features are usually sufficiently characteristic for accurate diagnosis. Confirmation by cardiac catheterization is required when the diagnosis is in doubt or surgical treatment is planned. The oxygen saturation in the right atrium is markedly higher than that in the superior vena cava, and the catheter tip may be advanced through the septal defect into the left atrium and thence to the left ventricle. In the ostium primum defect, injection of radio-opaque contrast medium into the left ventricle often reveals mitral regurgitation. When there are anomalies of the pulmonary veins (see Fig. 15.3C), the anomalous veins may be entered directly from the right atrium, or, occasionally, from connections to the superior or inferior venae cavae.

Closure of an ostium secundum defect is relatively easy, carries a low mortality rate and is advisable in all patients with pulmonary blood flow more than twice the systemic blood flow. Correction of the ostium primum type of defect, with its associated anomalies, is more difficult and carries a higher mortality rate. Surgery is usually undertaken if there are symptoms or when the shunt is large. The complete atrioventricular canal may need surgical treatment in the first few months of life because of symptoms or to prevent the development of pulmonary hypertension.

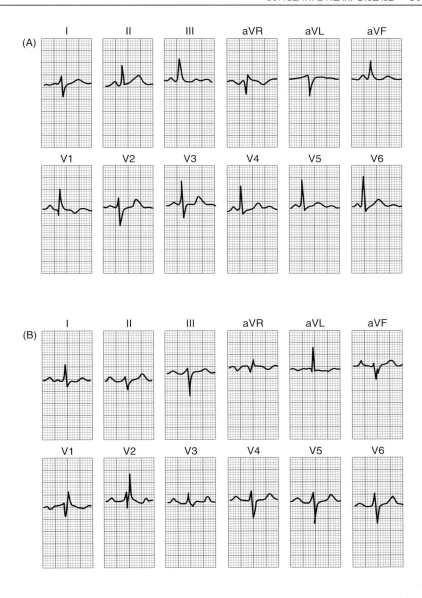

Fig. 15.4. (A) Ostium secundum atrial septal defect. The ECG typically shows an rSR′ pattern, with right axis deviation. (B) Ostium primum atrial septum defect. The ECG again shows an rSR′ pattern, but there is left axis deviation. In this example there is also PR prolongation.

VENTRICULAR SEPTAL DEFECT (VSD)

The ventricular septum consists of four components: the trabecular or muscular septum extending to the apex, the inlet or posterior septum lying between the atrioventricular valves, the outlet or infundibular septum subtending the great arteries, and the membranous septum which lies under the aortic root and abuts on to the other three components. Defects can arise in any one of these components, but the membranous septum is the most commonly affected.

Defects of the ventricular septum, which may be large in relation to the size of the heart at birth, tend to become smaller or to close in early childhood. If closure is insufficient to prevent a large shunt, the small pulmonary vessels may be damaged by being exposed to the ejectile force and pressure of left ventricular contraction. Irreversible pulmonary hypertension may be produced.

The effect of a ventricular septal defect depends upon its size and upon the impedance to blood flow imposed by the pulmonary arterial vessels. If the defect is small, the jet of blood from the high-pressure left ventricle to the low-pressure right ventricle has little haemodynamic effect. If the defect is large and the impedance of the pulmonary vessels low, a large shunt develops and the pulmonary blood flow becomes more than twice the systemic flow. If, on the other hand, there is a high pulmonary vascular resistance, the pulmonary blood flow is little or no more than the systemic and the pressure in both circuits is similar. If the pulmonary vascular resistance is very high, the shunt reverses.

In the patient with a small defect ('maladie de Roger'), there are no symptoms, but there is a loud 'tearing' pansystolic murmur accompanied by a thrill, maximal to the left side of the lower sternum.

A large left-to-right shunt at ventricular level is liable to produce cardiac failure in the second or third month after birth. The special problems associated with this type of abnormality are discussed under the section 'The diagnosis and management of the infant with heart failure and cyanosis' (p. 318). If a large shunt does not produce symptoms during infancy, there is usually little disturbance until late adolescence or early adult life. Breathlessness and fatigue may then develop and cardiac failure subsequently ensue. In the presence of a large left-to-right shunt with pulmonary blood flow greater than twice systemic, the pulse is usually small and the venous pressure normal, unless there is right heart failure. Both left and right ventricles may be hyperdynamic, and there may or may not be a systolic thrill between the apex and the left sternal edge. A pansystolic murmur is heard at this site, usually accompanied by a mid-diastolic murmur at the apex due to high flow through the mitral valve.

In patients with a high pulmonary vascular resistance, breathlessness, fatigue and cyanosis are likely to develop during the second or third decade with progression to effort syncope, recurrent haemoptysis or heart failure. The signs of the ventricular septal defect are then less obvious, although there may still be a systolic murmur between the apex and the left sternal edge. Right ventricular hypertrophy is evident; the pulmonary second sound may be accentuated and followed by the early diastolic murmur of pulmonary regurgitation.

The ECG in small defects is normal. When the left-to-right shunt is large there is usually evidence of biventricular enlargement, manifested by abnormally deep but narrow Q waves and tall R waves in the left chest leads and an rsr pattern in V1. In cases with a high pulmonary vascular resistance, the ECG pattern of isolated right ventricular hypertrophy develops.

The chest radiograph is normal with a small defect, but with a large left-to-right shunt there is some enlargement of the heart and, more specifically, prominence of the pulmonary vessels, left atrium and both ventricles.

With small defects, the cross-sectional echocardiogram is often normal. With larger defects, there is usually a 'drop-out' of septal echoes, and both left atrium and ventricle may be enlarged. Doppler and colour flow mapping can usually provide unequivocal evidence of a ventricular septal defect and, in association with echocardiography, permit an assessment of its size and the flow through it.

Correlation of these features usually provides sufficient evidence for accurate clinical diagnosis in spite of the various forms which defects of the ventricular septum may take. Further investigation may be advisable when the diagnosis is not clear-cut and is necessary if surgical treatment is contemplated. Cardiac catheterization usually demonstrates that the oxygen saturation of right ventricular blood is higher than that in the right atrium. However, if the defect is small or if there are equal pressures in the systemic and pulmonary circulations, no shunt of oxygenated blood may be demonstrable. The injection of radio-opaque contrast medium into the left ventricle may then be necessary for the angiocardiographic visualization of the defect.

The prognosis of ventricular septal defect depends upon the age of the patient, the size of the defect, and the pulmonary vascular changes. Large ventricular septal defects are an important cause of death in the infant; in those who survive, the defect usually becomes smaller or closes. After the first year, few affected children die, but death is likely to occur in those with major defects between the ages of 20 and 40. Patients with small defects usually live a normal life span, but are exposed to the risk of infective endocarditis.

In deciding upon the appropriate therapy for a patient with ventricular septal defect, the expected prognosis must be taken into account. In all patients precautions must be taken to avoid infective endocarditis. Because the outlook in small defects is excellent, surgery is not indicated. If there is a large left-to-right shunt, the defect should be closed. When the pulmonary vascular resistance is high, surgery is usually contraindicated as it cannot correct and may, indeed, worsen the pulmonary hypertension.

PERSISTENT DUCTUS ARTERIOSUS (Fig. 15.5)

During fetal life, the ductus arteriosus permits blood to flow from the pulmonary artery into the aorta. Within a few hours or days of birth, it narrows and then closes.

In a few infants, the ductus arteriosus remains open and permits a large flow of blood from the high-pressure aorta to the low-pressure pulmonary artery. This may cause heart failure and death in the first few weeks of life. More commonly the ductus arteriosus undergoes partial closure and the shunt from aorta to pulmonary artery is relatively small. This gives rise to no symptoms during the first few years of life and is usually detected at a routine physical examination. A persistent ductus arteriosus of this kind may eventually become harmful for three reasons. First, it may act as a focus for infective endarteritis. Secondly, the leak of blood from the aorta to the pulmonary artery and the consequent high pulmonary blood flow may lead to cardiac failure in adolescence or adult life. Thirdly, but rarely, severe pulmonary hypertension may develop.

The patient is usually in good general health. The pulse may be of normal volume if the duct is small, but if it is large, the diastolic leak from the aorta causes a collapsing pulse. Correspondingly, the diastolic blood pressure may be low. The heart may be of normal size, or the left ventricle enlarged. The most characteristic feature of the condition is the 'continuous murmur', situated in the second left intercostal space by the sternal edge but often loudest 5–7.5 cm above or to the left of this. This murmur continues from systole into diastole and is maximal about the time of the second sound (Fig. 15.6). It seldom lasts for the whole of systole and diastole and may occupy only the latter part of systole and the earlier part of diastole. In a few instances, particularly in infants, it may occur as a crescendo in late systole only. The murmur is due to flow of blood from the aorta through the persistent ductus arteriosus into the pulmonary artery in both phases of the cardiac cycle. If the shunt is large, the increased venous return from the lungs causes a mid-diastolic murmur at the apex as it crosses the mitral valve.

The ECG is usually normal but may show the deep Q and tall R waves of left ventricular hypertrophy. The chest radiograph may show enlargement of the left ventricle, aorta and pulmonary artery, and the

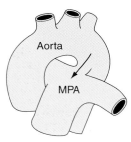

Fig. 15.5 Persistent ductus arteriosus. The shunt is from aorta to pulmonary artery because of the low resistance of the pulmonary circuit.

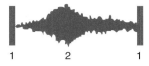

Fig. 15.6 The continuous murmur of a persistent ductus arteriosus.

features of increased pulmonary blood flow. The duct can sometimes be visualized by cross-sectional echocardiography. Enlargement of the left atrium and left ventricle on the M-mode echo confirms the presence of left ventricular volume overload.

The clinical diagnosis is usually easy because of the characteristic continuous murmur. Special investigation is seldom required even prior to surgical treatment. Care, however, is necessary to avoid confusion with the venous hum which is common in normal children. The hum is usually maximal to the right of the sternum below the right clavicle, diminishes or disappears when the child lies flat and can usually be abolished by compression of the jugular veins on the right side. Continuous murmurs due to other causes are rare and their maximum intensity is usually below and medial to the pulmonary area. When in doubt, because of the site or quality of the murmur or the lack of correlation with the electrocardiographic and radiological features, special investigation is necessary. At cardiac catheterization there is a 'step-up' in oxygen saturation in the pulmonary artery. This can be shown to result from a persistent ductus by the passage of the catheter through it into the descending aorta, or by the angiocardiographic delineation of the ductus by the injection of contrast medium into the arch of the aorta.

Surgical treatment of a persistent ductus arteriosus by division and suture carries little risk and is the correct management in almost all patients. An alternative procedure of closure is to use a catheter occluder, which is introduced via the femoral vein. An umbrella-like device with two spring-loaded discs is positioned in the duct and left there, and the catheter removed. These procedures should be performed, if possible, before the child starts school.

In symptomatic low birth weight premature infants, the ductus frequently causes life-threatening cardiac decompensation. Although immediate surgery is probably still the most successful mode of treatment, administration of indomethacin, a prostaglandin inhibitor, can induce duct closure medically. This method is, however, not always successful.

Obstructive lesions

COARCTATION OF THE AORTA

Coarctation of the aorta is a narrowing of the lumen, usually just beyond the origin of the left subclavian artery (Fig. 15.7). It is characteristically of severe degree and is commonly associated with a bicuspid aortic valve which may be or may become stenosed or allow regurgitation. The ductus arteriosus may also persist, particularly if the coarctation is proximal to its attachment to the aorta.

The systolic pressure in the aorta and its branches proximal to the coarctation is raised, but this may not be obvious in early childhood; diastolic hypertension is uncommon before adult lift and is seldom severe at rest. The hypertension may induce irreversible changes in the arterioles so that the blood pressure may not return to normal even after the removal of the coarctation.

Only a small volume of blood flows through the narrowed segment; much of the blood supply of the lower part of the body is by way of collateral vessels which attain great size. The blood pressure in the lower half of the body is lower than that in the upper half and the pulse wave takes longer to arrive.

The hypertension is eventually liable to cause left ventricular failure. Other risks include infection of the coarctation or of a bicuspid aortic valve, rupture or dissection of the ascending aorta, and cerebral haemorrhage. Cystic medial necrosis of the aortic wall, which is present in only a few patients with coarctation, is the deciding factor in rupture. Rupture of an intracranial aneurysm, which occurs in 5–10% of affected individuals, is the usual cause of subarachnoid haemorrhage.

Coarctation may produce no symptoms and is most often suspected during a routine medical examination when a systolic murmur is heard or hypertension detected. However, long segment narrowing in the pre-ductal area of the aorta is associated with heart failure in infancy. In such infants, commonly, the ductus is patent, and pulmonary hypertension is present; a VSD may coexist.

The blood pressure in the upper limbs is raised; that in the legs is normal or low. The femoral arterial pulse is small and delayed in com-

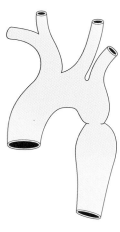

Fig. 15.7   Coarctation of the aorta. The constriction is usually in the descending aorta just below the left subclavian artery. Beyond the constriction, there is post-stenotic dilatation.

parison with the radial pulse. In adults, collateral vessels may be seen and felt along the borders of the scapulae and over the posterior chest wall. The left ventricle is occasionally enlarged. A systolic murmur is almost invariably heard over the area of the coarctation at about the level of the fourth intercostal space posteriorly, and tends to be louder than a systolic murmur which is often audible in the second intercostal spaces close to the sternum. A more continuous murmur may be heard over collaterals.

The ECG is usually normal; left ventricular hypertrophy is uncommon before adult years. The chest radiograph is seldom abnormal in childhood, but characteristically shows an abnormal aortic knuckle with an enlarged left subclavian artery and poststenotic dilatation of the aorta in adults. Another feature is notching of the undersides of the ribs due to the erosion by enlarged intercostal arteries (Fig. 15.8). The left ventricle may also be enlarged.

The diagnosis is usually made without difficulty on clinical grounds. It may be confirmed by intra-aortic pressure tracings above and below the coarctation and the precise anatomy can be outlined by aortography.

The correct treatment is surgical resection of the coarctation and restoration of the aorta by end-to-end anastomosis or, if necessary, by the insertion of a graft. This should be performed electively in childhood. None the less, hypertension may not be completely abolished or

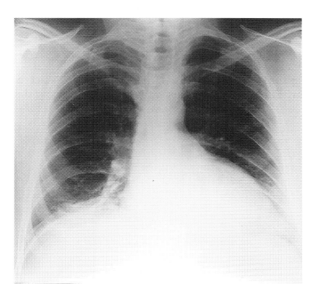

Fig. 15.8 Coarctation of the aorta. Chest radiograph in a patient with coarctation of the aorta. Prominent rib notching is apparent and the heart has a left ventricular configuration due to hypertension.

may recur later. Balloon angioplasty has been used with varying success in the treatment of coarctation, but is particularly effective in the 5–10% of patients who have a recurrence of the coarctation after surgery.

AORTIC STENOSIS

This condition is considered in Chapter 14.

HYPOPLASTIC LEFT HEART SYNDROME

This term is used to describe a number of disorders, such as mitral atresia and aortic atresia, in which the characteristic feature is virtual absence of left ventricular outflow. The diagnosis can usually be established by echocardiography, which reveals a small left ventricle and absent aortic valve. Life can be sustained if there is a large persistent ductus which allows blood to flow from the pulmonary artery to the aorta. Affected infants are intensely cyanosed and usually die within hours of birth. There is, as yet, no successful corrective operation; transplantation has been used successfully in some cases.

The abnormality can be detected at about the 18th week of pregnancy by fetal echocardiography; termination can then be considered.

PULMONARY STENOSIS

Pulmonary stenosis is almost invariably of congenital origin. Except when it is complicated by a ventricular septal defect (see 'tetralogy of Fallot', p. 312), the stenosis is usually confined to the valve cusps. These may be fused to form a cone-shaped structure with a narrow orifice. Beyond the obstruction the pulmonary artery is dilated; proximal to it the right ventricle is hypertrophied.

The obstruction to right ventricular emptying leads to a high right ventricular systolic pressure and a systolic pressure drop across the pulmonary valve (Fig. 15.9). In the more severe cases, right ventricular failure develops. If the foramen ovale is unsealed, or if there is an atrial septal defect, a right-to-left shunt with central cyanosis may develop as the right atrial pressure rises.

Although pulmonary stenosis may cause cardiac failure in the first few weeks of life, survival into late childhood or adult life is usual. Often the lesion is first detected on routine clinical examination in asymptomatic individuals, but some patients present with fatigue, breathlessness or syncope.

The arterial pulse may be normal or small. The jugular venous pulse is usually normal, but in severe grades it exhibits a large 'a' wave as the

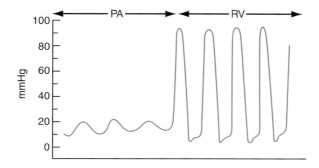

Fig. 15.9   The pressure pulse obtained as the catheter is withdrawn from pulmonary artery to right ventricle in pulmonary valve stenosis.

right atrium contracts forcibly in the face of the non-compliant hypertrophied right ventricle. On palpation, there is nearly always a systolic thrill in the second left intercostal space; the left parasternal heave of right ventricular hypertrophy can sometimes be felt. The first heart sound is normal, but it is often followed by an early systolic 'ejection' click and a loud midsystolic murmur best heard in the second left intercostal space. The second sound is normal in the mild case, but in the more severe it is split abnormally widely and the second (pulmonary) element is soft.

The electrocardiogram indicates the severity of the pulmonary valve stenosis for, in general, the greater the ECG features of right ventricular hypertrophy, the tighter the stenosis. The chest radiograph shows the post-stenotic dilatation of the pulmonary artery. In severe cases, right ventricular hypertrophy and diminution in the pulmonary vascular markings may be detected.

An accurate diagnosis can usually be made clinically. Cardiac catheterization provides confirmatory evidence; the systolic pressure difference across the pulmonary valve is a valuable index of severity, a drop of more than 50 mmHg suggesting severe stenosis (Fig. 15.9). Doppler ultrasonography provides reliable evidence of the severity of the stenosis, and is particularly valuable as a means of follow-up. Unless the foramen ovale is unsealed or there is an associated atrial septal defect, no intracardiac shunting can be detected.

A minor degree of pulmonary stenosis is compatible with a normal life span. When the stenosis is more severe, death is likely to ensue sooner or later from right ventricular failure; relief of the stenosis should not be delayed too long as irreversible fibrotic changes take place in the hypertrophied right ventricle. Balloon valvoplasty is an effective and safe method of enlarging the valve orifice but the long-term results are not yet known. Surgical valvotomy is a low risk alternative.

TRICUSPID ATRESIA

In this relatively uncommon disorder, there is absence of the normal atrioventricular connection on the right side. For life to be sustained in the extra-uterine state, an atrial septal defect and a ventricular septal defect must be present. Frequently there is associated pulmonary stenosis or pulmonary atresia and, more rarely, transposition of the great arteries. The left ventricle is large and the hypoplastic right ventricle receives blood by the VSD. Cyanosis in infancy is the rule. The ECG shows left axis deviation and left ventricular hypertrophy. Cross-sectional echocardiography reveals the absent connection and can also demonstrate the VSD and ASD.

Balloon septostomy or the surgical creation of an aortopulmonary shunt is life saving in the severely affected infant. In later childhood a conduit is inserted between the right atrium and the right ventricular outflow tract or pulmonary artery (Fontan procedure).

Combined obstructive and shunt lesions

PULMONARY STENOSIS AND VENTRICULAR SEPTAL DEFECT (TETRALOGY OF FALLOT)

When pulmonary stenosis coexists with a ventricular septal defect, the stenosis may be slight and shunting exclusively from left to right. In most cases, however, pulmonary stenosis is severe and the ventricular septal defect large, and there is a right-to-left shunt. These abnormalities are the major features of the 'tetralogy of Fallot', of which the other components are dextroposition of the aorta (with the aortic root overriding the defect) and right ventricular hypertrophy (Fig. 15.10). The pulmonary stenosis is situated in the infundibulum of the right ventricle and, often, at the pulmonary valve as well. The infundibular stenosis tends to become more severe with advancing age and there is a

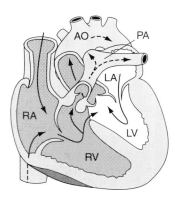

Fig. 15.10 Tetralogy of Fallot. Note infundibular pulmonary stenosis and ventricular septal defect, with right-to-left shunt at ventricular level.

progressive increase in the proportion of blood shunted from right to left.

In the most severe cases, symptoms start soon after birth. More frequently, cyanosis develops in the second half of the first year or not until later in childhood.

With increasing cyanosis, dyspnoea becomes more severe. The child is liable to sudden attacks of intense cyanosis, sometimes associated with syncope, for which spasm of the infundibulum of the right ventricle may be responsible. Children with the tetralogy of Fallot are liable to squat after exercise. It is believed that the squatting position, by compressing the abdominal aorta and the femoral arteries, increases the arterial resistance and therefore diminishes the right-to-left shunt at the ventricular level.

The child is often abnormally small and has central cyanosis with finger clubbing. The arterial pulses are small and venous pulses normal. Clinical evidence of right ventricular hypertrophy is slight. There is a loud systolic murmur accompanied by a thrill in the second or third left intercostal space unless the stenosis is so severe that virtually no blood traverses it. The second heart sound is single because the pulmonary valve component is inaudible. The electrocardiogram shows moderate right ventricular hypertrophy. The chest radiograph is characteristic in showing a 'boot-shaped' heart with a concavity on the left border in the place where the pulmonary artery is normally seen, and a prominent and elevated apex (Fig. 15.11). The pulmonary vascularity is decreased. Echocardiography shows that the aorta is large and overrides the septum, the normal continuity between the anterior aortic wall and septum being lost. Polycythaemia, secondary to the cyanosis, is usual.

The tetralogy of Fallot is the underlying lesion in 70% of children with central cyanosis over the age of 3. This frequency and the characteristic clinical, electrocardiographic and radiological features usually make the diagnosis easy in childhood. In infancy and also in later life, a confident diagnosis can less often be reached without further investigation.

On cardiac catheterization, a systolic pressure drop can be demonstrated between the body and the outflow tract of the right ventricle. Pressures in the right and left ventricles are identical. The oxygen saturation in the aorta is reduced. Injection of radio-opaque contrast medium into the right ventricle delineates the region of stenosis and demonstrates the shunt through the ventricular septal defect.

Patients with severe pulmonary stenosis and large ventricular septal defects often die in childhood and rarely reach middle age without surgery. Death may result from hypoxic episodes during childhood, from cerebrovascular accidents as a result of thrombosis promoted by polycythaemia, from infective endocarditis and from cerebral abscesses. Virtually all patients require surgery at some stage, but the type of surgery depends upon the severity of the lesion and the age.

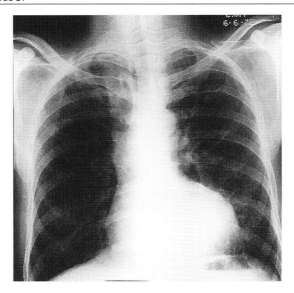

Fig. 15.11   Tetralogy of Fallot. The heart shadow is typically 'boot-shaped' with a concavity of the left heart border, instead of the normal pulmonary artery shadow. The apex is high and rounded. The lung fields are oligaemic.

Ideally, the abnormality should be totally corrected by relief of the pulmonary stenosis and by closure of the ventricular septal defect. In severely affected infants, some surgeons prefer to perform a palliative procedure first, such as the creation of a shunt between the aorta and pulmonary circulations, either directly or by anastomosing the subclavian artery to the pulmonary artery. This increases the proportion of blood going through the lungs and thus becoming oxygenated. The child can be given several years of comparatively good health before the corrective procedure is performed.

Severe hypoxic attacks should be treated with oxygen and morphine (0.1 mg/kg). The baby should be placed in the knee–chest position. Blood pCO_2 and pH should be estimated and sodium bicarbonate given intravenously as necessary. Propranolol is possibly of value.

HIGH PULMONARY VASCULAR RESISTANCE WITH RIGHT-TO-LEFT SHUNT THROUGH A SEPTAL DEFECT OR DUCTUS ARTERIOSUS (EISENMENGER SYNDROME)

Eisenmenger originally described a patient with a ventricular septal defect with central cyanosis in the absence of pulmonary stenosis. It is now known that the reason for the right-to-left shunt in such cases is the presence of a severe pulmonary vascular disease. Because the clinical pictures of pulmonary hypertension with right-to-left shunt are so similar, irrespective of whether the shunt is at atrial, ventricular or aorto-pulmonary level, the term Eisenmenger syndrome is employed to describe all three lesions.

The cause of the pulmonary vascular disease responsible for the pulmonary hypertension is unknown. Factors which may be involved include:

- lack of regression of the fetal type of pulmonary vasculature;
- prolonged exposure to high pulmonary blood flow;
- prolonged exposure to high pulmonary blood pressure;
- genetic predisposition.

Although irreversible pulmonary arterial changes may develop during early childhood, they more commonly occur during adolescence. Dyspnoea and fatigue, which are usually the first symptoms, are liable to develop in late childhood, adolescence or early adult life. Other complaints include syncope, angina pectoris, oedema and haemoptysis.

On examination the patient is usually cyanosed. When the shunt is through a ductus arteriosus, the venous blood is directed into the descending aorta and only the lower limbs become cyanosed ('differential cyanosis').

The arterial pulse is usually small, due to a low stroke volume; a large 'a' wave may be present in the venous pulse, due to forceful atrial contraction in the face of right ventricular hypertrophy. On palpation, one can detect right ventricular hypertrophy and the shock of pulmonary valve closure. On auscultation, the signs are mainly those of pulmonary hypertension: a loud second heart sound, a right ventricular fourth heart sound, a pulmonary early systolic ('ejection') click and, occasionally, the early diastolic murmur of pulmonary regurgitation and the pansystolic murmur of functional tricuspid regurgitation. In atrial septal defect, the second sound remains split on expiration (because only the right ventricle is overburdened). In ventricular septal defect, there is a single second sound, because the pressure in both ventricles is identical. In persistent ductus arteriosus, there is normal splitting of the second heart sound.

The ECG shows right atrial and right ventricular hypertrophy. On the chest radiograph there are large main pulmonary arteries but small peripheral arteries, together with right ventricular and right atrial enlargement. Cross-sectional echocardiography can reliably demonstrate the ventricular or atrial septal defects in these patients.

The diagnosis is suggested by the combination of central cyanosis and pulmonary hypertension in an adolescent or young adult. The Eisenmenger syndrome differs from the tetralogy of Fallot (the commonest cardiac cause of central cyanosis in this age group) in there being no pulmonary systolic thrill or loud murmur, in the greater severity of right ventricular hypertrophy, and in the large pulmonary arteries on the chest radiograph. The diagnosis can be confirmed by demonstrating by cardiac catheterization that the pulmonary artery pressure equals the systemic pressure, and by angiocardiographic delineation of the shunt. The progress of the Eisenmenger syndrome is usually slowly downhill, death commonly occurring between the ages of 20 and 40. The main causes of death are pulmonary infarction, right heart failure and arrhythmias and, less often, infective endocarditis. Pregnancy is particularly hazardous in these patients and should be avoided or terminated early.

No surgical treatment, other than heart–lung transplantation, is of value because the major defect is the irreversible change in the small pulmonary arteries. Temporary benefit may result from the conventional treatment of cardiac failure.

Displacement lesions

TRANSPOSITION OF THE GREAT ARTERIES (Fig. 15.12)

In transposition of the great arteries, the aorta arises from the right ventricle and the pulmonary artery from the left. As a consequence, there are separate systemic and pulmonary circulations; life cannot be sustained unless there is some communication between them. Usually there is one or more of the following:

- a patent foramen ovale;
- an atrial septal defect;
- a ventricular septal defect;
- a persistent ductus arteriosus.

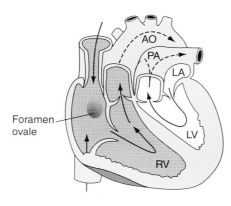

Fig. 15.12 Transposition of the great arteries. The aorta arises from the right ventricle and the pulmonary artery from the left. Life can be sustained only if communications exist between systemic and pulmonary circulations.

The infant is characteristically of normal size and well nourished. Cyanosis develops at birth or shortly thereafter. There is difficulty in completing feeds; increasing breathlessness, deep cyanosis, cardiac failure and death are usual within the first month.

On auscultation there may be a gallop rhythm and a systolic murmur.

The chest radiograph may show little abnormality at birth, but within a few days the heart becomes enlarged and the vascularity of the lung fields increased. The ECG shows little more than the right ventricular preponderance normal for this age group.

Echocardiography is an invaluable diagnostic tool. It permits observation of the aorta, arising from the right ventricle and lying anterior to the pulmonary artery, and also allows detection of other defects.

Transposition of the great arteries is the most common cardiac cause of cyanosis at birth and of overt heart failure in cyanotic congenital heart disease within the first few weeks of life. Accurate diagnosis at this stage is urgent; it is usually fatal to await the effects of medical treatment. Investigation should be undertaken within a matter of hours. Echocardiography is of diagnostic value in showing the abnormal connections of the great arteries. If it supports the diagnosis, it is usually then necessary to proceed to cardiac catheterization which not only enables the precise nature of the anomalies to be determined but is an essential preliminary to therapy.

In the acutely ill infant, great improvement can be achieved by producing a large defect in the atrial septum to allow mixing of the blood between systemic and pulmonary circulations (Rashkind procedure). This is done by introducing a catheter with a deflated balloon at its tip into the femoral vein and advancing it via the right atrium and foramen ovale into the left atrium. The balloon is then inflated and withdrawn abruptly so as to tear the atrial septum. This procedure is usually effective in the neonatal period and allows the child to live until the latter part of the first year of life when the venous return to the two ventricles is rerouted by the insertion of an intra-atrial baffle. This operation can be carried out with a low mortality rate. An alternative procedure – the 'switch' operation – is now the preferred choice for most cases in major centres. In this procedure, the surgeon detaches the aorta and pulmonary artery, and connects each to its appropriate ventricle.

EBSTEIN'S ANOMALY

In this disorder, the posteromedial part of the tricuspid valve ring is displaced towards the apex of the right ventricle. An atrial septal defect is usually present.

Dyspnoea, fatigue and arrhythmias are usual. Cyanosis may be present if there is an atrial septal defect. There are often scratchy tricuspid systolic, mid-diastolic and presystolic murmurs, arising from flow across the abnormal tricuspid valve. Tall P waves, a long PR interval and a low-voltage right bundle branch block pattern are the usual ECG features. The chest radiograph shows a large right atrium and clear lung fields. Echocardiography demonstrates the abnormal position and movement of the tricuspid valve cusp.

Death usually results from arrhythmias in childhood or early adult life, but may occur later from cardiac failure or hypoxaemia.

Partial correction, with prosthetic replacement of the tricuspid valve and repair of the atrial septal defect is indicated for the disabled case but this neither restores normal function nor prevents arrhythmias.

DEXTROCARDIA

Dextrocardia refers to all situations where the heart is in the right chest. The lung and abdominal situs or arrangement may be reversed or normal. When dextrocardia exists with complete right–left reversal of the lungs and viscera then the heart is usually normal, but the ECG can be very misleading if the condition is not recognized. When the heart is in the right chest and the other organs are normally sited, or if the heart is in the left chest (laevocardia) and the other organs reversed, then the chance of complex congenital cardiac lesions is high.

RIGHT-SIDED AORTA

In this condition, the aorta turns posteriorly and runs down on the right of the trachea and the oesophagus instead of arching upwards and to the left. It may continue to descend in this direction or may cross behind the trachea and oesophagus and attain the normal left-sided course.

As an isolated anomaly it is of no clinical significance. When associated with a congenital lesion of the heart, its detection may be of diagnostic assistance for it is found in 20–25% of patients with the tetralogy of Fallot. When associated with other arterial anomalies the trachea and oesophagus may be encircled and obstructive symptoms result.

The diagnosis and management of the infant with heart failure and cyanosis

The general paediatrician and the general practitioner have the responsibility of detecting heart disease in the newborn; an expert in neonatal cardiology should be contacted without delay if there is any evidence of cyanosis or heart failure. All too frequently, the clinical evidence of heart disease is overlooked until it is too late.

Central cyanosis is a serious finding in the newborn. If it persists after exposure to oxygen therapy, and there is no evident respiratory or cerebral cause, congenital heart disease should be suspected. If the cyanosis is indeed due to congenital heart disease, the prognosis without treatment is poor. Echocardiography should be undertaken immediately. The findings of this investigation may suggest that cardiac catheterization is required; this can be combined with therapy (e.g. the Rashkind procedure, see p. 317).

The commonest causes of cardiac failure, with or without cyanosis, in the newborn are ventricular septal defect, persistent ductus arteriosus, hypoplastic left heart, coarctation of the aorta and transposition.

The early signs of heart failure are tachypnoea, tachycardia, gallop rhythm and enlargement of the liver. Cyanosis is often present as well. The venous pressure is a poor guide to heart failure in infants. Crepitations and rhonchi are common and should not be attributed to pulmonary disease until left ventricular failure has been excluded. Oedema, which is most likely to affect the backs of the hands and feet, is a late sign, and is common in the absence of heart failure in premature infants.

Tachycardia may be difficult to assess because the pulse rate is normally fast in infants, but it seldom exceeds 140/min during sleep in the healthy baby or in those with respiratory disease. If the rate is in excess of 210/min, there is a supraventricular tachycardia requiring urgent treatment. If the heart rate is less than 50/min, heart block is almost certainly present.

Thirty per cent oxygen should be given to all infants who are cyanosed or in cardiac failure. The air should be humidified. Measurement of the blood gases and the correction of acidosis is an essential part of the proper management of heart failure in infancy. Frusemide starting with an oral dose of 2 μg/kg is first choice in severe failure. Digoxin may also be of value starting with 40–60 μg/kg by mouth or 40 μg/kg intramuscularly. Good nursing, temperature and humidity control, supportive frames or suspension in the propped-up position and tube feeding are essential in the early stages of treatment. Sedation with trimeprazine or promethazine may be required.

These medical measures are quite often successful in correcting cardiac failure due to a ventricular septal defect or persistent ductus arteriosus. The cyanotic infant is in a precarious state and may be dependent on a patent ductus; deterioration takes place as the ductus closes. This can usually be prevented by the intravenous infusion of prostaglandins.

Further reading

Anderson, R. H., Macartney, F. J., Shinebourne, E. A. & Tynan, M. (1987) *Paediatric Cardiology.* Edinburgh: Churchill Livingstone.
Perloff, J. K. (1987) *The Clinical Recognition of Congenital Heart Disease,* 3rd edn. Philadelphia: Saunders.

Hypertension and Heart Disease

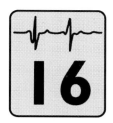

Hypertension is a major risk factor for cardiovascular morbidity and mortality. It accelerates the process of atherosclerosis in the coronary, cerebral and renal arteries, as well as increasing the workload of the heart. As a result, the hypertensive patient is at risk of developing myocardial infarction, stroke, renal failure and congestive cardiac failure. In total, hypertension is probably directly or indirectly responsible for 10–20% of all deaths.

For reasons that will become apparent, it is impossible to define hypertension. For practical purposes, the blood pressure may be regarded as abnormally high if it persistently exceeds 150/95 mmHg in a quietly resting individual. This does not imply that individuals with raised pressure necessarily require treatment. The presence of other risk factors and evidence of target organ damage from hypertension must be taken into account before initiating treatment that is likely to be life-long.

The concept of normal blood pressure

Within populations, blood pressure, like height and weight, is normally distributed. There is, therefore, no clear separation between hypertension and normotension. Within individuals, the level of arterial pressure is determined by the cardiac output and peripheral vascular resistance, two factors that vary widely from individual to individual, and within one individual at different times. Marked variations have been observed in individuals in whom the blood pressure is continuously monitored throughout the day. The mean pressure during sleep may be 30 mmHg lower than it is in the waking state. Factors that transiently increase pressure include anxiety and cold. Exercise leads to a brisk rise in systolic pressure but little change in the diastolic pressure. A transient doubling of systolic pressure may occur at the climax of coitus.

Certain identifiable factors are associated with persistently high blood pressure. Thus, at least in Western societies, both diastolic and systolic pressure increase with age. The blood pressure averages about 80/60 mmHg at birth and rises slowly throughout childhood. The resting blood pressure in the adolescent is often in the region of 120/70 mmHg, whilst in middle age 140/80 mmHg is more common. The systolic pressure often continues to rise into old age as the aorta becomes increasingly rigid. However, in many individuals and throughout some societies (e.g. in some Pacific islands) hypertension is virtually non-existent and there is no rise with age. In the younger age groups, males, on average, have higher pressures than females, but this tendency is reversed after the age of 45. Obese individuals tend to have pressures higher than can be accounted for by recording errors due to increased arm circumference.

The variability of arterial pressures within one individual and between individuals makes it impossible to define normality. It has been established, however, that the higher the pressure even within the 'normal' range, whether systolic or diastolic, the more likely the individual is to develop life-threatening cardiovascular disease processes including coronary artery disease, cerebrovascular disease and renal disease.

Classification of hypertension (Table 16.1)

Normal adult blood pressure has been defined as a systolic blood pressure equal to or below 140 mmHg together with a diastolic (fifth Korotkoff phase) equal to or below 90 mmHg.

Hypertension may be regarded as 'mild' if the diastolic pressure is between 90 and 104 mmHg, 'moderate' if between 105 and 114 mmHg, and 'severe' if above this. Hypertension is said to be in the *malignant* or accelerated phase if there is widespread arterial fibrinoid necrosis. The diastolic pressure is very high (often above 130 mmHg) with retinal haemorrhages and exudates and frequently papilloedema.

Although the unqualified term 'hypertension' generally refers to elevation of the diastolic blood pressure, it is also possible to define systolic hypertension. A systolic pressure above 160 mmHg is regarded as abnormal, even when the diastolic pressure is within normal limits.

Table 16.1   Definitions of hypertension

Diastolic pressure (mmHg)	
<85	Normal
85–90	High normal
90–104	Mild hypertension
105–114	Moderate hypertension
>115	Severe hypertension
Systolic pressure (mmHg)	
<140	Normal
140–159	Borderline isolated systolic hypertension
>160	Isolated systolic hypertension (disastolic < 90 mmHg)

AETIOLOGY OF HYPERTENSION

In 95% of patients with high blood pressure, no specific cause can be identified. This condition is termed 'essential' or 'primary' hypertension. In approximately 5% of hypertensive patients, a specific cause can be identified and the hypertension is termed 'secondary'. Although secondary hypertension accounts for a small minority of all hypertensive patients, it is important to identify this condition because specific and potentially curative treatment may be available.

Essential hypertension

Although no single cause has been identified for this condition, a number of factors have been shown to influence the development of essential hypertension:

Genetic influences. The influence of heredity is unquestioned, hypertension being many times more common in the families of hypertensive patients than in those of normotensive individuals. Although some have suggested that hypertension is due to a single dominant gene, most of the evidence points to the influence of many genes.

Dietary influences. There is an undoubted relationship between weight and blood pressure. Weight loss in the obese substantially lowers the blood pressure. Very low salt intake appears to protect against hypertension, but there is little evidence to incriminate excessive sodium chloride intake as a cause of high blood pressure. A high potassium intake may be protective. There is some evidence that a high intake of saturated fats may raise blood pressure. High alcohol consumption has been identified as a risk factor for hypertension, as has cigarette smoking, at least in regard to the malignant phase.

Physical activity. Physical exercise can reduce blood pressure in hypertensive subjects. This suggests that inactivity may play a role in the genesis of hypertension in some individuals.

Hormonal changes. Hormonal changes are implicated in a number of causes of secondary hypertension. The possibility that hormonal changes might also be involved in the pathogenesis of essential hypertension has attracted particular interest. Attention has concentrated on the adrenergic and renin–angiotensin systems, but there is as yet no clear evidence indicating a primary role for either system in the genesis of essential hypertension.

Haemodynamic changes. A slight sinus tachycardia and a high cardiac output may be found in early hypertensives before there is a rise in peripheral resistance. These features may result from an excessive adrenergic influence. There is good evidence that baroreceptors are reset in hypertension, as bradycardia is not induced by the rise in pressure.

Secondary hypertension

The most common causes of secondary hypertension are renal disease, adrenal disease, coarctation of the aorta and drug-related hypertension (Table 16.2).

Renal disease

All forms of parenchymal renal disease can be associated with significant hypertension. These include acute and chronic glomerulonephritis, chronic pyelonephritis and polycystic kidney disease.

Renal artery stenosis as a cause of hypertension deserves special consideration. In this condition, the stenosis may be unilateral or bilateral and may take the form of a fibromuscular narrowing in young patients or atheromatous narrowing in older patients, who will often have evidence of atherosclerosis elsewhere. Renal artery stenosis results in ischaemia of the kidney with high circulating levels of

Table 16.2   The causes of secondary hypertension

Renal
   Acute glomerulonephritis
   Chronic glomerulonephritis
   Chronic pyelonephritis
   Polycystic kidneys
   Renal artery stenosis
   Diabetic nephropathy

Endocrine
   Adrenal
   Primary aldosteronism
   Cushing's syndrome
   Phaeochromocytoma
   Acromegaly
   Exogenous hormones
   Oral contraceptives
   Glucocorticoids
   Mineralocorticoids – liquorice

Coarctation of the aorta

Pregnancy

Neurological

Raised intracranial pressure

---

angiotensin II. High levels of angiotensin II then lead to hypertension by two different mechanisms (Fig. 16.1). Hypertension in these patients is often relatively resistant to drug treatment. Angiotensin-converting enzyme (ACE) inhibitors, by preventing the release of angiotensin II, will lower the blood pressure markedly but should be avoided in patients suspected of having renal artery stenosis because they reduce renal perfusion and may result in renal infarction. If a patient has bilateral renal artery stenoses, the introduction of an ACE inhibitor can precipitate acute renal failure.

Abdominal ultrasonography provides a simple non-invasive means of assessing renal anatomy in patients with a suspected renal cause for hypertension. In patients with chronic nephritis, kidney size is reduced. In patients with pyelonephritis, there is likely to be dilatation of the calyceal system. In unilateral renal artery stenosis, kidney size is reduced on the side of the stenosis. If renal artery stenosis is suspected, then renal arteriography remains the investigation of choice although the diagnosis can now often be made using either spiral computed tomography (CT) or magnetic resonance imaging (MRI). If the patient is shown to have either unilateral or bilateral renal artery stenosis, then renal revascularization either by renal artery angioplasty or by a surgical approach should be considered. If there is doubt as to whether a renal artery lesion is the cause of hypertension, bilateral renal vein sampling of plasma renin activity may be helpful; high levels of renin

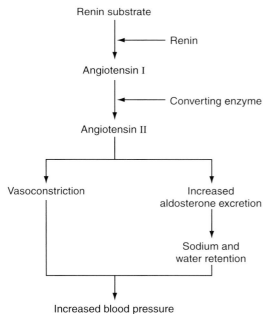

Fig. 16.1 The renin–angiotensin system.

activity coming from the affected site would suggest that the stenosis is significant and that revascularization would probably improve blood pressure control.

Endocrine disease

Cushing's syndrome. This results from cortisol excess and may be due to hyperplasia of the adrenal cortex, adrenal tumours, or to the excessive administration of glucocorticoids or adrenocorticotrophic hormone (ACTH). Adrenal hyperplasia is often the result of increased ACTH production by a pituitary microadenoma.

Hypertension, which occurs in more than 50% of cases, may be severe and proceed to the malignant phase. Other features of the syndrome are muscle weakness, osteoporosis, purple cutaneous striae, obesity of the trunk, a 'buffalo' hump, a 'moon' facies and diabetes mellitus. There may also be hirsutism, amenorrhoea, a liability to spontaneous bruising, and dependent oedema.

Diagnosis. The diagnosis should be suggested by the combination of hypertension, diabetes and truncal obesity. Investigations include:

- excessive 24-h urinary free cortisol excretion;
- failure to suppress plasma cortisol levels following dexamethasone administration;
- the ACTH levels are valuable in determining the cause, being high with pituitary tumours and low if the adrenal is responsible;
- CT or MRI imaging of the adrenal glands.

Management. Treatment depends upon the aetiology of the condition. Surgical removal of one or both adrenal glands or of a pituitary tumour may be necessary.

Primary aldosteronism. Aldosterone, which is secreted by the zona glomerulosa of the adrenal cortex, promotes sodium reabsorption and potassium excretion in the distal tubules of the kidney. Normally, aldosterone secretion is largely regulated by angiotensin, but in primary aldosteronism there is an overproduction of aldosterone as a result of an adrenal cortical adenoma (Conn's syndrome) or bilateral hyperplasia; angiotensin and, therefore, plasma renin levels are abnormally low. The condition occurs most often in young and middle-aged females. Because of the mode of action of aldosterone, the symptoms and signs are related to sodium retention, hypokalaemia and hypertension. Frequently, the patient presents with mild to moderate hypertension, but the predominant complaints are those of muscle weakness, headache, thirst and polyuria. The hypertension is seldom severe and malignant changes are rare. There is usually hypokalaemia, with a serum potassium level of less than 3.0 mmol/litre, and a serum sodium concentration that is normal or high. Characteristically, there is a metabolic alkalosis and a low serum chloride level. The diagnosis should be suspected in patients with hypertension and hypokalaemia, particularly if this is associated with hypernatraemia. However, hypokalaemia is not uncommon in other hypertensive patients, particularly if they have been treated with diuretics. Furthermore, patients with malignant hypertension develop 'secondary aldosteronism' with low serum potassium. These patients usually do not have a high serum sodium.

Diagnosis. The diagnosis is suggested by:

* hypokalaemia, persisting after stopping diuretic therapy;
* excessive urinary potassium loss;
* elevated plasma aldosterone levels;
* suppressed renin levels which fail to rise on assumption of an upright posture;
* CT or MRI imaging is now the investigation of choice in establishing the presence of an adenoma and differentiating this from hyperplasia.

Management. Adenomas should be removed surgically. Patients with hyperplasia should be treated medically with spironolactone or amiloride, which antagonize the actions of aldosterone.

Phaeochromocytoma. Phaeochromocytoma arises in chromaffin tissue, usually in the adrenal gland. It is sometimes described as the '10% tumour'. This is because 10% are said to arise outwith the adrenal gland, 10% are malignant and 10% are bilateral. The tumours usually secrete noradrenaline (norepinephrine), but adrenaline (epinephrine) may predominate.

Phaeochromocytomas may produce either paroxysmal or persistent hypertension. The paroxysms are associated with the sudden onset of bilateral headache, and with perspiration, palpitation and pallor (features often regarded as neurotic). The attacks usually last from a few minutes to an hour. If the hypertension is persistent, the clinical picture is that of severe hypertension, often of the malignant variety. Because of the hypermetabolic state induced by the phaeochromocytoma, the patients are rarely obese.

Diagnosis. The diagnosis should be suspected in any severe case of hypertension, particularly if the hypertension is paroxysmal. The diagnosis is confirmed by:

* excessive excretion of the catecholamine metabolite vanilmandelic acid (VMA) in the urine is a useful screening test;
* urine and plasma catecholamine levels;
* CT to localize the tumour.

Management. Phaeochromocytomas should be removed surgically. This is a potentially hazardous procedure and requires close control of the blood pressure and careful anaesthesia. Beta-adrenergic blocking drugs should not be used alone because unopposed alpha-adrenergic activation may aggravate hypertension and lead to serious complications such as stroke. This can be avoided by the initial use of an alpha-adrenergic blocking drug. The non-competitive alpha-antagonist phenoxybenzamine is frequently chosen. Once alpha-adrenergic blockade is fully established, beta-blockade can be added.

Coarctation of the aorta

This is a congenital condition associated with a narrowing of the lumen of the aorta just beyond the origin of the left subclavian artery. It is described in more detail in Chapter 15.

Drug-related causes

The oral contraceptive pill may lead to a small rise in arterial pressure but this is now much less common than 30 years ago when higher doses of oestrogen were used. It is wise, however, to check the blood pressure within a few months of starting the oral contraceptive pill. Other drugs that may be associated with hypertension include steroids (see under Cushing's syndrome), carbenoxolone and liquorice.

PATHOPHYSIOLOGY OF HYPERTENSION

The high blood pressure in essential hypertension is due to increased peripheral vascular resistance as a result of widespread constriction of the arterioles and small arteries. The cardiac output and the viscosity of the blood are normal. In the earlier stages, the hypertension is largely explicable on the basis of increased arteriolar muscle tone, but subsequently structural alterations take place in the arterioles. These changes may account for the fact that hypertension tends to beget further hypertension, and the removal of the cause of hypertension does not necessarily lead to a fall in the blood pressure to normal.

In the heart, there are two major consequences of sustained hypertension. The increased work of the heart imposed by the higher resistance results in hypertrophy of the myocardial cells. As this process progresses, the myocardial hypertrophy may outstrip the coronary blood supply; this occurs particularly in the subendocardial layers which are the most vulnerable to ischaemia. Just as in the peripheral vessels, fibrous tissue is then deposited in the subendocardium leading to reduced ventricular compliance and, ultimately, to heart failure. The second effect of hypertension is to accelerate the development of atherosclerosis. This occurs not only in the coronary arteries but also in the cerebral arteries, particularly those of the basal ganglia, and in the renal arteries. The mechanism of this action is less clear but may be related to long-standing mechanical stresses; in experimental situations, hypertension, like cigarette smoking and hypercholesterolaemia, has been shown to induce dysfunction of the endothelial layer of the coronary arteries which, in turn, is thought to herald the development of atherosclerosis.

There are racial differences in the pathophysiological effects of hypertension on the heart. In negro patients, 'pressure' effects with the development of severe left ventricular hypertrophy and subsequent left ventricular failure are more common than in caucasian patients, who are more likely to present with the clinical consequences of atherosclerosis.

Examination and investigation of the hypertensive patient

Most patients with hypertension are asymptomatic, the high blood pressure usually having been noted during an incidental clinical examination. A proportion will present with a major complication of hypertension such as stroke or myocardial infarction, but only a small number will present with symptoms directly attributable to hypertension such as breathlessness or headache.

Examination and investigation should be directed towards the detection of an underlying cause of hypertension (see Secondary hypertension) and the assessment of end-organ damage, which may influence the decision to treat the patient. Blood pressure levels should be recorded after the patient has been lying quietly for 5 min.

Examination of the hypertensive patient.   Clinical examination should take note of:

Signs suggestive of secondary hypertension

- features of endocrine abnormalities, particularly Cushing's syndrome;
- multiple neurofibromatoma – present in 5% of patients with phaeochromocytoma;
- inappropriate tachycardia, suggesting catecholamine excess;
- abdominal or loin bruits, suggesting renal artery stenosis;
- renal enlargement (suggestive of polycystic kidney disease);
- radiofemoral delay, due to coarction of the aorta.

Signs suggestive of end-organ damage

- a forcible and displaced apex beat due to left ventricular hypertrophy;

- accentuation of the aortic component of the second sound;
- added heart sounds. A fourth sound may be audible, reflecting decreased ventricular compliance. As failure develops a third sound may occur;
- fundal examination to detect hypertensive retinopathy.

Fundoscopy.   Examination of the optic fundus is of great importance in the evaluation of patients with hypertension, for it is only in the retina that the state of the arterioles can be directly observed. The grading introduced by Keith, Wagener and Barker is widely used:

- grade 1 – increased tortuosity of the retinal arteries with increased reflectiveness, termed silver wiring;
- grade 2 – grade 1 with the addition of compression of the veins at arteriovenous crossings (AV nipping);
- grade 3 – grade 2 with the addition of flame-shaped haemorrhages and 'cotton wool' exudates;
- grade 4 – grade 3 with the addition of papilloedema – the optic disc is pink with blurred edges and the optic cup is obliterated.

Investigation of the hypertensive patient.   Routine investigation of all hypertensive patients should include:

- *chest radiography.* Cardiac enlargement is usually a sign of left ventricular dilatation.
- *an ECG.* This is usually normal in patients with mild hypertension but may show evidence of left ventricular hypertrophy. This is characterized by tall R waves in the lateral chest leads and deep S waves in the antero-septal leads. In severe hypertrophy, or if there is accompanying ischaemic heart disease, the T waves in the lateral chest leads become flattened and then inverted, and the ST segment may show down-sloping depression in the same leads. This is the so-called 'left ventricular hypertrophy and strain' pattern (Fig. 16.2) which carries a high risk of major events including sudden death (30–40% 5-year mortality rate).
- *urinalysis.* Proteinuria, hyaline and granular casts may be found when there is renal disease or malignant hypertension. There is little or no protein in the urine of patients with benign essential hypertension.
- *urea and electrolyte.* A raised level of urea suggests renal impairment, which may be the cause or an effect of hypertension. A low serum potassium concentration in the absence of diuretic therapy might suggest Conn's or Cushing's syndrome.
- *lipids.* Although not directly related to the blood pressure, an increased level of cholesterol is a powerful risk factor for cardiovascular events, which may require specific treatment and which should be monitored in all hypertensive patients.

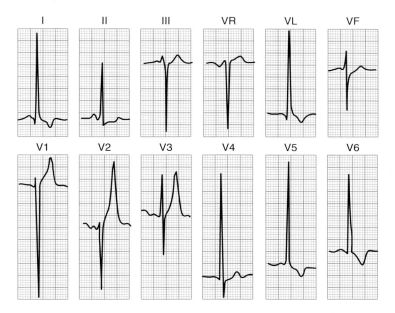

Fig. 16.2 ECG showing left ventricular hypertrophy and 'strain' in a patient with severe hypertension. This pattern is characterized by large voltages in the chest leads and the presence of ST segment depression and T wave inversion in leads V5 and V6.

The following additional investigations may also be helpful:

- *24-h ambulatory blood pressure monitoring.* In this technique, the patient wears a sphygmomanometer cuff for a period of 24 h while going about their normal activities. The cuff is connected to an automatic inflation device and to a recorder which records the blood pressure at regular intervals, usually every 15–30 min. Opinion is divided as to the usefulness of this technique. Blood pressure levels are generally lower during ambulatory recordings than during single clinic visits. The finding of high clinic readings and substantially lower ambulatory readings is sometimes used to reassure patients that they do not have 'sustained' hypertension, and the phrase 'white coat hypertension' has been coined. However, the benefits of treating hypertension have all been based on clinic blood pressure readings and there are no comparable data showing what levels of ambulatory blood pressure are 'safe' and unlikely to benefit from treatment.
- *echocardiography.* Echocardiography is much more sensitive than the ECG in detecting left ventricular hypertrophy. In patients with borderline hypertension, therefore, the finding of

echocardiographic left ventricular hypertrophy, which is associated with an increased risk of cardiovascular events, might influence the clinician in favour of starting the patient on antihypertensive medication.

- *detailed investigation of suspected secondary hypertension.* This may involve CT or MRI of the adrenal glands, renal angiography and 24-h urine collections for catecholamines.

It is impractical to screen all hypertensive patients for secondary causes of hypertension. Selection of patient groups for further investigation is arbitrary, but investigation is particularly appropriate in the following groups:

- young patients under 40 years of age;
- patients with malignant hypertension;
- patients resistant to antihypertensive therapy;
- patients with unusual symptoms (such as sweating attacks or weakness) which might suggest an underlying cause;
- patients with abnormal renal function, proteinuria or haematuria;
- patients with hypokalaemia off diuretic therapy.

The nature and scale of further investigations will be determined by the index of suspicion of a secondary cause for hypertension.

THE DECISION TO TREAT

Almost all patients with untreated malignant hypertension die within 1 year. Death is usually due to uraemia but heart failure and cerebrovascular accidents are common. In these patients, and in those with moderate to severe hypertension, there is clear evidence that treatment prolongs life.

The situation in patients with mild essential hypertension is more complicated. If the diastolic blood pressure is greater than 100 mmHg on multiple readings over a period of 3–4 months, then treatment is probably indicated. If the diastolic pressure is in the range of 95–100 mmHg, treatment should be started if there is evidence of end-organ damage. This might include left ventricular hypertrophy by ECG or echo criteria, evidence on blood testing of renal dysfunction, or clear-cut changes on fundoscopy. In the absence of evidence of structural change, it is reasonable to keep the blood pressure under review.

Other risk factors should also be taken into account when deciding whether to initiate therapy. Factors such as age, sex, hypercholesterolaemia, cigarette smoking and diabetes are not simply additive but multiplicative in terms of the risk to the individual. Patients with multiple risk factors, therefore, are more likely to benefit from antihypertensive treatment than those with the same level of blood pressure but no other risk factors.

In deciding when to initiate treatment, two patient groups require specific mention. These are the elderly (patients over 70 years of age) and those with isolated systolic hypertension (systolic blood pressure greater than 160 mmHg and diastolic blood pressure less than 95 mmHg). In the past, these groups of patients were thought not to benefit from antihypertensive therapy. However, recent studies have demonstrated that both elderly patients and those with isolated systolic hypertension (who are also likely to be elderly) derive very considerable benefit from treatment. Indeed, recent studies have demonstrated not only a reduction in stroke risk, but also a significant reduction in cardiac death in elderly patients. This is possibly because the absolute number of events (strokes, myocardial infarctions and deaths) is much higher in the elderly than in younger hypertensive patients.

In patients with mild to moderate hypertension, treatment has effectively eliminated death from cardiac failure and has reduced the incidence of fatal and non-fatal strokes. The effect on the incidence of myocardial infarction has been less impressive. If data from the major hypertensive studies are pooled together (so-called meta-analysis technique; see Chapter 23), then treatment can be shown to reduce the risk of myocardial infarction by about 14%. Although the percentage reduction in myocardial infarction is less than that in stroke death, this none the less represents a large absolute number of lives saved, as myocardial infarction is a much commoner cause of death in hypertensive patients than stroke.

Treatment of hypertension

Malignant hypertension, demonstrating retinal haemorrhages and exudates, requires urgent hospitalization and treatment. Patients with severe hypertension (diastolic > 120 mmHg) require early initiation of treatment. In most patients in whom there is evidence of target organ damage, early drug therapy will be required.

In all hypertensive patients, attention should be paid to non-pharmacological interventions that will reduce blood pressure and obviate the need for drug therapy in mild hypertensives, particularly if there is no evidence of end-organ damage. These include:

- weight reduction;
- regular exercise;
- reduction of alcohol consumption.

All hypertensive patients should be strongly advised against smoking and given dietary advice to reduce cholesterol intake and to reduce overall coronary risk.

Drugs used in the treatment of hypertension

There are a large number of drugs in current use for the treatment of hypertension, and new ones are continually being added. It is only possible to mention those which, at present, seem to be of greatest value. Every physician should be familiar with the use of four or five of these drugs as patients vary from one another in their response to therapy and no one drug can be regarded as superior in all respects to others.

Although the aim should be to make the blood pressure 'normal', it is not necessary to reduce the blood pressure rapidly in most patients and many drugs can take weeks or even months before the full hypotensive effect is seen. Too rapid a reduction in blood pressure may impair the circulation to the heart, brain or kidneys and precipitate myocardial infarction, stroke or renal failure.

An important consideration is the effect of treatment on the quality of life particularly in patients with mild hypertension, only an unidentifiable minority of whom will gain benefit from antihypertensive drugs.

The principal classes of drugs used are described below.

Beta-adrenoceptor blocking drugs. Beta-blockers are effective antihypertensive drugs whose mode of action remains uncertain. They are more effective when combined with a diuretic or other antihypertensive drugs but are often sufficient on their own and produce no marked orthostatic effects. To improve patient compliance, it is best to use a preparation that needs to be given only once or twice per day (atenolol 50 mg once or twice daily, or bisoprolol 5 mg once daily). These drugs may exacerbate obstructive airway disease, heart failure and intermittent claudication, and should probably be avoided in patients with these conditions. Minor side-effects, such as fatigue and cold extremities, are relatively common and disappear on stopping the drug.

Thiazide diuretics. These drugs have been used widely in the treatment of essential hypertension for many years. Their mechanism of action remains unclear. Initially, plasma volume and cardiac output may be reduced, but these values later normalize. Much has been made of the undesirable metabolic effects of thiazides which include hypokalaemia, hyperuricaemia, hypercholesterolaemia and hyperglycaemia. With the currently used low doses of thiazides, these effects are small and of doubtful significance. In their favour, only the thiazides, along with the beta-blockers, have been shown to reduce stroke risk in patients with mild to moderate hypertension.

ACE inhibitors. These drugs block the enzyme that converts angiotensin I to angiotensin II (see Fig. 16.1). They cause a fall in blood pressure by reducing systemic vascular resistance, without having any major effect on heart rate and cardiac output. The fall in systemic vascular resistance is probably mainly due to a reduction in plasma angiotensin II levels, but there is also a secondary fall in aldosterone concentration.

ACE inhibitors are effective in all grades and types of hypertension, but their action is potentiated by diuretics. A small rise in plasma urea and creatinine values is normal with ACE inhibitors but a marked increase may indicate unsuspected renal artery stenosis and is an indication for stopping the drug and considering renal angiography. Hyperkalaemia can occur because of the anti-aldosterone effects; therefore, concomitant use of ACE inhibitors and potassium-sparing diuretics is not recommended. Profound hypotension may occasionally be induced on first commencing treatment but this is usually seen only in patients who are already hypovolaemic as a result of high-dose diuretic therapy. This can be avoided by omitting diuretics on the day of starting the ACE inhibitor and also by starting with a small dose.

Cough is a particularly troublesome side-effect, occurring in some 5% of patients. Other side-effects include taste disorders, nausea, diarrhoea, rashes, cough, neutropenia, proteinuria and angioneurotic oedema.

Calcium-blocking drugs. These drugs have become increasingly used in the treatment of hypertension over the last 10–15 years. The dihydropyridine group, including nifedipine, nicardipine and amlodipine, all act predominantly by relaxing vascular smooth muscle and hence lowering peripheral vascular resistance. Side-effects with these agents include headache, flushing and ankle swelling.

The phenylalkylamine calcium channel blockers, such as verapamil and diltiazem, act more on the myocardium and conducting tissue. These are free from the vasodilator side-effects of the dihydropyridine class but do have negative inotropic effects and may potentiate heart failure.

Alpha-blockers. This class includes prazosin, terazosin and doxazosin. These drugs have marked arteriolar and venous vasodilating effects and the initial dose may produce profound postural hypotension. For this reason, the first dose should be taken on retiring to bed and the dosage gradually increased over a period of several weeks.

Angiotensin receptor antagonists. These are new agents which act by blocking the angiotensin II receptor. They appear to be effective in lowering blood pressure and are relatively free from side-effects. Unlike the ACE inhibitors, they do not cause cough, possibly because they do not interfere with bradykinin degradation.

Other vasodilator agents. Drugs such as hydralazine and minoxidil are not now used as first-line therapy but may still be useful in combination with other agents when multiple drugs are required to control blood pressure. Diazoxide and nitroprusside are very effective vasodilators but are generally used only in hypertensive emergencies.

Choice of therapy for the individual patient

All drugs cause side-effects in some people. This is a particular problem in the treatment of hypertension where patients are usually asymptomatic before the commencement of medication. The unexpected development of side-effects will often cause the patient to stop taking the medication and it is generally better to warn patients that side-effects may occur. Finding a treatment regimen that is acceptable to both patient (in terms of side-effects) and doctor (in terms of blood pressure control) involves a degree of 'trial and error' and may take 6–12 months.

As a first choice, many clinicians would use either a thiazide diuretic, such as bendrofluazide 2.5 mg once daily, or a long-acting beta-blocker, such as atenolol 50–100 mg once daily or bisoprolol 5 mg once daily. Thiazides and beta-blockers are favoured because both have been shown to reduce stroke risk in patients with mild to moderate hypertension. Other classes of drug, such as the ACE inhibitors and the alpha-blockers, have theoretical advantages over the more established drugs; thus alpha-blockers may have beneficial effects on lipid levels and the development of atherosclerosis, whereas ACE inhibitors may be more effective than other agents in producing regression of left ventricular hypertrophy. Although it is generally assumed that these drugs will reduce major vascular events such as stroke, this has not yet been tested in large-scale randomized studies.

The choice of medication is also determined by coexisting disease and the side-effect profile of a given agent. In patients with angina, for example, a beta-blocker would be a logical choice to treat both the angina and hypertension, whereas diuretics and ACE inhibitors would be preferable in patients with impaired left ventricular function. Beta-blockers should be avoided in patients with asthma or severe heart failure, and diuretics should be avoided in those patients with gout. ACE inhibitors should be used with caution in patients with impaired renal function.

If the response to a single drug is inadequate, a second agent should be added. Particularly useful combinations include:

- beta-blocker plus diuretic;
- beta-blocker plus dihydropyridine calcium antagonist;
- ACE inhibitor plus diuretic.

If a two-drug regimen does not give adequate blood pressure control, a third or fourth agent can be added. If the patient has not already been investigated for secondary hypertension, this should be considered if the hypertension appears to be resistant to drug treatment. It is also important to remember that non-compliance is common in the treatment of hypertension, and this should be suspected if the blood pressure fails to fall despite the use of multiple drugs.

A patient embarking on antihypertensive treatment should be aware that drug treatment is usually for life and that regular monitoring of the blood pressure will be required. Finally, the physician should bear in mind that the purpose of blood pressure reduction is to reduce the risk of a major vascular event. As hypertension is only one of a number of risk factors for cardiovascular disease, it follows that all risk factors should be addressed in the hypertensive patient; this may well include advice about diet, smoking, regular exercise and perhaps also the prescription of cholesterol-lowering agents.

Further reading

Cunningham, F. G. & Lindheimer, M. D. (1992) Hypertension in pregnancy. *New England Journal of Medicine* **326**: 927.
Frolich, E. D. et al. (1992) The heart in hypertension. *New England Journal of Medicine* **327**: 998.
Kaplan, N. M. (1990) *Clinical Hypertension*, 5th edn. Baltimore: Williams & Wilkins.
Sever, P., Beevers, G., Bulpitt, C. et al. (1993) Management guidelines in essential hypertension. *British Medical Journal* **306**: 983.
Williams, G. H. (1988) Converting enzyme inhibitors in the treatment of hypertension. *New England Journal of Medicine* **319**: 1517.

Diseases of the Aorta

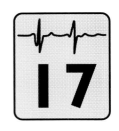

The aortic wall is composed of an endothelial lining or intima, a media containing smooth muscle and elastic tissue, and a fibrous adventitia. The media is largely responsible for the elasticity of the aortic wall, and the adventitia for its strength and resistance to rupture.

Dissecting aneurysm

A dissecting aneurysm (Fig. 17.1) results from the entry of blood into the media, either as a consequence of the rupture of vasa vasorum or from a tear of the aortic intima. No histological abnormality is seen in the media of most cases although cystic changes are sometimes present. Dissecting aneurysm is an important complication of the Marfan syndrome and of pregnancy, but the majority of cases occur in middle-aged or elderly men with systemic hypertension. The dissection usually starts either in the ascending aorta, a short distance above the aortic valve, or just beyond the origin of the left subclavian artery. The blood dissects a channel between the intima and the adventitia and usually advances distally. In so doing, it may occlude branches of the aortic arch and the descending aorta, including the renal and iliac arteries. If the dissection spreads proximally, the aortic valve may be involved, producing aortic regurgitation and, occasionally, occlusion of a coronary artery. The aneurysm usually ruptures externally into the pericardium, pleural cavity, mediastinum or retroperitoneal tissues, but sometimes it perforates the intima and the dissection 're-enters' the aortic lumen. Occasionally, the dissection becomes chronic without perforation.

Dissecting aneurysms usually present with the sudden onset of a 'tearing' pain of extreme severity. The site of the pain depends upon the location of the dissection and moves as the dissection progresses. The pain may start in the anterior or posterior chest or in the abdomen, but nearly always affects the upper back at some stage. Intervals of freedom from pain may occur; with recurrences, the pain may involve the

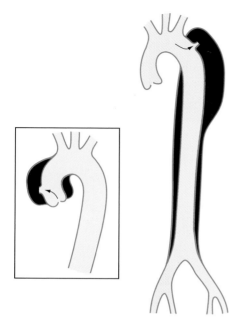

Fig. 17.1 Dissecting aneurysm of the aorta. This usually starts either a short distance above the aortic valve (left) or just below the origin of the left subclavian artery (right).

neck, arms, chest, trunk or legs. Occasionally, the pain is slight; breathlessness or syncope may then be the presenting symptom.

Classification

Dissecting aneurysms are most simply classified into two types:

- type A – involvement of the ascending aorta with or without extension into the descending aorta;
- type B – involvement of the descending aorta without involvement of the ascending aorta.

Type A dissections account for about two-thirds of cases and type B for one-third.

Clinical features

On examination, the patient appears pale and sweaty and has a tachycardia; although there may be the appearance of shock, the blood pressure is usually within normal limits, having fallen from hypertensive levels. Other signs depend on which branches of the aorta are occluded. Thus, one or more of the arteries to the limbs may become impalpable. Other complications include aortic regurgitation, tamponade, hemiplegia, mental disturbances, haematuria, bloody diarrhoea and haemothorax.

Investigation

The ECG is of little diagnostic value, but pre-existing hypertension may have caused left ventricular hypertrophy. The appearances of myocardial ischaemia or myocardial infarction may be present if there has been encroachment on a coronary artery. The chest radiograph shows an increase in the width of the mediastinum. The presence of aortic dissection can be confirmed in a number of ways:

- oesophageal echocardiography – this technique is proving of particular value in the diagnosis of aortic dissection (Fig. 17.2);
- computed tomography (Fig. 17.3);
- magnetic resonance imaging;
- aortic angiography.

Management

The value of the type A/type B classification (see above) lies in the differentiation of management between the two types of dissecting aneurysm. As a general rule, type A dissections are best managed by early surgery, whereas type B dissections can be managed medically.

In *type A dissections*, there is a strong likelihood of further dissection and death unless surgical repair is undertaken. Patients should first be stabilized medically. Blood pressure should be lowered to reduce the strain on the aorta; beta-blockers are preferred for this purpose. Labetolol, which combines the properties of an alpha- and beta-blocker, is particularly useful in the management of aortic dissection. In occasional patients a nitroprusside infusion may be required to control blood pressure.

The choice of surgical procedure depends on the extent of dissection. If the dissection involves the aortic root, it may be necessary to insert a Dacron tube graft with resuspension or replacement of the aortic valve and reimplantation of the coronary arteries.

In *type B dissections*, the risks of surgery are generally considered to exceed the risks of medical management. Antihypertensive therapy should be continued long term to guard against risks of recurrent dissection.

Atypical aortic dissection

In recent years, the advent of new imaging techniques has led to the recognition of two additional conditions closely related to aortic dissection.

- *intramural haematoma* is a haemorrhage contained within the aortic media. The initiating event is believed to be rupture of the

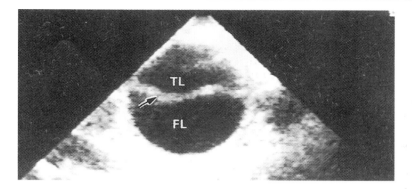

Fig. 17.2 Aortic dissection. Transoesophageal echocardiogram showing the descending aorta in cross section. A flap is demonstrated (arrowed) separating the true lumen (TL) from the false lumen (FL).

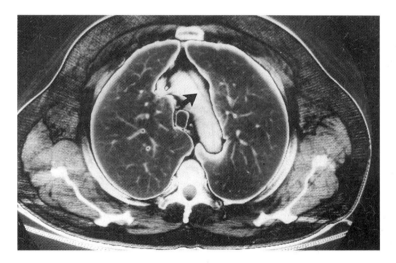

Fig. 17.3 Computed tomogram of an aortic dissection. Arrow points to detached flap in aorta.

vasa vasorum. The condition is distinguished from traditional dissection by the lack of an associated intimal tear. Intramural haematoma may regress with time or may progress to aortic dissection. Because of a high incidence of progression, intramural haematomas should be managed in a similar fashion to conventional dissection;

- *penetrating atherosclerotic ulcer* is a communication into the media from the aortic lumen which may extend for a few centimetres but which does not develop a false lumen. Such ulceration occurs almost exclusively in the descending aorta. The natural history is unclear but a substantial proportion progress to transmural rupture and for this reason surgery should be considered.

Aortic trauma

Rupture of the aorta is a common cause of death following automobile accidents. Following sudden deceleration of the body, the heart and horizontal portion of the aortic arch continue to move forwards. The descending aorta is fixed to the spine by intercostal arteries. As a consequence a tear can arise in the aorta at the junction of the fixed descending aorta and the mobile aortic arch.

The diagnosis should be suspected in any chest injury that involves sudden deceleration of the body. A chest radiograph will commonly show widening of the upper mediastinum. In contradistinction to aortic dissection, computed tomography (CT) and transoesophageal echocardiography may fail to detect the localized nature of an aortic tear, and aortography remains the investigation of choice. Treatment is surgical repair.

Saccular and fusiform aortic aneurysms

These are localized distensions of the wall of the aorta, being fusiform if the whole circumference of the vessel is involved and saccular if only part of it is affected.

Atherosclerotic aneurysms, which are usually situated in the descending aorta, result from atrophy of the media and adventitia with fibrous replacement. Syphilis, formerly the major cause of aortic aneurysms, has become uncommon. Syphilitic aneurysms usually affect the ascending aorta and the aortic arch, as a result of inflammatory changes in the aortic wall and subsequent fibrosis and calcification (see p. 359). Fusiform aneurysms are also seen in association with the Marfan syndrome and coarctation of the aorta. A distinctive type of aneurysm is that of the sinus of Valsalva, which will be considered separately.

Clinical features

The clinical features resulting from an aneurysm of the thoracic aorta depend upon its size and site. When the aneurysm is in the ascending aorta, there is often associated aortic regurgitation which leads to cardiac failure. As the aneurysm enlarges and encroaches upon neighbouring structures, there may be pain as a result of erosion of ribs and sternum. A pulsating mass may be seen in the front of the chest and obstruction of the superior vena cava may occur. When the aneurysm is situated in the aortic arch, wheezing, cough and hoarseness may arise from compression of the trachea, bronchus or recurrent laryngeal nerves. Aneurysms of the descending aorta are most likely to produce symptoms as a result of encroachment on the vertebrae, ribs or spinal nerves.

Investigations. Often, however, an aneurysm of the thoracic aorta is first diagnosed in an asymptomatic patient by the radiographic demonstration of a localized dilatation of the aorta. The diagnosis can be confirmed by angiography, although CT and transoesophageal echocardiography are also of value.

Management

Asymptomatic patients with relatively small aneurysms may survive for many years. However, the prognosis is generally poor and the patient with symptoms is unlikely to survive more than 1–2 years.

Most patients with aneurysms of the aorta have severe associated disorders such as hypertension, ischaemic heart disease or cerebrovascular disease, and death more often results from one of these than from the aneurysm. Perhaps only one-third of the patients die from aortic rupture; before surgery is undertaken, the cardiovascular and cerebral circulations must be carefully evaluated. The optimal timing of surgical repair is uncertain. In general, surgical repair should be considered when an aneurysm measures 6 cm or more in diameter. However, surgery may be indicated earlier in aneurysms showing a rapid rate of expansion. Marfan's syndrome is also an indication for considering earlier surgery, as these patients are particularly susceptible to dissection and rupture. In patients at high operative risk, surgery is likely to be deferred until the aneurysm is 7 cm or larger.

In general, surgery involves resection of the aneurysm and replacement with a prosthetic graft. In aneurysms involving the ascending aorta with significant aortic regurgitation, the aortic valve is frequently replaced as part of the surgical repair. A composite graft comprising a Dacron tube with a suspended prosthetic aortic valve is sewn directly into the aortic annulus and the coronary arteries reattached to the Dacron graft.

Aneurysm of the sinus of Valsalva

This is most commonly caused by a congenital localized absence of the aortic media, but can result from syphilitic aortitis or infective endocarditis. The aneurysm forms a thin-walled sac which in most

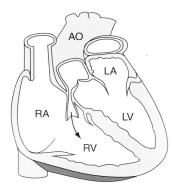

Fig 17.4 Aneurysm of sinus of Valsalva rupturing into right atrium.

instances protrudes into the right ventricle or right atrium (Fig. 17.4). No symptoms or signs are produced until the aneurysm ruptures. When it does so a fistula is formed between the aorta and the relevant chamber. Congenital aneurysms of the sinus of Valsalva are often associated with other congenital lesions, particularly a ventricular septal defect.

Sudden death sometimes occurs; more often rupture causes the abrupt onset of chest pain and breathlessness. These symptoms subside over a period of days or weeks. Cardiac failure develops subsequently, but is very variable in its rate of progression.

On examination the patient may have a collapsing pulse due to the aortic diastolic leak, and there is usually a continuous systolic and diastolic murmur, resembling that of a persistent ductus arteriosus, but loudest over the sternum at the level of the third or fourth interspace.

The ECG may be normal initially, but the signs of right ventricular hypertrophy or right bundle branch block may develop later. The chest radiograph shows cardiac enlargement with pulmonary plethora. The aneurysm may be demonstrated by echocardiography, and the shunt by Doppler ultrasonography. The definitive diagnosis is made by showing the leak on aortography, and by the demonstration of a left-to-right shunt on cardiac catheterization.

The ruptured sinus of Valsalva should be treated by repair of the aortic wall.

Further reading

Cigaroa, J. E., Isselbacher, E. M., DeSanchio, R. W. & Eagle, K. A. (1993) Diagnostic imaging in the evaluation of suspected aortic dissection. *New England Journal of Medicine* **328**: 35.

Isselbacker, E. M., Eagle, M. A., Desanctis, R. W. (1997) Diseases of the Aorta. In Braunwald, E. (Ed.) *Heart Disease*, 5th edn. Philadelphia: Saunders.

Liddicoat, J. E., Bekassy, S. M., Rubio, P. A., Noon, G. P. & DeBakey, M. E. (1975) Ascending aortic aneurysms. *Circulation* **52 (Suppl. I)**: 202.

Disorders of the Lungs and Pulmonary Circulation

18

PULMONARY EMBOLISM

Pulmonary thrombo-embolism can cause or aggravate heart disease, and is a common and serious complication of cardiac disorders. Pulmonary embolism, pulmonary thrombosis and pulmonary infarction are related conditions:

- *pulmonary embolism* results from the obstruction of the pulmonary arterial vessels by thrombus or by material, such as fat or air, originating in some other site;
- *pulmonary thrombosis* implies the formation of clot *in situ*;
- *pulmonary infarction* is the necrosis of a wedge of lung tissue resulting from pulmonary arterial occlusion.

Pulmonary embolism is usually a consequence of thrombophlebitis or phlebothrombosis in the leg veins but may also follow thrombosis of the pelvic veins, or clot formation in the right atrium in patients with right-sided cardiac failure, particularly if there is atrial fibrillation. Deep vein thrombosis is often asymptomatic, but the leg may be warm, tender, slightly dusky and swollen by oedema. Thrombosis is most likely to occur when there has been stasis in the veins, especially in association with childbirth, abdominal surgery, acute myocardial infarction and right-sided cardiac failure. There is a slightly increased risk in women taking oral contraceptives. Pulmonary thrombosis is uncommon except as a complication of pre-existing disease of the pulmonary arteries.

Prevention

Pulmonary embolism can be prevented by measures which prevent the development or progression of venous thrombosis. Simple measures to encourage venous flow such as the use of leg exercises and elastic stockings in those confined to bed are important and effective ways of doing so. Once thrombosis has been diagnosed treatment should be initiated with heparin, unless there are contraindications. A bolus of 5000 units may be given, followed by a continuous infusion of the drug. The dosage should be controlled by the activated partial thromboplastin time (APTT). Oral warfarin should be started at the same time. The international normalized ratio (INR) should be maintained between 2.0 and 3.0, unless there is recurrent thrombo-embolism when between 3.0 and 4.5 would be appropriate. Heparin may be stopped after 5–7 days. Warfarin should be continued for 3 months for calf thrombosis and 6 months for iliofemoral thrombosis.

Clinical features

The nature of the clinical presentation with pulmonary embolism depends on the size of the embolus:

- *a small embolus* may present with non-specific features such as dyspnoea or tiredness;
- *a medium-sized embolus* may cause the occlusion of a segment of the pulmonary arterial tree, causing pulmonary infarction. This may result in pleuritic pain, haemoptysis, a low-grade pyrexia and dyspnoea;
- *massive pulmonary embolism* results from the occlusion of two-thirds or more of the pulmonary arterial bed. This causes right-sided failure, a low cardiac output and a rise in venous pressure.

The physical signs of pulmonary emboli vary with the size of the embolus. Small and even medium-sized emboli may be devoid of any abnormal clinical signs. Following pulmonary infarction, signs of a pleural effusion and pleural rub may be present.

Large emboli may cause:

- hypotension and shock;
- tachycardia;
- cyanosis;
- elevation of the jugular venous pulse;
- accentuation of the pulmonary component of the second heart sound due to pulmonary hypertension;
- right ventricular third and fourth heart sounds;
- occasionally continuous, systolic and diastolic murmurs due to turbulent flow caused by the embolus.

Massive pulmonary embolism should be suspected in any patient who suddenly develops the features of shock, syncope, acute dyspnoea or chest pain, particularly if the subject has evidence of a venous thrombosis or has been confined to bed during the preceding days.

Investigations. Investigations of patients with suspected pulmonary embolism include:

- chest radiography
- ECG;
- blood gases;
- ventilation–perfusion scan;
- pulmonary angiography.

The chest radiograph is seldom helpful, although it may show enlarged proximal pulmonary arteries and small peripheral ones.

The ECG. In cases of mild to moderate pulmonary embolism the ECG is usually normal, except for demonstrating sinus tachycardia. In cases of severe pulmonary embolism, characteristic ECG features may be observed (Fig. 18.1):

- $S_1 Q_3 T_3$ pattern. A narrow Q wave and inverted T wave in lead III, accompanied by an S wave in lead I, all due to changes in the position of the heart caused by dilatation of the right ventricle and atrium;
- P pulmonale;
- right bundle branch block;
- 'right ventricular strain' pattern with T inversion in the leads of V1 to V4;
- atrial arrhythmias.

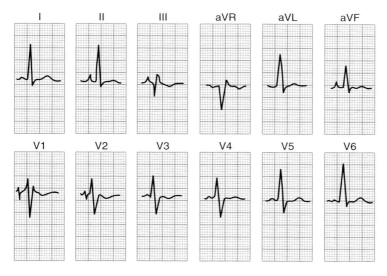

Fig. 18.1 ECG appearances in pulmonary embolism. Note tall, peaked P waves, partial right bundle branch block (rSr in VI), S in lead I, Q and negative T in III, and inverted T waves in VI to V3.

The differential diagnosis from acute myocardial infarction may be extremely difficult. The ECG is of considerable value, but the patterns associated with massive pulmonary embolism are often misinterpreted as being those of a combination of inferior and anteroseptal infarction. The appearance of Q waves and negative T waves in lead III (but not in lead II) in association with inverted T waves from V1 to V4 strongly suggests pulmonary embolism.

Blood gases. Characteristically pulmonary embolism causes a reduced arterial pO_2 due to shunting of blood through underventilated parts of the lung. Simultaneously pCO_2 is normal or reduced due to hyperventilation.

Pulmonary scintigraphy, using radioactive technetium, is a sensitive technique for detecting perfusion abnormalities. A perfusion deficit might be due either to impaired blood flow to that segment of lung or to primary pulmonary problems, such as effusion or collapse. To improve the specificity of the method, it is generally combined with a ventilation scan using radioactive xenon gas. The demonstration of a non-perfused but ventilated zone is strongly suggestive of pulmonary embolism.

Venous ultrasonography or contrast venography provide useful circumstantial evidence in cases in which the diagnosis remains uncertain following a ventilation–perfusion scan. In 70% of cases of pulmonary embolism, evidence of venous thrombosis can be demonstrated, even though this is evident clinically in less than 2%.

Pulmonary angiography can be undertaken in cases of diagnostic doubt or in cases of massive pulmonary embolism if surgery is considered. Contrast material is injected via a catheter inserted in the pulmonary artery. The procedure is potentially hazardous, but risks can be reduced by selective injections into each lung in turn or by using digital subtraction angiography to enable the volume of contrast injected to be reduced.

Management

In the majority of patients the haemodynamic consequences of pulmonary emboli are not severe. The primary objective of treatment is the prevention of further emboli. Patients are treated initially with intravenous heparin (5000 units bolus, followed by an infusion of 15 000 units/12 h, adjusted according to the patient's activated partial thromboplastin time). Warfarin therapy is commenced and heparin discontinued after 5–7 days. Heparin should be maintained for at least 2 days after achieving a therapeutic INR. The target INR therapeutic range for the management of pulmonary embolism is generally 2.0–3.0. Warfarin should be maintained for 3–6 months, depending on the likelihood of recurrence.

In exceptional patients who have recurrent pulmonary emboli while on warfarin, an inferior vena caval filter device can be considered. This device, inserted percutaneously via a catheter, traps clots preventing migration to the lungs.

In patients with massive pulmonary embolism, sufficient to cause severe haemodynamic compromise, two approaches are possible:

- thrombolytic therapy;
- surgical embolectomy.

Streptokinase may be administered either into a peripheral vein or directly into the pulmonary artery. A large loading dose (usually 600 000 units over 30 min) is given initially, followed by a smaller maintenance dose (100 000 units hourly), monitoring clotting parameters.

Surgical embolectomy is an alternative to thrombolytic therapy. The operation requires cardiopulmonary bypass and experienced cardiac surgeons. Embolectomy is indicated in patients with a contraindication to thrombolysis or who continue to deteriorate despite thrombolysis. The operation is rarely used but in occasional patients may be life-saving.

Recurrent pulmonary emboli and thrombo-embolic pulmonary hypertension

Recurrent pulmonary embolization, which is usually associated with chronic or recurrent venous thrombosis, may appear as massive emboli, as pulmonary infarction or be silent. Eventually, the vascular obstruction may become so widespread as to cause a substantial increase in the resistance of the pulmonary arteries and lead to pulmonary arterial hypertension. Once this has become established, the prognosis is poor and most patients die within a period of 5 years. The process may sometimes be reversed or prevented from progression by permanent anticoagulant therapy.

PULMONARY HYPERTENSION

The pulmonary arterial pressure is determined by the pressure in the pulmonary capillaries, the pulmonary blood flow and the resistance of the pulmonary arteries (especially the arterioles).

The small pulmonary arteries of the fetus have a thick muscular media and the pulmonary vascular resistance of the non-aerated lung is high. This muscular layer regresses over the first 2–3 months of life. As a consequence the pulmonary vascular resistance and arterial pressure start to fall shortly after birth and within a few weeks have declined to normal adult levels.

The pulmonary arteries in the adult are relatively thin-walled, the smaller vessels having considerably less muscle in their walls than corresponding systemic arterioles. The resistance to flow is much lower and the pressure in the pulmonary artery (about 20/10 mmHg) is approximately one-seventh that in the aorta. It is believed that many of the capillaries in the lung are closed at rest, particularly those of the upper parts of the lungs. When the cardiac output increases, as on exercise, the vascular resistance falls as capillaries open and small arteries dilate. As a consequence, blood flow through the lungs can increase threefold before any rise in pressure occurs.

Aetiology

Pulmonary arterial hypertension (greater than 30/15 mmHg) may result from:

- an increase in pulmonary capillary pressure;
- an increase in pulmonary blood flow;
- an increase in pulmonary vascular resistance.

Elevated pulmonary capillary pressure.   Passive pulmonary hypertension due to a raised pulmonary capillary pressure occurs in all conditions in which the left atrial pressure rises, such as mitral stenosis and left ventricular failure. The pulmonary artery pressure rises in proportion to the pulmonary capillary pressure.

Increased pulmonary blood flow.   Pulmonary hypertension due to increased flow develops in disorders in which there are left-to-right shunts. These include septal defects and persistent ductus arteriosus. In atrial septal defect, a large pulmonary blood flow of 10–15 litres/min may be unassociated with pulmonary hypertension because there is a compensatory vasodilatation with a fall in vascular resistance. In many cases of ventricular septal defect and persistent ductus arteriosus, there is no vasodilatation, and the resistance remains normal. The pulmonary arterial pressure may therefore rise even with comparatively small shunts. With large shunts, pulmonary arterial pressure may reach systemic levels.

Increased pulmonary vascular resistance.   There are a number of causes of increased pulmonary vascular resistance (Table 18.1). These diverse causes lead to increased pulmonary vascular resistance through three basic mechanisms:

- *pulmonary vasoconstriction.* Hypoxia is a potent pulmonary vasoconstrictor and is a factor in the pulmonary hypertension that occurs in respiratory disease;
- *blockage* of the pulmonary arteries or arterioles by thrombosis and embolism, as in thrombo-embolism and schistosomiasis;
- *arterial medial hypertrophy.* Proliferation of the muscular medial layer of the small pulmonary arteries which are the main deter-

Table 18.1   Causes of increased pulmonary vascular resistance

Cor pulmonale
Chronic thrombo-embolism
Eisenmenger's syndrome (p. 314)
Collagen vascular diseases
Schistosomiasis
Primary pulmonary hypertension

minants of the pulmonary vascular resistance. The muscular proliferation may progress to fibrosis. Medial hypertrophy plays a major role in primary pulmonary hypertension and in Eisenmenger's syndrome.

Combinations of the three mechanisms are common. In mitral stenosis, for example, the initial phase of passive pulmonary hypertension is often complicated by vasoconstriction and by the obliterative changes of pulmonary embolism. In many cases of ventricular septal defect, both high blood flow and pulmonary vascular disease contribute to pulmonary hypertension. In emphysema, obliteration of the vascular bed and hypoxia are contributory factors.

Clinical features of pulmonary hypertension

Independent of causation, certain clinical features are characteristic of severe pulmonary hypertension. The symptoms include:

- dyspnoea;
- fatigue;
- syncope;
- haemoptysis;
- chest pain;
- symptoms of right-sided cardiac failure.

Abnormal features on clinical examination may include:

- elevation of the jugular venous pulse with a prominent 'a' wave;
- features of tricuspid regurgitation;
- a forceful right ventricular heave along the left sternal edge;
- a right ventricular fourth-heart sound at the lower left sternal edge;
- a loud pulmonary component to the second sound, which may be followed by an early diastolic murmur of pulmonary regurgitation (Graham Steell murmur).

Investigation.   The chest radiograph may show enlargement of the proximal pulmonary arteries, right ventricle and right atrium. The peripheral lung fields appear oligaemic.

The ECG demonstrates features of right ventricular hypertrophy:

- tall peaked P waves in lead II due to right atrial enlargement;
- right axis deviation;
- a predominant R wave in lead V1;
- inverted T waves in leads V1–V3.

Management

Both management and prognosis of pulmonary arterial hypertension depend upon its aetiology and on its severity. Passive pulmonary hypertension responds well if the underlying disorder can be corrected (e.g. mitral stenosis). Pulmonary hypertension due to high pulmonary arterial flow can usually be reversed by the correction of the underlying congenital abnormality. Increased pulmonary arterial resistance due to vasoconstriction can often be diminished by relieving hypoxia or by the successful treatment of mitral valve disease. When pulmonary hypertension is due to severe pulmonary vascular disease, as in the Eisenmenger syndrome, the prognosis is poor and life is usually sustained for only a few years. In these cases, cardiac failure is progressive in spite of treatment and the only hope may lie in heart–lung transplantation.

Primary ('unexplained') pulmonary hypertension

Pulmonary hypertension is said to be primary when the aetiology cannot be determined. It is possible that small pulmonary emboli are responsible for some cases. The condition, which is rare, is most common in young women; the first symptoms are usually fatigue and exertional dyspnoea. The diagnosis is made by exclusion in patients found to have the clinical features of pulmonary hypertension. Lung biopsy can aid diagnosis, but is potentially hazardous. Characteristic 'plexiform' lesions are present in the arterioles in approximately 70% of cases.

The prognosis is poor; death is likely to occur within 5 years. Thrombosis may contribute to the progression of hypertension and anticoagulants are recommended; oral contraceptives and pregnancy must be avoided. Vasodilator therapy may prove of value in some patients, but may cause deterioration in others if there is a greater fall in systemic than pulmonary resistance. For this reason patients should be carefully monitored on first commencing therapy. Some success has recently been claimed using high doses of the calcium antagonist, diltiazem. Prostacyclin may also be of value, but is very expensive and needs to be given parenterally.

In patients failing to respond to conventional treatment, combined heart and lung transplantation should be considered.

PULMONARY HEART DISEASE

The understanding of pulmonary heart disease (cor pulmonale) has been made difficult by problems of nomenclature. Here it is defined as heart disease secondary to disorders of ventilation and respiratory function. Right-sided heart failure due to pulmonary arterial disease or secondary to left-sided heart failure is not included in this definition, and is considered in the section on pulmonary hypertension (above).

The prevalence of pulmonary heart disease varies greatly between one geographical area and another. There is abundant evidence that heavy cigarette smoking and air pollution are major factors in the production of chronic bronchitis; cor pulmonale is commonest in those exposed to these influences. It is predominantly a disease of middle-aged and elderly men, and is uncommon in young men or in women of any age.

Pathogenesis of heart failure in lung disease

Lung disease causes heart disease mainly because of its effects on the pulmonary vessels. Due to a number of different mechanisms, there is an increase in pulmonary vascular resistance, leading to pulmonary hypertension, right ventricular hypertrophy and right heart failure.

These mechanisms include:

- *pulmonary arteriolar constriction* due to low alveolar oxygen tension in areas of underventilated lung;
- *anatomical reduction of the pulmonary vascular bed* from rupture of alveolar walls and from fibrotic or thrombotic obliteration of capillaries;
- *compression of pulmonary capillaries* by high intra-alveolar pressures when there is air trapping.

Pulmonary hypertension is seldom severe in pulmonary disease except when there is superadded respiratory infection.

Abnormalities in the blood gases nearly always precede the appearance of heart failure due to lung disease. Hypoxaemia is almost invariable. Even if the arterial oxygen tension is normal at rest, it is reduced on exercise. The hypoxaemia results either from disturbances in the ventilation–perfusion relationship or from interference with the diffusion of oxygen through the alveolar wall.

The carbon dioxide tension is raised when the heart failure is secondary to chronic obstructive airways disease and alveolar hypoventilation. If there is a rapid rise in carbon dioxide tension, the pH is low, but in the chronic stage of the disease the renal retention of bicarbonate maintains a normal or near normal acid–base balance.

These blood gas abnormalities are responsible for many of the characteristics of pulmonary heart disease:

- *polycythaemia* and increased blood volume due to hypoxaemia;
- *peripheral vasodilatation*, due to high carbon dioxide tension, producing a large pulse and warm extremities;
- *cerebral vasodilatation*, due to high carbon dioxide tension, which leads to a raised cerebrospinal fluid pressure, with tremor, confusion and papilloedema;
- *impaired myocardial function* due to hypoxaemia.

The more advanced symptoms of carbon dioxide retention occur mainly, if not exclusively, in patients receiving oxygen in high concentration. Such treatment is dangerous if there is carbon dioxide retention because it abolishes the hypoxaemia which is a major stimulus to respiration.

Clinical features of pulmonary heart disease

Diseases causing pulmonary heart disease cover the full spectrum of pulmonary disease including obstructive airways disease, emphysema, pulmonary fibrosis, pulmonary infiltration (e.g. sarcoidosis), pulmonary resection, skeletal abnormalities and disorders of the respiratory muscles.

The patient is commonly a cigarette-smoking middle-aged man with a long history of morning cough and sputum. There may have been recurrent attacks of winter bronchitis. These symptoms are slowly progressive until breathlessness becomes disabling. Overt cyanosis and peripheral oedema are usually late features but are sometimes the first clear manifestation of pulmonary disease. Recent worsening of cough and the production of purulent sputum is common.

The clinical features reflect pulmonary hypertension and right ventricular failure and include:

- dyspnoea;
- cyanosis;
- features of carbon dioxide retention;
- an elevated jugular venous pulse, possibly with signs of tricuspid regurgitation;
- peripheral oedema and hepatic enlargement.

Investigations.   The ECG is often normal but may show P pulmonale, right axis deviation, right ventricular hypertrophy, right bundle branch block, or an rS pattern across the chest. In emphysema the QRS complexes are often small.

The radiological appearances depend upon the nature of the lung disease. When there is emphysema with an increased total lung volume, one may see a low diaphragm and a narrow heart. Enlargement of the main pulmonary artery and its major branches occurs when there is pulmonary hypertension. The radiograph is, however, often normal.

Pulmonary function tests usually demonstrate a forced expiratory volume in 1 s (FEV_1) below 1.5 litres and a peak expiratory flow rate less than 200 litres/min. Blood gas analysis will usually show an arterial $pO_2 < 6$ kPa (46 mmHg).

Differential diagnosis. The pulmonary origin of cardiac failure is often overlooked, particularly when it coexists with known ischaemic, rheumatic or hypertensive heart disease. This is particularly the case with hypertension; mild hypertension is often blamed for heart failure which is secondary to chronic bronchitis and emphysema. The history of chronic cough with sputum and wheezing should suggest the possibility, as should poor chest movement and the presence of rhonchi. The diagnosis is usually best made by studies of ventilation and blood gases; carbon dioxide retention makes it almost certain that there is a pulmonary component in heart failure.

Prognosis and treatment

The prognosis is poor once cardiac failure has complicated pulmonary heart disease. Treatment may overcome individual attacks, but the subject is liable to further episodes with recurrent infection, and is unlikely to survive more than two or three such attacks over a period of a few years.

When a patient is seen in cardiac failure due to pulmonary heart disease, the major objects of treatment should be to combat respiratory infection, correct hypoxaemia and carbon dioxide retention, and relieve airways obstruction. Acute chest infections should be promptly treated with antibiotics. Beta$_2$-agonists, such as salbutamol, may have some benefit in reducing pulmonary hypertension. Corticosteroids may be of benefit in patients with reversible airways obstruction. Some patients may also benefit from the provision of long-term domiciliary oxygen. This has been shown to lower mortality in patients with chronic obstructive airways disease and persistent hypoxaemia, although improvement in pulmonary hypertension has not been convincingly demonstrated.

Diuretics are widely used for the control of right heart failure. Digoxin may also be of value.

Further reading

American Heart Association (1996) Management of deep vein thrombosis and pulmonary embolism. A statement for healthcare professionals from the Council on Thrombosis, American Heart Association. *Circulation* **93**: 2212.

Flenley, D. (1981) *Respiratory Disease*. London: Baillière Tindall.

Fuster, V., Steele, P. M., Edwards, W. D., Gersh, B. J., McGoon, M. D. & Frye, R. L. (1984) Primary pulmonary hypertension. *Circulation* **70**: 580.

Goldhaber, S. Z. (1997) Pulmonary hypertension. In Braunwald, E. (Ed.) *Heart Disease*, 5th edn. Philadelphia: Saunders.

Rich, S., Braunwald, E., Grossman, W. (1997) Pulmonary hypertension. In Braunwald, E. (Ed.) *Heart Disease*, 5th edn. Philadelphia: Saunders.

Systemic Disorders and the Heart

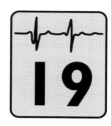

INFECTIONS AND THE HEART

Infections can affect the circulation in a variety of ways:

- direct invasion of endocardium, myocardium and pericardium;
- toxic myocarditis;
- acute circulatory failure due to toxic effects on the vasomotor centre or peripheral vessels, or to dehydration.

Infective endocarditis and pericarditis are considered in Chapters 12 and 14 and will not be discussed in detail here.

Diphtheria

Diphtheria causes an acute myocarditis in approximately 20% of subjects. Acute circulatory failure may occur in the first few days but the major cardiovascular effects are more common at the end of the first and during the second week. The presence of acute myocarditis is suggested by gallop rhythm, cardiomegaly, ECG abnormalities, heart block or cardiogenic shock.

ECG abnormalities often precede the clinical signs of myocarditis, the commonest change being flattening or inversion of the T waves. All grades of heart block may occur.

Nearly all infants with acute diphtheritic myocarditis die; the mortality rate in adults is less than 25%. In those who recover from the acute attack, residual cardiac damage is almost unknown.

Diphtheria should be prevented by immunization. If it occurs, the patient requires treatment with antitoxin and penicillin. Electrical pacing may be required for heart block; conduction disorders are seldom, if ever, permanent.

Tuberculosis

Tuberculosis may cause pericarditis, with or without subsequent constriction (see p. 230). It may also be responsible for heart disease secondary to pulmonary fibrosis. Tuberculous myocarditis is very rare.

Virus infections

Viruses cause both pericarditis and myocarditis. Coxsackie viruses of group B are probably the commonest organisms affecting the heart; most infections are subclinical. The clinical picture is usually one of fever, malaise and muscular pains, accompanied by evidence of pericarditis and, if there is myocarditis, tachycardia, gallop rhythm, cardiomegaly and cardiac failure. The ECG usually shows non-specific abnormalities, but there may be ST and T wave changes suggesting pericarditis or myocardial infarction. Blood levels of myocardial enzymes (such as creatine kinase) may be raised transiently. The diagnosis can be made by isolating the organism from the stool or by demonstrating a rise or fall in serum antibodies. Rest is desirable during the acute phase, and return to vigorous activity should be progressive. The patient nearly always recovers completely, but there may be residual myocardial damage and recurrences are not unusual. Myocarditis may also be associated with infectious mononucleosis, acute anterior poliomyelitis and many other virus infections.

AIDS (acquired immune deficiency syndrome)

Cardiac involvement is becoming more common in patients with AIDS as the prognosis in relation to other complications improves. It may take many forms, including myocarditis, endocarditis, pericarditis, dilated cardiomyopathy and Kaposi's sarcoma. Manifest heart disease is apparent in about 20% of patients and heart failure develops in at least 10%.

Trypanosomiasis (Chagas' disease)

Myocarditis due to infection by *Trypanosoma cruzi* is common in South America, where about 20 million people are believed to be infected. It is transmitted by the bite of infected reduviid bugs. These live in the roofs and walls of houses, and drop down on to the face of a sleeping person below. There are two major forms, acute and chronic. Acute Chagas' disease, which occurs predominantly in childhood, may be asymptomatic but can produce tachycardia, cardiomegaly and cardiac failure. Much more important is the chronic form which leads to cardiac failure of insidious onset. It particularly affects men between the ages of 20 and 40. The left ventricle is enlarged, and there may be dyspnoea, chest pain and palpitation. Eventually, right-sided heart failure develops; this is frequently complicated by thrombo-embolic events. Arrhythmias are almost invariable and complete heart block common. The ECG usually shows right bundle branch block. Death is often sudden due to ventricular fibrillation or asystole. Echocardiography shows the features of a dilated cardiomyopathy. Chagas' myocarditis should be suspected when patients who have lived in the tropical or subtropical areas of America develop arrhythmias, cardiac failure and right bundle branch block. A complement fixation test is useful in diagnosis. Treatment is essentially directed at the complications of heart failure, arrhythmias and heart block.

Toxoplasmosis

Toxoplasma gondii can give rise to a myocarditis which may complicate either the disseminated form of the disease, in which there is hepatitis, pneumonia and meningo-encephalitis, or the less acute form which resembles infectious mononucleosis with lymphadenopathy the most obvious abnormality. The myocarditis usually gives rise to tachycardia and may cause heart failure, pericarditis and arrhythmias. Complete recovery is unusual.

Syphilis

Cardiovascular syphilis used to be an important cause of death, but is now uncommon. It seldom affects the myocardium, although gummata can occur. The organism localizes in the aorta soon after the primary infection, but a latent period of 10–25 years elapses before clinical evidence of aortitis develops.

The initial lesion involves the vasa vasorum of the aorta which become obliterated. The muscle and elastic tissues of the media necrose and are replaced by scar tissue which becomes calcified. The lesions predominantly affect the ascending aorta. The process may involve the mouths of the coronary arteries producing stenosis. Damage to the aortic valve ring produces dilatation with aortic regurgitation. Aortic stenosis does not occur. Aneurysms of either saccular or fusiform type may be formed.

The symptoms and signs of syphilitic disease depend mainly on whether there is coronary artery involvement, aortic valve disease or aneurysm formation. Coronary artery stenosis leads to angina pectoris and, rarely, myocardial infarction. Syphilitic aortic regurgitation may cause the clinical features of left-sided cardiac failure. Because syphilitic aortic aneurysms affect predominantly the ascending aorta and arch, the major symptoms are those of chest pain due to erosion of bone, cough and dyspnoea due to pressure on the trachea and bronchi, and hoarseness from paralysis of the left recurrent laryngeal nerve. The aneurysm may be visible in the second or third right intercostal spaces, and a systolic thrill may be palpable in this area. There is often a loud systolic murmer over the aneurysm and the second heart sound may be accentuated.

The ECG appearances depend on the nature of the complications and are not specific. A chest radiograph shows a dilated aorta (see Fig. 5.5), often with linear calcification.

Syphilitic aortitis should be suspected if the aorta is conspicuously dilated or aneurysmal, or if there is aortic regurgitation unassociated with stenosis. The diagnosis is confirmed by serological tests specifically directed against the treponemal antigen.

The prognosis is quite good in asymptomatic syphilitic aortitis, survival for 10–20 years being probable. The patient is unlikely to live more than 2–3 years if there is angina due to coronary stenosis or left ventricular failure due to aortic regurgitation.

Syphilitic cardiovascular disease does not develop if early syphilis is adequately treated. It is uncertain whether treatment of established cardiovascular syphilis is effective in preventing progression. It is customary to give 600 mg aqueous procaine penicillin intramuscularly daily for 20 days, or benzathine penicillin G 2.4 million units intramuscularly weekly for 3 weeks, to control the infection. Surgery may be necessary for relief of coronary ostial stenosis, for the correction of aortic regurgitation, or for the repair of an aneurysm.

ENDOCRINE AND METABOLIC DISEASES

Hyperthyroidism

Hyperthyroidism (thyrotoxicosis) is a syndrome due to an excess of the circulating thyroid hormones T4 and/or T3. This may result from diffuse hyperplasia of the thyroid gland (Graves' disease) or single or multiple hyperactive nodules. Thyroid overactivity is associated with increased oxygen consumption, heat production, and peripheral vasodilatation. The raised cardiac output which occurs in response to these demands, and to the direct effect of thyroid hormone on the heart, is achieved mainly by tachycardia and increased myocardial contractility rather than by an enlarged stroke volume.

The heart has to support the burden of a greatly enhanced cardiac output when its own metabolic requirements are increased. The normal heart may, in these circumstances, be unable to supply an adequate circulation; a diseased heart is likely to fail.

Clear manifestations of cardiac abnormality, such as cardiomegaly or heart failure, usually imply that the hyperthyroidism has aggravated underlying heart disease. This is most commonly ischaemic but it may be hypertensive or rheumatic. Occasionally, hyperthyroidism is the sole cause of heart failure.

Most of the cardiovascular features of hyperthyroidism can be accounted for by the hypermetabolic state, but it is difficult to attribute the common complication of atrial fibrillation to this cause. This arrhythmia may be due to a direct toxic effect of the thyroid hormone on the myocardium.

Cardiac symptoms are common in hyperthyroid patients, even in the absence of cardiac disease. Palpitation is particularly frequent, and is usually attributable to the combination of sinus tachycardia and a vigorous cardiac action. Atrial fibrillation may be responsible for irregular palpitation.

Breathlessness is also common, and can be due to hyperventilation, anxiety or left ventricular failure. Hyperthyroidism may aggravate angina pectoris in those with coronary artery disease.

Sinus tachycardia is almost invariable if there is not atrial fibrillation, and persists during sleep. The pulse is of large volume and may have a collapsing character. The systolic blood pressure is frequently high, whilst the diastolic is normal or low. The apical impulse is vigorous, but not usually displaced. The heart sounds are loud and there is often a pulmonary midsystolic murmur, due to high flow. Cardiac enlargement and the signs of left- or right-sided heart failure may develop if the thyroid disease is of long standing or if there is coexistent cardiac disease.

The classical features of hyperthyroidism such as weight loss, moist warm extremities, tremor, lid retraction, exophthalmos and goitre are usually present, but all these signs may be slight or absent in the older patient. There are no distinctive features on the ECG or chest radiograph.

Hyperthyroidism can be recognized easily if the characteristic features are present, but the diagnosis can be difficult if the abnormalities are largely confined to the cardiovascular system. It should be suspected whenever sinus tachycardia, atrial fibrillation or cardiac failure is unexplained.

The diagnosis of hyperthyroidism is established by finding abnormally high blood levels of T4 and/or T3 (after allowance has been made for their binding proteins).

Hyperthyroidism may be treated by antithyroid drugs (such as carbimazole, methimazole and propylthiouracil), radio-iodine or partial thyroidectomy. Radio-iodine is the most suitable therapy for most patients with thyrotoxic heart disease (except for women of childbearing age), but surgery may be indicated if the gland is large or if there is a danger of tracheal compression.

When the rapid control of the tachycardia of hyperthyroidism is necessary, a beta-adrenoceptor blocking drug should be given.

The atrial fibrillation of thyrotoxicosis is difficult to slow adequately with digitalis alone; a beta-blocker should be added if not contraindicated. When thyroid overactivity is controlled, d.c. shock is usually effective in restoring sinus rhythm.

Heart disease in hyperthyroidism usually responds well to therapy unless it has been untreated for several years.

Hypothyroidism

Hypothyroidism is associated with reduced levels of circulating T3 and T4, most often as a result of inflammatory destruction of the thyroid. It may, however, be secondary to reduced thyroid-stimulating hormone (TSH) secretion by the pituitary or hypothalamus, or to drugs such as amiodarone.

Hypothyroidism affects the cardiovascular system in several ways:

- the reduced level of body metabolism is associated with a low cardiac output, a diminished peripheral blood flow, a reduction in venous return, and sinus bradycardia;
- the deficiency of thyroid hormone seems to be responsible for interstitial oedema and mucoid infiltration of the myocardium, and for a pericardial effusion;
- the hypercholesterolaemia characteristically present may be responsible for premature coronary atherosclerosis and ischaemic heart disease;
- 'myxoedema coma' is associated with hypotension and bradycardia.

The patient with hypothyroidism seldom has cardiac symptoms, except for dyspnoea and angina pectoris due to coexistent coronary disease. The symptoms and signs of cardiac failure rarely, if ever, occur in the absence of some additional form of heart disease.

The pulse rate is usually between 50 and 60/min. The sluggish apex beat is difficult to feel and the heart sounds are soft.

The ECG is abnormal in showing low voltage of all components of the PQRST complexes; the T waves are flattened or inverted. The chest radiograph shows a large cardiac shadow; echocardiography often reveals that this is due to a pericardial effusion.

Hypothyroidism is usually suspected because of the general sluggishness, the cold and thickened skin, the husky voice, the coarse but scanty hair and the slow pulse, but minor forms of the disorder may easily escape detection. Blood levels of T4 and T3 are low. The most sensitive test for primary hyperthyroidism is the high serum level of TSH, but this is not raised if hypopituitarism is responsible.

Treatment with thyroid substances is effective but may provoke angina pectoris. For this reason, in those suspected of having coronary disease, small doses (e.g. thyroxine 0.0125 mg daily) should be used initially and the dose should be increased very cautiously, if necessary, but not beyond 0.15 mg. The serum TSH level can be useful as a marker of the adequacy of replacement therapy. The addition of a beta-adrenoceptor blocking drug may protect the patient from angina but often fails, in which case the coronary artery bypass surgery may be required.

Acromegaly

In acromegaly, hypersecretion of growth hormone from a pituitary adenoma results in overgrowth in many tissues and organs, including the heart. Hypertension and accelerated atherosclerosis occur.

Diabetes

Diabetes is a metabolic disorder due to the reduced availability or effectiveness of insulin. In type I (insulin-dependent diabetes or IDDM), there is a defective secretion of insulin by the pancreas, probably consequent upon infective or auto-immune damage to the islet cells. Most cases of type II diabetes (non-insulin-dependent diabetes or NIDDM) are probably genetic in origin; in this form of the disease, the tissues are relatively resistant to the actions of insulin. In both types, blood glucose is raised and there is glycosuria, but the major and most dangerous complications are predominantly cardiovascular – affecting the coronary, renal, retinal and peripheral circulations.

Diabetic patients are particularly prone to coronary heart disease, but there is also a diabetic form of cardiomyopathy. Diabetes is also commonly associated with hypertension.

Diabetes is managed with diet, insulin and hypoglycaemic agents. The actual regimen depends on the type of diabetes, and skilled advice is required with regard to diet. The use of hypoglycaemic drugs such as the sulphonylureas is controversial because of some evidence of adverse cardiac side-effects.

Carcinoid syndrome

Malignant carcinoid tumours with metastases in the liver may be associated with pulmonary stenosis and regurgitation, and with tricuspid stenosis or regurgitation, the valve cusps being fixed by fibrosis. The cardiac lesions are probably due to the actions of kinins or of 5-hydroxy-tryptamine (5HT, serotonin) secreted by the tumour. These substances are also responsible for the flushing attacks, telangiectasia, diarrhoea and bronchospasm characteristic of this syndrome.

The cardiac findings in the carcinoid syndrome are those of the particular valve lesion and of right-sided heart failure. The diagnosis is established either by identification of the tumour at laparotomy or by the detection in the urine of large quantities of 5-hydroxy-indole acetic acid (5-HIAA), a breakdown product of 5-HT.

Treatment is unsatisfactory, the diarrhoea may be controlled by codeine, and the flushing by ketanserin (a 5-HT blocker); cardiac failure is treated on conventional lines, valve replacement occasionally being necessary.

Haemochromatosis

In this disorder, which is mainly encountered in older males, there is excessive iron storage associated with cirrhosis of the liver, diabetes and pigmentation of the skin, and a substantial proportion of patients die from a cardiomyopathy, which may be restrictive, but is usually of the dilated congestive type. Treatment of the failure may be temporarily effective as may repeated venesection, but the prognosis is poor.

Gout

There is a statistical association between hyperuricaemia and coronary artery disease, but there is no definite evidence of an increased incidence of coronary disease in those with clinical gout. Gout may be provoked by diuretics; it may occur in severe cyanotic congenital heart disease in association with secondary polycythaemia. It occasionally causes an acute pericarditis.

Glycogen storage disease

In this autosomal recessive disorder, excessive glycogen is deposited in skeletal and cardiac muscle. Breathlessness, feeding difficulties and muscular weakness usually develop about the third month of life and the progression of cardiac failure is relentless. The ECG and the chest radiograph demonstrate biventricular enlargement. Death occurs before the age of 3 years – usually within the first year of life.

Overweight and obesity

Overweight is associated with heart disease in a number of ways:

- overweight is a risk factor for both coronary heart disease and hypertension;

- fat arms in obese patients may cause falsely high blood pressure recordings;
- a specific Pickwickian syndrome of hypoventilation with carbon dioxide retention, hypoxia, somnolence, polycythaemia and right-sided heart failure is sometimes caused by obesity. The obesity is directly responsible for the hypoventilation because it restricts respiratory movement; improvement can be achieved by weight loss;
- overweight is associated with sleep apnoea;
- obesity is important in patients with cardiac disease of any type because the demands on the heart are increased. Weight reduction is an essential component in the prevention and treatment of angina pectoris, hypertension and cardiac failure.

Beriberi

This disease is due to thiamine deficiency, which is usually the result of a diet with a high proportion of polished rice in Eastern countries but is associated with alcoholism in North America and Europe. The deficiency leads to a lack of co-carboxylase which is necessary for the oxidation of pyruvic acid to acetyl coenzyme A. The citric acid cycle is inhibited and the accumulation of lactate and pyruvate may lead to peripheral vasodilatation and impaired cardiac function. The characteristic haemodynamic features are those of a low peripheral vascular resistance and a high cardiac output. Cardiac failure eventually occurs and, in the later stages, the cardiac output may fall.

The clinical features of beriberi heart disease include palpitation, fatigue, breathlessness and peripheral oedema. In some cases there may be acute circulatory failure with hypotension and syncope. There is usually sinus tachycardia with a large pulse and right-sided cardiac failure. The heart is enlarged and there may be a gallop rhythm and systolic murmurs.

The neurological features are those of an ascending peripheral neuritis, commonly accompanied by mental confusion. Paraesthesiae occur in the hands and feet and there is weakness of the legs. The calf muscles are tender and areas of anaesthesia occur.

Neither the ECG, which usually shows non-specific T wave changes, nor the chest radiograph, which reveals cardiomegaly, is helpful in diagnosis. This is usually achieved by obtaining a history of nutritional deficiency or of alcoholism, and by finding evidence of both peripheral neuritis and cardiac failure. Laboratory tests show increased serum pyruvate and lactate levels and a low red blood cell transketolase level.

Most cases respond quickly to thiamine chloride, 50 mg intramuscularly per day. Subsequently, thiamine should be given orally in a dose of 10–20 mg.

Alcoholic cardiomyopathy

Heavy alcohol consumption, even in the absence of nutritional deficiency, can lead to cardiomyopathy. The patients are often middle-aged men who are excessively fond of both food and alcohol. The initial symptom is either breathlessness or palpitation, due to ectopic beats or atrial fibrillation. The ECG may show low, dimpled T waves. In the early stages, abstinence may reverse the picture, but otherwise there is progression with increasing cardiac failure to death.

Treatment consists of complete abstinence from alcohol and use of conventional measures for controlling atrial fibrillation and cardiac failure.

MISCELLANEOUS DISORDERS

Rheumatoid arthritis

This is accompanied by valve disease rather more often than would be expected by chance, although by no means as frequently as is rheumatic fever. Acute pericarditis and pericardial effusion are quite common; pericardial constriction is rare.

Ankylosing spondylitis (rheumatoid spondylitis)

This is associated with aortic regurgitation due to focal destruction of the elastica and media of the aorta.

Reiter's disease

This is characterized by urethritis, seronegative arthritis and conjunctivitis. It is sometimes complicated by pericarditis, myocarditis and aortic regurgitation.

Systemic lupus erythematosus

This often affects the heart, although cardiac symptoms and signs seldom dominate the clinical picture. Acute or chronic pericarditis, with or without effusion, is usually the most obvious evidence of cardiac involvement. Myocarditis sometimes develops, and may be due to disease of the small coronary vessels. Endocarditis also occurs, with large warty excrescences which may involve any of the four heart valves. These lesions seldom give rise to clinical heart disease, but may act as a focus for infective endocarditis.

Polyarteritis

This may result in myocardial infarction, or in cardiac failure without evidence of infarction. The heart failure may be, in part, the result of hypertension which is common in this disorder. Pericardial effusions occasionally occur.

Scleroderma

This may lead to cardiac failure either by producing a cardiomyopathy, usually of the constrictive type, or as a result of pulmonary heart disease secondary to diffuse pulmonary fibrosis.

Pseudoxanthoma elasticum

This is a familial disease affecting connective tissue associated with calcification and proliferation of the media of the coronary and peripheral arteries which may give rise to ischaemic heart disease and hypertension. The skin, particularly in certain areas such as the elbow creases and back of the neck, takes on a crêpe-like appearance with much redundant tissue. Characteristic dark 'angioid' streaks occur in the fundi.

Sarcoidosis

Sarcoidosis can affect the heart primarily, but cardiac sarcoid more often follows lung or more general involvement. It may cause heart failure, syncope due to arrhythmias and heart block, and sudden death.

The Marfan syndrome

This familial autosomal dominant disorder of connective tissue may result in many skeletal, cardiovascular and other abnormalities. These include great height, long limbs with spidery fingers (arachnodactyly), a high arched palate and dislocation of the lens. Defects in the synthesis, secretion and assembly of fibrillin seems to be involved; the gene for fibrillin is closely identified with the site of the Marfan gene on chromosome 15.

A weakness of the aortic media is common and leads to dilatation, aneurysm formation, and dissection. Aortic regurgitation may follow dilatation of the valve ring. Mitral valve disease may result in cusp prolapse and regurgitation.

These abnormalities can be evident in childhood but may not develop until the fifth decade.

There is no specific treatment, but contact sports and isometric exercise should be avoided. The risk of dissection can be reduced by the use of beta-blockers. Surgery may be required for the valve disorders and for progressive enlargement of the aorta, urgently for dissection.

Cardiac tumours

Cardiac tumours are rare. The commonest is the *myxoma* which occurs most frequently in the left atrium, but occasionally in the other chambers. It varies from 1 to 8 cm in diameter, and is usually attached by a pedicle to the atrial septum. Because its position may vary with posture, transient or complete obstruction of the mitral valve may result. The tumour may prolapse into the left ventricle and cause mitral regurgitation. The haemodynamic effects of left atrial myxoma usually resemble those of mitral stenosis. The tumour may also be responsible for embolic phenomena, and can produce constitutional effects such as fever, weight loss, anaemia, finger clubbing, raised sedimentation rate and abnormal serum protein levels. The obstruction of the mitral valve may lead to dyspnoea and, rarely, syncope or vertigo related to posture. Variable mitral systolic and diastolic murmurs may be heard, and there may be a loud first sound and opening snap. The diagnosis should be suspected in patients with signs of mitral stenosis, who have a history of syncope, or variable murmurs, or unexplained fever with a high ESR. The diagnosis can be most readily established by echocardiography which demonstrates a mass within the left atrium (Figs 19.1A and B). The tumour should be removed under cardiopulmonary bypass.

Trauma

Traumatic lesions of the heart may be due to penetrating chest injuries as, for example, from gunshot wounds or stabbing, or from non-penetrating injuries produced by blows to the chest such as steering wheel accidents.

Penetrating injuries

Penetrating injuries may cause lacerations of any of the heart chambers or great vessels, and death may ensue from haemorrhage or cardiac tamponade. If the victim does not die within a few hours, late complications may occur due to infective pericarditis, valve damage or

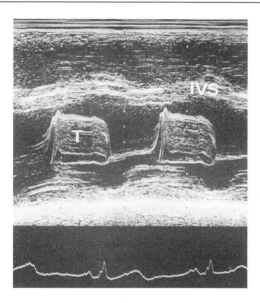

Fig. 19.1A Parasternal M-mode echocardiogram of a left atrial myxoma. Multiple echoes are seen behind the anterior mitral valve leaflet in diastole as the tumour prolapses downwards towards the left ventricle. IVS = interventricular septum. T = tumour.

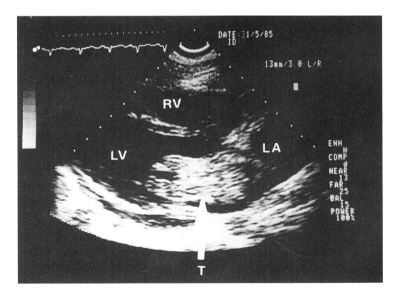

Fig. 19.1B Cross-sectional echocardiogram of myxoma. There is a large tumour (T) situated in the mitral valve orifice.

intracardiac shunts. The diagnosis is usually not difficult and can be deduced from the site of the injury, the evidence of blood loss or cardiac tamponade, or ECG abnormalities.

The chest radiograph may be valuable in locating foreign bodies in or around the heart; echocardiography is useful in detecting pericardial fluid. Pericardial aspiration may relieve tamponade, but for the other serious complications, immediate surgery is usually necessary.

Non-penetrating injuries

A substantial proportion of blunt chest injuries seen in hospital have some cardiac damage. This may take the form of myocardial 'concussion' in which there is functional impairment but no structural damage, or 'contusion' in which there is myocardial necrosis. Myocardial infarction may occur from direct trauma to the muscle, or as a consequence of injury to a coronary artery. In either case, any of the complications of infarction may be seen, including arrhythmias, rupture, and aneurysm formation. In addition, valves and chordae tendineae may be ruptured, and haemopericardium and tamponade may occur. Aortic transection is relatively common, particularly in acceleration accidents.

Unless tamponade or murmurs develop, cardiac damage may not be suspected. Chest radiography, ECG and cross-sectional echocardiography should be undertaken in all cases of severe blunt chest trauma. Aortic damage is probably best located by computed tomography. The patient may require surgical treatment for tamponade, aortic rupture or valve regurgitation.

Physical activity and the athlete's heart

Regular exercise has beneficial effects in preventing coronary heart disease and hypertension, but changes in trained athletes may simulate heart disease. Amongst these are cardiac hypertrophy and bradycardia. Occasionally minor degrees of heart block occur, and in extreme cases, there may be dizziness and syncope. Other symptoms may include palpitation and musculoskeletal chest pain. Undue breathlessness may be due to exercise-induced bronchospasm.

The ECG and echocardiogram may both show the characteristic features of left ventricular hypertrophy, but the abnormalities are usually minor and of no significance.

Sudden death in young athletes attracts great media attention but is very rare. It is usually due to myocarditis or cardiomyopathy, but in older athletes it is more often a result of coronary heart disease.

ANAEMIA AND THE HEART

Anaemia imposes increased demands upon the heart and, at the same time, impairs its function. It aggravates the symptoms of the patient with heart disease and has important circulatory effects even in the individual with a normal heart.

The haemodynamic effects of anaemia probably result mainly from a decrease in blood viscosity and from tissue hypoxia, which is responsible for peripheral vasodilatation. As a consequence, the peripheral arterial resistance is diminished, the diastolic pressure falls and the pulse pressure widens. Ventricular afterload is decreased. The stroke volume and cardiac output are increased when the haemoglobin falls below 7 g/100 ml blood, and both respond to exercise to a greater degree than normal. The hypoxia produces coronary vasodilatation when this is possible, but in the patient with coronary heart disease the ability to dilate is restricted. If anaemia is both severe and prolonged, fatty degeneration of the myocardium takes place.

For the reasons described, anaemia may precipitate or aggravate cardiac failure in the patient with pre-existing heart disease, and it may induce or exacerbate angina in those with coronary heart disease.

It is rare for either heart failure or angina to develop in anaemic patients with normal hearts, but signs and symptoms may occur in such patients which mimic those of heart disease. Dyspnoea, tachycardia and peripheral oedema are common in patients with chronic and severe anaemia.

Anaemia may produce:

- the warm skin and bounding arterial pulse of the high output state;
- a venous hum in the neck;
- cardiac enlargement in the advanced case;
- very commonly, a systolic murmur in the second or third left intercostal space close to the sternum. This is probably due to turbulence resulting from increased flow and reduced blood viscosity;
- a loud third heart sound;
- in very severe cases, a short mitral mid-diastolic murmur, due to increased flow.

The ECG is usually normal, but non-specific ST and T wave changes may occur and the ST depression of myocardial ischaemia may develop.

The clinical features of anaemia are usually readily corrected either by appropriate drug therapy, or by blood transfusion. Rapid transfusion is dangerous, particularly if there is heart failure; in this situation, it is advisable to use packed cells. If whole blood only is available, a diuretic such as intravenous frusemide 40 mg should also be given.

PREGNANCY AND THE HEART

Pregnancy imposes a substantial load on the heart and circulation. The cardiac output and blood volume increase from the sixth week onwards, until, about the 30th week, they are some 30–50% above normal levels at which they remain during the rest of pregnancy. During the last 8 weeks, the inferior vena cava may be obstructed by the uterus when the subject is supine; as a consequence, the cardiac output may fall when this position is assumed. Other factors affecting the cardiovascular system are an increased metabolic rate, a corresponding rise in oxygen consumption, the arteriovenous shunt in the uterus and an elevation in the venous pressure due to the increased blood volume.

Cardiovascular symptoms and signs of normal pregnancy

Dyspnoea, orthopnoea and syncope are not uncommon in the normal pregnant woman. The circulatory changes of pregnancy produce characteristic signs:

- the hands are warm and the pulse is large;
- a tachycardia is present and the venous pressure slightly raised;
- the apex beat is vigorous and may be displaced outwards, partly as a consequence of cardiomegaly and partly by the high diaphragm;
- the high flow almost always produces a soft pulmonary midsystolic murmur and a third heart sound. These are often mistaken for cardiac disease;
- the ECG often shows an axis shift and minor ST segment and T wave changes.

Heart disease in pregnancy

The circulatory burden of pregnancy frequently reveals pre-existing heart disease for the first time. Symptoms may start at about week 12 and tend to progress until they may become severe from week 24 onwards. A period of particular danger occurs after delivery, when the sudden reabsorption of blood from the uterus into the circulation may precipitate pulmonary oedema.

Rheumatic heart disease

Mitral stenosis is the most serious lesion encountered. Patients with tight mitral stenosis may become breathless in early pregnancy and progress to pulmonary oedema or right-sided cardiac failure. Even those with less severe lesions may develop symptoms during the last months or shortly after delivery. Patients with mild mitral stenosis, mitral regurgitation and aortic regurgitation usually tolerate pregnancy well, but may become increasingly breathless.

The management of rheumatic heart disease in the pregnant woman depends upon a number of factors including her age, parity, and religious beliefs, the stage of the pregnancy, the nature of the lesion, and the response to treatment. In the patient with severe mitral stenosis, pregnancy should be avoided or deferred until mitral valvotomy has been performed. If such a patient becomes pregnant, a decision should be made before week 16 as to whether valvotomy should be undertaken or the pregnancy terminated. As pregnancy progresses beyond this time, both termination and valvotomy become more hazardous. If the patient is seen for the first time at a later stage of pregnancy, she should be managed medically, for with adequate bed rest, digitalis and diuretics, the maternal mortality rate is low.

Patients with rheumatic valve lesions other than mitral stenosis should be managed medically or have the pregnancy terminated.

Prosthetic heart valves. Prosthetic heart valves pose a special problem in pregnancy. Warfarin, particularly in the first trimester, may induce congenital abnormalities, but the discontinuation of anticoagulants exposes the patient to an increased risk of thrombo-embolism. Heparin may be preferable for this early phase as well as for the last few weeks of pregnancy. The British Society for Haematology has recommended 10 000 units subcutaneously 12-hourly or 7000 units 8-hourly up to 16 weeks and from 36 weeks to delivery, with warfarin as an alternative from 16 to 36 weeks. If possible, prosthetic valves should not be inserted in women who are likely to become pregnant.

Congenital heart disease

Patients who were born with congenital heart disease are being seen with increasing frequency in pregnancy, but the cardiac abnormality is usually mild or has been corrected by surgery prior to conception. Pregnancy is tolerated well if there is an uncomplicated septal defect or persistent ductus arteriosus. Severe pulmonary hypertension of whatever aetiology is extremely hazardous, with a 25–50% risk of maternal death during the pregnancy or in the puerperium; termination in early pregnancy is to be strongly recommended.

Infective endocarditis

Normal pregnancy rarely gives rise to infective endocarditis even in those with abnormal valves. Routine antibiotic prophylaxis is probably best reserved for patients with prosthetic valves.

Cardiomyopathy

Cardiomyopathy ('peripartal') of unknown aetiology sometimes develops during later pregnancy or the puerperium. Although about one-third of patients recover permanently, there is a risk of progression and of recurrence during subsequent pregnancies.

Termination of pregnancy

With good medical preparation and skilled anaesthesia there is little risk in terminating a pregnancy in the presence of cardiac disease. This procedure is indicated in women with advanced heart disease and severe symptoms in early pregnancy, if they are not suitable candidates for mitral valvotomy. Termination should also be considered for those with less severe disease who would find the care of an additional child burdensome.

Sterilization

This should be considered in patients with heart disease who have completed their families or in whom further pregnancies would be harmful. It should not be undertaken lightly. The religious beliefs of the patient must be respected, the risk of psychological disturbance considered, and the possibility of surgical correction of the cardiac lesion borne in mind.

Contraception

Patients with cardiac disease may wish or need to practise contraception. Advice should be proffered to those for whom pregnancy is temporarily inadvisable.

Oral methods of contraception have the major advantage of reliability. The combined oestrogen and progestogen pill increases the risk of arterial and venous thrombosis, and exacerbates systemic hypertension and pulmonary hypertension. It should, therefore, be avoided in women known to have or be at high risk of these conditions. Women over 35 who smoke should not take the combined oral contraceptive because of the greatly increased risk of cardiovascular disease. Less information is available on the progestogen-only pill, but the risks seem to be substantially less. Intra-uterine devices are better avoided in congenital and valvar heart disease because of the risk, albeit small, of infective endocarditis.

Further reading

Braunwald, E. (1996) *Heart Disease*, 5th edn. Philadelphia: Saunders.
Julian, D. G., Camm, A. J., Fox, K. M., Hall, R. J.C. & Poole-Wilson, P. A. (1994) *Diseases of the Heart*, 2nd edn. London: WB Saunders Company.

Psychological Aspects of Heart Disease

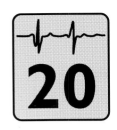

The relationship between psychological factors and heart disease is complex. Many anxious individuals believe, erroneously, that they have heart disease; anxiety and depression often complicate and aggravate organic heart disease.

PSYCHOLOGICAL FACTORS IN THE GENESIS OF HYPERTENSION AND CORONARY DISEASE

The blood pressure rises acutely on emotion; it is therefore reasonable to speculate that there is a relationship between chronic emotional stress and sustained hypertension. This would be very difficult to establish and, as yet, the evidence is equivocal. None the less, hypertensives and their normotensive children appear to have exaggerated responses to emotional stimuli, and relaxation techniques are antihypertensive in some individuals.

There has been much interest in psychological factors in coronary heart disease. Rosenman and Friedman described a 'specific overt behaviour pattern' which they designated type A, characterized by aggression, ambition, impatience and preoccupation with deadlines. They reported a high incidence of coronary disease in such individuals and have also claimed that they could be trained out of these habits after myocardial infarction, with beneficial results. Some have confirmed their observations; others have not. If what they say is true, it is surprising that coronary disease is now commonest amongst manual workers. Other psychological characteristics have been related to coronary disease – perhaps the most persuasive evidence points to suppressed anger and hostility as risk factors. There is certainly little to suggest the view that stressful occupations (traditionally doctors and lawyers) lead to coronary disease.

On the other hand, there can be no doubt of the importance of emotional stress in precipitating episodes of angina pectoris. Rarely, there is strong circumstantial evidence that emotional stress has been a contributory factor in causing myocardial infarction or fatal arrhythmias.

ANXIETY STATE AND THE HEART

Individuals with an anxiety state often have complaints suggestive of heart disease. A large number of labels have been applied to the complex of symptoms of such patients, including 'effort syndrome', 'cardiac neurosis' and 'neurocirculatory asthenia'. It was particularly common in the armed services during war-time, and has therefore been called 'soldier's heart', but it also occurs frequently in civilians.

Breathlessness, palpitation and fatigue are almost invariable, and are usually accompanied by feelings of faintness and dizziness. Chest pain is less common, but is often the reason for referral to a physician.

The breathlessness may be related to exertion, but also occurs at rest. Frequent complaints are that 'I can't take a deep breath' or 'I can't get enough air'. The palpitation is usually the awareness of a sinus tachycardia, but can be due to ectopic beats which cause the patient to think that his or her heart is about to stop.

The chest pain of anxiety state is usually situated in the left submammary region but may be elsewhere in the left chest and may radiate to the left arm. It is sometimes provoked by effort, but tends to come on after exercise rather than during it; it can develop at rest and at night time. It often takes the form of a persistent ache lasting for hours or days; sharp momentary stabs of pain are also frequent. The patient will often say that the pain is 'in his heart'. The muscles in the area may be tender, and in some cases the pain can be abolished by infiltration with local anaesthetics.

Whilst recounting the history, the patient gives an impression of distress, and is tense or rather withdrawn in manner. Sighing respiration is common and there may be hyperventilation. Sinus tachycardia is usual, and palpation reveals a hyperdynamic heart. The hands are often sweaty but cool; there may be a coarse tremor.

The ECG confirms sinus tachycardia and may show non-specific flattening or slight inversion of T waves.

The diagnosis can usually be made from the characteristic symptoms and from observing the patient. The poor relationship of the breathlessness and pain to exertion, and the site, character and duration of the chest discomfort differentiate the syndrome from angina pectoris. The palpitation can be distinguished from that of paroxysmal tachycardia by the lack of sudden onset and by the relationship to emotion.

The prognosis with regard to the relief of symptoms is poor if it is a chronic condition or if there is a serious personality derangement. If the complaints have occurred in response to an obvious emotional stress, the outlook is relatively good. When anxiety about the heart has been induced by the thoughtless or ill-informed comments of physicians, it is particularly difficult to eradicate.

Psychiatric treatment is necessary for the more severe cases, but strong reassurance by the physician may be effective in those patients in whom cardiac symptoms predominate, particularly when an unfounded fear of organic heart disease provoked them. The patient should be instructed to embark upon a programme of gradually increasing physical activity. Sometimes, it may be necessary to give tranquillizers such as diazepam 2–5 mg three times a day. Propranolol in a dose of 10 or 20 mg four times a day is helpful if the palpitation of sinus tachycardia is distressing.

Psychological disturbances in patients with heart disease

Many individuals equate heart disease with total disability and death. Patients with cardiac disorders may regard themselves and be considered by others as 'invalids', even though the lesion may be of little importance or be correctable.

Fear of sudden death is common in those who experience angina and palpitation. Anxiety and depression are important causes of symptoms and disability in patients who have sustained a myocardial infarction or have undergone coronary surgery (see Chapter 9). Headache in hypertensive patients is usually due to tension and only rarely to the high blood pressure.

Excessive anxiety can be prevented by thoughtful management of the patient and his relatives. Frankness should be combined with optimism. One must be careful in one's choice of words; if such terms as angina, murmur or heart failure are to be used, they must be explained in such a way that they do not cause alarm.

Advanced heart disease can cause confusion and delirium as a result of hypoxia or hypotension or, when associated with pulmonary disease, carbon dioxide retention. Similar symptoms may arise from lignocaine overdosage, or following cardiac surgery. Depression may result from a number of cardiac drugs including methyldopa. Fatigue is common in patients on beta-blocking drugs. These psychological disturbances, which are secondary to medical disorders, should be treated by correcting the underlying cause.

Surgery and the Heart

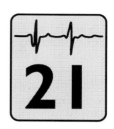

ANAESTHESIA AND GENERAL SURGERY IN PATIENTS WITH HEART DISEASE

Anaesthesia is potentially hazardous in patients with heart disease. Problems may arise due to the direct cardiovascular effect of the anaesthetic agent or indirectly through autonomic reflexes. The interplay of these factors can produce profound effects on blood pressure, cardiac output and heart rhythm and may lead to myocardial ischaemia, myocardial infarction and serious arrhythmias. However, with modern anaesthetic agents and skilled anaesthetic management, these risks can be minimized.

The period of induction of anaesthesia is a time of particular risk. Induction agents generally lower blood pressure. In addition vagal reflexes initiated by endotrachael intubation may result in bradycardia, heart block or even asystole. These problems can once again be minimized with good anaesthetic management.

Although regional anaesthesia, for example with a spinal or epidural anaesthetic, avoids direct cardiac depressant effects, this does not necessarily reduce the risks of the procedure, as these techniques are particularly prone to hypotension, which may provoke myocardial ischaemia.

Ischaemic heart disease

Ischaemic heart disease is a major determinant of operative mortality. Hypotension may provoke serious arrhythmias or result in myocardial infarction. The risks are greatest in patients with a recent myocardial infarction. Operation within 3 months of infarction carries a 30% risk of reinfarction or cardiac death. From 3 to 6 months, this risk falls to 15%, and thereafter to 5%.

Elective surgery should therefore be avoided in the first 6 months following a myocardial infarction. If surgery is unavoidable, risks can be reduced by invasive monitoring and careful regulation of oxygenation, electrolytes and volume status.

In patients with symptoms of stable angina, surgery is in general well tolerated. Once again hypotension should be avoided. Severity of ischaemia can be assessed non-invasively before operation by exercise testing. Maximum workload achieved on exercise testing is an important prognostic indicator – patients who can achieve higher workloads have fewer post-operative complications.

Patients undergoing surgery for peripheral vascular disease pose a particular problem for two reasons. Firstly, this patient population has a high incidence of serious underlying coronary disease. Secondly, patients may be incapable of performing an exercise stress test because of the development of claudication. Dipyridamole thallium imaging (p. 80) has proved of particular value in this patient group as a means of predicting post-operative complications. Patients with a positive dipyridamole thallium scan should undergo coronary angiography to determine the need for a coronary revascularization procedure prior to their peripheral vascular surgery.

Antianginal therapy should, in general, be maintained preoperatively. For beta-blockers in particular, there is a risk of rebound phenomena if the drugs are discontinued. Oral medication should be continued up to and including the morning of the operation. Postoperatively, oral medication should be resumed as soon as possible. If there is a delay in resuming oral medication, parenteral alternatives should be considered.

Hypertension

Patients with hypertension are at increased risk of major peri-operative cardiac complications. This risk is related to associated ischaemic heart disease and left ventricular impairment. Where possible, hypertension should be controlled pre-operatively. Anti-hypertensive medications should be continued up to the time of operation.

Congestive heart failure

Congestive heart failure is a major determinant of peri-operative risk. Both the symptomatic functional class, determined according to the New York Heart Association functional criteria (p. 40), and the presence of clinical signs of heart failure, such as a third sound or pulmonary crepitations, are predictive of outcome. When such features are present, treatment regimens should be optimized before undertaking elective surgery. Care should be taken to avoid excessive diuresis which may cause hypovolaemia and hypotension.

Arrhythmias

The risks associated with surgery in patients with arrhythmias are related to the risks of the underlying heart disease, rather than to the arrhythmias *per se*. There is, therefore, no evidence that simple suppression of ventricular ectopics, for example, will lower risk. The best approach for such patients is careful intra-operative and post-operative monitoring, with management of any haemodynamically compromising rhythm disturbances as they occur.

Conduction defects are a source of concern during anaesthesia, because of the possibility of progression to complete heart block. Temporary pacing is required for patients in established complete heart block or with Mobitz II second-degree AV block (p. 204). Pacing is in general not required for Mobitz I second-degree AV block (Wenckebach) or for patients with bifascicular block.

In patients with an implanted permanent pacemaker, special care is needed in the use of electro-cautery. There is a danger that the electrical fields caused by diathermy may cause inappropriate suppression of a demand pacemaker. Bipolar diathermy is preferable to unipolar. When unipolar diathermy is used, the indifferent electrode should be placed as far from the pacemaker generator as possible. A magnet should be available in the theatre to convert the pacemaker to fixed rate, if pacemaker inhibition should occur.

Valvular heart disease

Major surgery should, if possible, be avoided in patients with severe heart valve disease; it is better to defer general surgery until the valve lesion has been corrected. However, if prosthetic valve surgery is contemplated, it may be preferable to carry out general surgery first in order to avoid operating on a patient receiving anticoagulants.

Short-term withdrawal of anticoagulants in patients with valve prostheses is relatively safe. Oral treatment can be discontinued a few days before surgery, and patients maintained on intravenous heparin until the day of surgery. Heparin should then be resumed as early as is considered safe post-operatively, and maintained until the adequate anticoagulation on oral therapy is established once again.

In emergency operations, clotting can be restored to normal using fresh frozen plasma. Vitamin K reversal is best avoided, as this creates difficulties in re-establishing anticoagulant control post-operatively.

Estimation of risk

Attempts have been made to quantify the cardiac risk in patients undergoing general surgical procedures (Table 21.1). The most important factors in this risk table are a history of myocardial infarction in the last 6 months, and signs of heart failure. Patients can be stratified into four risk groups according to the number of points scored.

Such tables are a useful adjunct in predicting cardiac risk, but they are not a substitute for clinical judgement.

Table 21.1   Multifactorial index score to estimate cardiac risk

Criteria	Point score
History: Age > 70 years	5
Myocardial infarction in last 6 months	10
Examination: S_3 or raised jugular venous pressure	11
Significant aortic stenosis	3
Electrocardiogram: Rhythm other than sinus	7
> 5 ventricular ectopic beats/min	7
General: Any of the following:	
Respiratory failure, K^+ <3.0 mmol, HCO_3 <20 mmol, renal failure,	
liver dysfunction, immobilization	3
Surgery: Abdominal, thoracic, aortic	3
Emergency	4
Total possible	53

Group	Points total	Non-fatal complications (%)	Cardiac death (%)
I	0–5	0.7	0.2
II	6–12	5	2
III	13–25	11	2
IV	>26	22	56

Source: Goldman, L., Caldera, D. L., Nussbaum, S. R. *et al*. (1977) Multifactorial index of cardiac risk in noncardiac surgical procedures. *New England Journal of Medicine* **297**: 845.

SURGERY FOR HEART DISEASE

Indications and contraindications

Most types of congenital and rheumatic heart disease are amenable to surgical treatment (for discussion of individual lesions see Chapters 14 and 15). Surgery also has a major part to play in the management of ischaemic heart disease, infective endocarditis, pericardial constriction and in diseases of the aorta. In deciding whether surgery is necessary in an individual case, one must weigh up the prognosis of the patient without surgery and the risks of morbidity and mortality imposed by surgery. For example, most patients with atrial septal defects or persistent ductus arteriosus are asymptomatic, but have a life expectancy reduced to about 40 years. Surgery in childhood is justified in these cases because the mortality is very low. At the other end of the scale, severe aortic stenosis carries a very poor prognosis and surgery should be undertaken in spite of a mortality which commonly exceeds 5%.

Types of cardiac surgery

Cardiac surgery may be 'closed' or 'open'. In closed heart surgery, the circulation continues through the patient's heart throughout the operation, and the interior of the heart is not inspected. The operations are relatively simple and safe but are limited in scope to such procedures as mitral and pulmonary valvotomy, pericardectomy for pericardial constriction, division of persistent ductus arteriosus, resection of coarctation and shunt operations for tetralogy of Fallot. In experienced hands, the mortality of these operations is low, but post-operative complications include systemic embolism (after mitral valvotomy), arrhythmias, pulmonary collapse and infection, pulmonary embolism and the post-cardiotomy syndrome.

Cardiopulmonary bypass

The vast majority of cardiac operations in the adult require cardio-pulmonary bypass. In cardiopulmonary bypass, the heart and lungs are completely excluded from the circulation. Venous blood is drained by gravity into an oxygenator through cannulae inserted into the inferior and superior venae cavae. A pump is used to recirculate the blood through a cannula positioned in the aorta (Fig. 21.1). When operations are undertaken on the mitral valve, the aortic valve prevents regurgitation into the left ventricle of the blood pumped into the aorta by the artificial heart–lung apparatus. When operations are being carried out on the aortic valve, the aorta must be cross-clamped below the origin of the innominate artery to permit a dry surgical field. The ischaemic myocardium is protected during cross-clamping by a combination of cooling and electromechanical dissociation. Electromechanical dissociation can be achieved either by instilling a potassium-containing, crystalloid, cardioplegic solution into the aortic root (and hence into the coronary tree), or by fibrillating the heart so that contraction ceases. Cross-clamping is also necessary during the construction of coronary anastomoses in coronary artery bypass grafting.

With total cardiopulmonary bypass, the cerebral circulation is maintained, and operations on the open heart lasting up to 5 h can be performed. The potential risks are considerable; the major hazards are cerebral air embolism, trauma to blood by the pump-oxygenator, and electrolyte and acid–base disturbances. The lungs often become abnormally stiff in the post-operative phase, and pulmonary atelectasis and infection are common. If perfusion has been inadequate, renal failure may occur. In the first few days after operation, arrhythmias are frequent.

Open heart surgery with total bypass is suitable for all surgically treatable lesions. Because of the risks involved, it should be under-

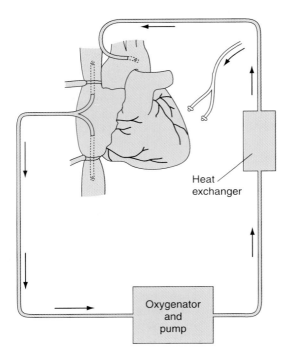

Heat exchanger

Oxygenator and pump

Fig. 21.1 Cardiopulmonary bypass. Venous blood drains from cannulae in the venae cavae into an oxygenator, and is then returned to the femoral artery or aorta by a pump. The temperature of the perfusing blood can be controlled with a heat pump.

taken only by an experienced team of surgeons, anaesthetists and ancillary staff. In the best hands, the mortality rate of the bypass technique itself is less than 1%.

Medical management of patients undergoing cardiac surgery

Pre-operative medical assessment and risk evaluation

The overall medical condition of the patient should be assessed, paying particular attention to major determinants of outcome and complications of surgery. These include:

- *left ventricular function.* This is the most important single determinant of outcome following cardiac surgery;
- *pulmonary function.* Patients with severe respiratory impairment are likely to require prolonged ventilatory support following surgery;
- *renal function.* Patients with renal impairment are likely to suffer further deterioration of renal function following surgery with a possible need for dialysis in the post-operative period;

- *cerebrovascular disease*. Patients with cerebrovascular disease are at increased risk during cardiopulmonary bypass and are at high risk of developing or extending a stroke due to cerebral ischaemia. Other risk factors include the need for emergency operation, age, repeat operation, diabetes and peripheral vascular disease.

In many cases these risk factors cannot be modified, but form part of the overall assessment of the risks and benefits of surgery. Where risk factors are modifiable (e.g. treatment of a chest infection), the patient's condition should be optimized before surgery.

Postoperative management

Ventilation.   Most patients require 6–24 h on a ventilator following cardiac surgery, but substantially longer periods may be required with underlying pulmonary disease.

Low output states.   Low cardiac output is common particularly in patients with poor pre-existing left ventricular function. In others intra-operative myocardial infarction may contribute to a low cardiac output. Such patients require prolonged haemodynamic monitoring, including measurements of pulmonary and systemic arterial pressures together with cardiac output. Filling pressures (preload) should be optimized with administration of intravenous fluid or blood as appropriate. Many patients will require inotropic support (see p. 172), while in a few circulatory support with an intra-aortic balloon pump (see below) may be necessary.

Hypertension.   Post-operative hypertension is common, particularly in patients with a previous history of hypertension. It is important that hypertension should be treated, both to reduce cardiac workload (afterload) and to reduce the risk of post-operative bleeding.

Arrhythmias.   Post-operative arrhythmias occur frequently. Atrial flutter and atrial fibrillation are the commonest and may occur during the patient's stay on intensive care or during subsequent postoperative convalescence. There is no single management strategy and optimal management will depend on the patient's haemodynamic status. Possibilities include d.c. cardioversion, pharmacological cardioversion or pharmacological control of ventricular rate. Management strategies should take consideration of the need for prior anticoagulation to minimize embolic risk in patients with a duration of atrial fibrillation of more than 24 h. Sinus rhythm should be the goal in all patients, although in some patients a decision may be taken to delay this for 6 weeks following surgery until the risks of recurrent atrial fibrillation have diminished. In such cases anticoagulation is essential.

Intra-aortic balloon pumping (counterpulsation)

Mechanical support may be given to the circulation by a balloon introduced via a femoral artery into the descending thoracic aorta which is
inflated in diastole and deflated in systole by an external pump (Fig.
21.2). This reduces afterload and increases coronary and peripheral
diastolic blood flow. It greatly improves the patient with poor cardiac
performance, particularly immediately after cardiopulmonary bypass
surgery. It is of value in cardiogenic shock, as after myocardial infarction, only if it allows the patient to survive until some corrective
surgical procedure can be undertaken.

The replacement of heart valves *(see also Chapter 14)*

Valve replacement has proved highly successful in the management of
serious valvular disease. In appropriately selected patients, valve
replacement ameliorates or abolishes symptoms and causes striking
haemodynamic improvement.

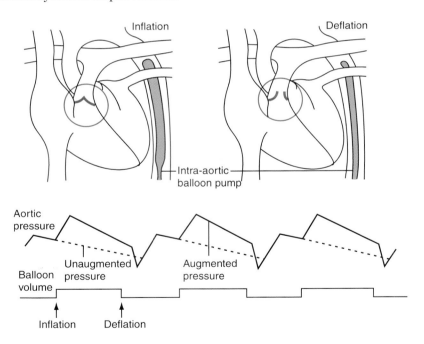

Fig. 21.2   Intra-aortic balloon pump. The balloon is inflated in diastole, following aortic valve
closure. Balloon inflation augments aortic pressure without adding to cardiac workload. The
balloon is deflated in late diastole. The resulting reduction in aortic pressure reduces left
ventricular afterload.

Replacement valves are of two types, mechanical and tissue. Mechanical prostheses take a variety of forms (Fig 21.3):

- ball valves (e.g. Starr–Edwards);
- tilting disc valves (e.g. Bjork–Shiley);
- bi-leaflet valves (e.g. St Jude).

Most tissue valves are isolated, sterilized animal valves (heterografts). The Carpentier–Edwards prosthesis (Fig. 21.4), for example, is prepared from pig valves.

Choice of prosthesis – mechanical or tissue?

Mechanical tissue prostheses differ in their types of complications and in the need for anticoagulants. For tissue valves, the thromboembolic

(A)
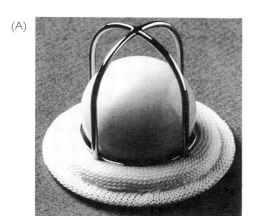

(B)
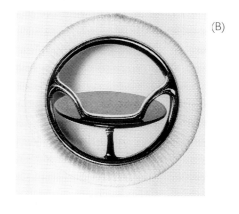

(C)
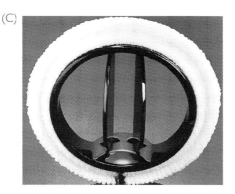

Fig. 21.3 Mechanical valve prostheses. (A) Starr–Edwards; (B) Bjork–Shiley; (C) St Jude.

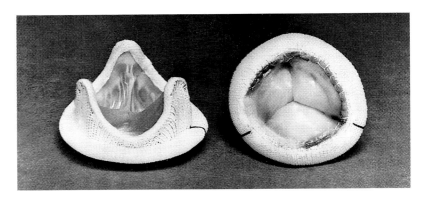

Fig. 21.4 Carpentier–Edwards tissue prosthesis.

complication rate is low and there is no requirement for long-term anti-coagulation. However, tissue valves are prone to failure due to a stiffening and subsequent tearing of the valve leaflets. Over a 10-year period 20–30% of patients require repeat valve replacement for this reason.

For mechanical valves the incidence of thromboembolic complications is greater. Consequently patients require long-term anticoagulation. This in itself carries a small risk of serious haemorrhagic complications. Set against this disadvantage, the incidence of valve failure is very much lower for mechanical valves than for tissue valves. Hence the likelihood of reoperation for valve failure is considerably less.

Prosthesis selection needs to be tailored to the individual patient. In a young individual with no contraindication to anticoagulation, a mechanical prosthesis is preferable. In patients in whom anticoagulants are contraindicated, tissue prostheses will be preferred. In elderly patients, in whom anticoagulants are relatively contraindicated and who are unlikely to live long enough to require a second valve replacement, tissue prostheses are once again preferable.

Complications of prosthetic valves

Thromboembolism. The annual incidence of thromboembolic events in a patient with a metal prosthesis receiving anticoagulant therapy is approximately 1–2%. The risk of thromboembolism is generally greater following mitral than following aortic replacement. The risk of embolic problems is related to the adequacy of anticoagulant control. The international normalized ratio (INR) should be maintained between 3 and 4.5.

Anticoagulant-related complications. The risk of serious haemor-rhagic complications related to anticoagulation is of the order of 1% per annum. For tissue valves, this is greater than the thromboembolic risk and for this reason anticoagulants are unnecessary, unless there is some additional indication for anticoagulation, such as atrial fibrillation.

Primary valve failure. Valve failure is rare with mechanical prostheses. On the rare occasions when failure does occur, it is generally sudden and results in disastrous haemodynamic consequences, frequently resulting in the death of a patient.

In contrast, primary valve failure is common with tissue valves. The incidence of valve failure in 10 years is approximately 20–30% but an accelerated rate of failure is probable after this time. Failure is gradual and generally provides forewarning, allowing valve replacement to be undertaken before serious haemodynamic consequences ensue.

Endocarditis. Endocarditis is a particularly serious complication in prosthetic valves, because eradication of the infection with antibiotics alone is difficult. Endocarditis frequently results in the development of a paraprosthetic leak, with consequent haemodynamic deterioration. Prosthetic valve endocarditis is further discussed on page 389.

Physical findings

Prosthetic valves produce characteristic clicks. These are particularly evident in patients with mechanical prostheses. A mitral prosthesis causes a 'first sound' and 'opening snap', and an aortic prosthesis an 'ejection click' and 'aortic second sound'. Ejection murmurs are common in the case of aortic prostheses and do not indicate any abnormality of function. Regurgitant murmurs, by contrast, are always abnormal, indicating either a valvar or para-valvar leak.

Valve repair as an alternative to replacement

Despite the great success of valve replacement, the problems and complications of prosthetic valves are well recognized. In recent years there has been an increasing emphasis on conservative surgery, when feasible, as an alternative to replacement.

The mitral valve presents the greatest scope for conservation. In patients with mitral stenosis, mitral valvotomy remains the operation of choice for patients with a non-calcified valve and minimal regurgitation. The subsequent incidence of complications is much lower than would be expected for valve replacement.

Valve conservation is also possible for some regurgitant mitral lesions. Best results have been achieved in patients with mitral prolapse, although results are also encouraging in patients with ruptured chordae. Techniques include remodelling of the mitral annulus by leaflet plication, incorporation of a prosthetic ring and chordal shortening procedures.

Conservative procedures have also proved successful in the management of tricuspid disease – this generally involves the insertion of a ring prosthesis.

Further reading

Bonchek, L. J. (1981) Current status of cardiac valve replacement. *American Heart Journal* **101**: 96.
Goodwin, J. F. (1986) Cardiac transplantation. *Circulation* **74**: 913.
Schroeder, J. S. & Hunt, S. A. (1986) Cardiac transplantation: where are we? *New England Journal of Medicine* **315**: 961.

Practical Guidelines for the Management of Cardiac Emergencies

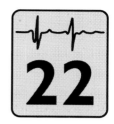

22

ACUTE MYOCARDIAL INFARCTION

The patient should be placed on a cardiac monitor and venous access established. A 12-lead ECG should then be performed. If this confirms acute myocardial infarction, the following treatment should be given.

Pain relief

Pain relief in acute myocardial infarction is of the utmost importance. Patients should be given diamorphine 5 mg i.v., accompanied by an anti-emetic such as cyclizine 50 mg i.v. In frail or elderly patients, or patients with a history of respiratory problems, it may be advisable to reduce the dosage of diamorphine to 2.5 mg. Conversely, in some individuals, 5 mg will not be enough to ensure pain relief and this dose may need to be repeated.

Aspirin

Aspirin is of proven benefit in reducing mortality in acute myocardial infarction. A 300 mg tablet of soluble aspirin should be given as quickly as possible. There are few absolute contraindications to aspirin. In the majority of instances, the relative contraindication of a history of peptic ulceration can be overlooked, as the benefits of treatment outweigh the risk.

Thrombolysis

A streptokinase infusion should be commenced as quickly as possible. Streptokinase (1.5 million units) is dissolved in 100 ml of saline, to be infused over 60 min. Hypotension is frequently encountered during the infusion, but in general resolves rapidly following temporary interruption of the infusion, which can then be resumed. Anaphylaxis can occur, but it is rare.

Table 22.1   Contraindications to thrombolytic therapy

Absolute contraindications
   Suspected aortic dissection
   Previous subarachnoid or intracerebral haemorrhage
Major contraindications
   Active bleeding
   Recent major surgery or serious trauma within 2 weeks
   Severe gastrointestinal haemorrhage within 2 weeks
Minor contraindications
   History of cerebrovascular accident with residual disability
   Use of anticoagulant
   Known bleeding diathesis
   Systolic blood pressure >180 mg – try to lower systolic blood pressure with nitrates before
     commencing thrombolysis
   Haemorrhagic diabetic retinopathy
   Active peptic ulceration
   Oesophageal varices or severe liver disease
   Prolonged cardiopulmonary resuscitation
   Possible pregnancy

Adapted from: Vincent, R. (1995) Myocardial infarction: thrombolysis after infarction. *Prescribers Journal* **35** (3): 140.

Contraindications. There are few absolute contraindications to thrombolysis (Table 22.1). Most contraindications are relative and must be considered in relation to the potential benefits of treatment. In general the potential benefits of treatment are greatest in large infarcts treated early and are greater in anterior than in inferior infarcts.

Streptokinase should not be used in a patient who has had previous streptokinase treatment more than 5 days and less than 2 years previously. In these patients tissue plasminogen activator (tPA) should be considered as an alternative.

tPA may also be considered as an alternative to streptokinase either for the treatment of selected patients or for the treatment of all patients (see Chapter 9, p. 136).

Supportive management

If the patient is short of breath, oxygen therapy may be indicated. If there is evidence of failure, a diuretic should be given. Arrhythmias should be treated if these are haemodynamically compromising.

CARDIAC ARREST

Basic life-support

The term basic life support refers to the simple resuscitative measures which any individual can undertake, without the use of specialist equipment, to restore an adequate ventilation and circulation following a cardiac arrest. It comprises:

- initial assessment
- airway maintenance
- mouth to mouth ventilation
- chest compression

The purpose of basic life-support is to maintain the circulation until more definitive treatment of the arrest, generally in the form of a defibrillator, is available. The majority of cardiac arrests occur outside hospital and in this setting the provision of basic life-support pending the arrival of a defibrillator is of the utmost importance to improve the chances of a successful outcome.

The following sequence of basic life-support measures have been proposed by the United Kingdom Resuscitation Council.

Check responsiveness

The subject should be gently shaken while asking 'What's the problem?' or 'Are you all right?'. If there is no response the rescuer should shout for help and continue with the resuscitative measures below.

Check the airway

It is necessary to open the airway by tilting the head backwards and lifting the chin. Any obvious obstructions such as dentures or vomitus should be removed.

Check for breathing and initiate respiration

The rescuer should look for chest movements, listen at the victim's mouth for breath sounds and feel at his mouth for any air movements. If he is not breathing help should be summoned, even if this means leaving the victim to call for help. Mouth to mouth resuscitation should be commenced with two *effective* rescue breaths. The chest should be seen to rise and fall with each breath. While pinching the subject's nose and maintaining chin lift, the rescuer should blow steadily into the victim's mouth for $1\frac{1}{2}$–2 s. If resuscitation aids are available, these should be used. An airway should be inserted and a bag valve mask unit substituted instead of mouth to mouth respiration.

Assess for signs of circulation

After two effective breaths the rescuer should check for signs of a circulation, by checking the carotid pulse. If a pulse is detected the rescuer should continue rescue breathing until the victim breathes on his own. When he does so he should be turned on his side into the recovery position to help to safeguard his airway.

If no pulse is detected within 10 s chest compression should be commenced. For external cardiac massage the patient must be lying on a firm surface, either on the floor or on a board placed behind his chest. The heel of one hand should be placed on the lower part of the sternum and the heel of the other hand placed immediately on top of it. The sternum should then be rhythmically depressed, by about 3–5 cm, 100 times per minute. The action should be forceful and must be applied only to the sternum. Pressure by the fingers or the hand on the ribs may lead to fractures which may cause serious respiratory embarrassment or damage the liver and spleen. If the cardiac compression is effective, pulses can be felt in the carotid or femoral arteries and the pupils become smaller. Rescue breathing should be combined with chest compression. After every 15 compressions, two effective breaths should be administered.

After every minute of cardio-pulmonary resuscitation, chest compressions and breathing should be briefly interrupted to check for the return of a pulse and spontaneous respiration.

Advanced life-support

Basic life-support is a holding measure until definitive treatment of the patient's underlying rhythm disturbance can restore cardiac output. Out-of-hospital ambulance paramedics equipped with defibrillators can provide definitive treatment. In hospital, this is the role of the cardiac arrest team.

Guidelines for the sequence of resuscitative procedures in advanced life support have been suggested by the United Kingdom Resuscitation Council. Patients can be divided into three categories according to their presenting arrhythmia in cardiac arrest

- ventricular fibrillation
- apparent asystole
- electro-mechanical dissociation

Although the specific treatment given to the patient will differ according to the mode of arrest, there is a considerable overlap of the general procedures which should be applied during advanced life-support. The most recent guidelines emphasise these common features and advocate a single algorithm (Fig. 22.1).

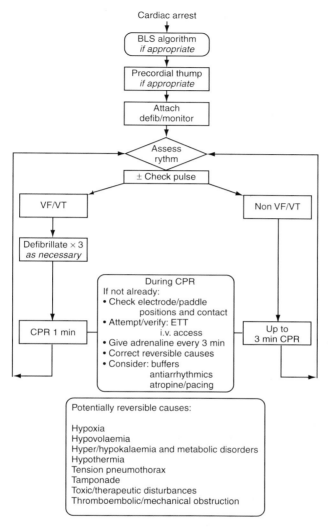

Fig. 22.1 Algorithm for advanced life support management. BLS = Basic life support. Reproduced with permission from Robertson, C. E. (1997) *British Journal of Anaesthesia* **79**: 172.

The route of access to this algorithm will vary from patient to patient. In some basic life-support may have been ongoing for some time. In others, for example those monitored on a coronary care unit, clinical and electrocardiographic detection of arrest are likely to be simultaneous.

In patients who have had a witnessed collapse, a precordial thump is advocated prior to the attachment of monitor/defibrillator leads or if there is any delay in the administration of the first defibrillating shock. With many defibrillators application of the paddles to the chest wall enables an ECG strip to be recorded, categorising the underlying rhythm disturbance. In other instances, the rhythm should be established by attaching the patient to a cardiac monitor.

If ventricular tachycardia or ventricular fibrillation is confirmed, a defibrillator shock should be given as rapidly as possible. The patient should receive up to three shocks in rapid succession of 200 J, 200 J and 360 J. If these do not restore sinus rhythm cardio-pulmonary resuscitation should be commenced and continued for 1 minute before the rhythm is again assessed and a further sequence of three shocks aplied, assuming the patient continues in ventricular fibrillation.

While the sequential loops of the left-hand side of the algorithm are continuing, other resuscitative measures should be put in place. These should include attempts to secure the airway with an endotracheal tube, the establishment of intravenous access and the administration of intravenous adrenaline. 1 mg of adrenaline should be administered every 3 minutes throughout the resuscitation.

In patients with refractory ventricular fibrillation, consideration should be given to the administration of additional drugs such as sodium bicarbonate (50 mmol i.v.). Antiarrhythmic drugs such as lignocaine (100 mg i.v.), bretylium (400 mg i.v.) or amiodarone (300 mg i.v.) should also be considered. Changing the defibrillator paddle positions or substituting an alternative defibrillator may also be apropriate.

Apparent asystole

True asytole is uncommon early in cardiac arrest. When asystole does occur it is generally the result of prolonged arrest and indicates a very poor prognosis. On occasions it is possible to be misled, if the gain control has been turned back on the monitor, and to interpret ventricular fibrillation as asystole. For this reason, unless the physician is certain that the underlying rhythm is true asystole, the patient should be defibrillated.

In cases of true asystole, patients should be given 3 mg of atropinine i.v., in addition to the standard advanced life-support algorithm. Emergency pacing should be considered if facilities are available for this.

Electro-mechanical dissociation

Electro-mechanical dissociation is frequently a late event in cardiac arrest and indicates a poor prognosis. When electro-mechanical dissociation is the presenting feature it suggests the possibility of an underlying left ventricular rupture and it is unlikely that the patient will be resuscitated. However there are also other causes of electro-mechanical dissociation which should not be overlooked, as these disorders are potentially remediable. Treatable causes of electro-mechanical dissociation include

- hypovolaemia
- pneumothorax
- cardiac tamponade
- pulmonary embolism
- drug overdose or intoxication
- hypothermia
- electrolyte imbalance

Appropriate treatment depends on recognition of the specific underlying cause.

Management post-arrest

After resuscitation from a cardiac arrest the patient should be carefully monitored, preferably on a coronary care unit. If the patient remains unconscious it will certainly be necessary to protect the airway and it may be necessary to provide ventilatory support. Blood gases should be checked frequently. Electrolytes should also be checked and hypokalaemia corrected. Following an arrest due to ventricular fibrillation potassium should be maintained in the high normal range.

MANAGEMENT OF TACHYARRHYTHMIAS

For all tachyarrhythmias, if the patient is severely compromised haemodynamically, cardioversion is the most appropriate treatment. In less severely compromised patients, drug management may be considered. Drug selection is determined by the nature of the arrhythmia. A simple diagnostic algorithm to aid in the diagnosis of a number of common arrhythmias is presented in Fig. 22.2.

Ventricular tachycardia

Rapid ventricular tachycardias cause cardiac arrest and management is similar to ventricular fibrillation. In less severely compromised patients, intravenous drug treatment should be considered, before resorting to cardioversion. Lignocaine is the drug of first choice. It is relatively non-toxic and is unlikely to cause haemodynamic deterioration or to exacerbate the arrhythmia. In patients failing to respond to lignocaine, cardioversion is the safest option. Alternatively, another

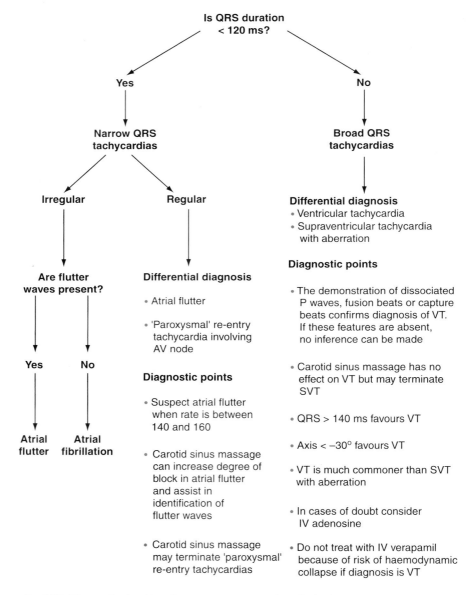

Fig. 22.2 Diagnostic algorithm for some common tachyarrhythmias.

class I antiarrhythmic agent can be administered. Flecainide (up to 2 mg/kg i.v. over 10 min) is one possibility but care needs to be taken because of the drug's negative inotropic effects and potential pro-arrhythmic action.

Undiagnosed broad complex tachycardias

The majority of broad complex tachycardias are ventricular in origin. A minority are supraventricular, with accompanying bundle branch block. The diagnostic features of ventricular tachycardia are described on p. 200. If the diagnosis remains in doubt, the patient should be given intravenous adenosine. This terminates the majority of supraventricular tachycardias and is without effect on ventricular tachycardias (Table 22.2).

Adenosine should be administered as a series of increasing intravenous boluses, successive doses being determined by response of the arrhythmia. The recommended initial bolus dose for adults is 3 mg over 2 s. If the tachycardia does not terminate within 1–2 min, a second bolus dose of 6 mg should be given. If after a further 1–2 min, this too is unsuccessful a third bolus dose of 12 mg should be given.

Transient side-effects, particularly chest discomfort and dyspnoea, are common. Occasionally there may be excessive bradycardia and heart block, but this generally lasts only a few seconds. Adenosine is best avoided in patients on therapy with dipyridamole and may be ineffective in patients receiving theophylline. Adenosine can provoke bronchospasm in predisposed individuals and is contraindicated in asthmatics.

Torsades de pointes tachycardia

This arrhythmia is generally a manifestation of drug toxicity or metabolic disturbance. It is frequently multifactorial in origin. Episodes causing collapse and loss of consciousness may require d.c. shock, although the arrhythmia generally takes the form of recurrent, self-terminating episodes of tachycardia. The precipitating cause should be identified and corrected. Correction of hypokalaemia is particularly important. In many cases, bradycardia contributes to the genesis of the arrhythmia. This should be treated by pacing, at a rate of 90–100 beats/min. Atrial pacing is satisfactory but is more prone to lead displacement than ventricular pacing, which is more commonly chosen. If pacing cannot be easily instituted, then an isoprenaline infusion should be considered as an alternative.

Atrial fibrillation

If the patient is severely compromised haemodynamically, cardioversion may be appropriate. However, in many cases atrial fibrillation occurs because the patient is ill in other ways and in these circumstances the arrhythmia is likely to recur after cardioversion. If cardioversion is undertaken, the initial shock strength should not be less than 100 J.

In many cases drug treatment of the arrhythmia is appropriate. A number of options are possible. These options are alternatives – different antiarrhythmic drugs should not be combined:

Table 22.2 Response to adenosine

Arrhythmia	Response
'Paroxysmal' supraventricular tachycardia	Termination
Atrial fibrillation, atrial flutter	Transient increase in AV block
Ventricular tachycardia	No effect
Atrial fibrillation in Wolff–Parkinson–White syndrome	No effect on ventricular rate, but increased pre-excitation

- digoxin 1 mg i.v. in 100 ml saline over 2 h (or 0.5 mg orally repeated after 2 h). Digoxin limits the ventricular response rate but has no direct action to restore sinus rhythm;
- flecainide up to 2 mg/kg i.v. over 10 min. Flecainide is effective in restoring sinus rhythm in the majority of patients with acute onset atrial fibrillation. However the drug should be used with caution because of its negative inotropic effects and potential pro-arrhythmic action;
- amiodarone 300 mg i.v. over 30 min followed by up to 1200 mg in 24 h. Amiodarone is effective in restoring and maintaining sinus rhythm. The drug has the disadvantage of causing thrombophlebitis when given via a peripheral line and should hence be administered via a central line.

It should be appreciated that many cases of atrial fibrillation terminate spontaneously without the need for any treatment. This is particularly true following myocardial infarction. Episodes of atrial fibrillation related to alcohol abuse are also, in general, self-limiting and specific antiarrhythmic treatment is unnecessary.

When intervening either pharmacologically or with cardioversion to restore sinus rhythm, the possibility of systemic embolism should be considered. There is a risk of thrombus formation in the fibrillating atria, particularly during prolonged episodes of fibrillation, with subsequent embolism on restoring sinus rhythm. If atrial fibrillation is not causing haemodynamic compromise, a safer approach may be to control the ventricular response rate and anticoagulate the patient with warfarin, prior to elective cardioversion in 1 month.

Atrial flutter

The same agents used for ventricular rate control in atrial fibrillation can also be used for rate control in atrial flutter. However, pharmacological treatment is less often successful in restoring sinus rhythm and hence cardioversion may be more appropriate. The initial shock strength should be 25 J and this succeeds in reverting the majority of patients. In some patients it is possible to terminate the arrhythmia by atrial pacing.

Paroxysmal supraventricular tachycardia

This term encompasses a number of different arrhythmias, due to re-entry tachycardia involving conduction through the AV node (Chapter 11, p. 184). Carotid sinus massage will terminate a proportion of these arrhythmias and should be attempted before drug therapy. If the patient is severely compromised cardioversion is appropriate, in which case a 25-J shock is generally sufficient. In most instances the patient is sufficiently well to consider drug treatment. Intravenous adenosine (see p. 399 for dosage) is an appropriate treatment (Fig. 22.3). Verapamil 5 mg i.v. over 30 s (repeated after 1 min if necessary) is an alternative.

Atrial fibrillation in Wolff–Parkinson–White syndrome

Patients are frequently severely compromised haemodynamically. Cardioversion may well be necessary (100-J shock). In patients well enough to consider drug treatment, flecainide (up to 2 mg/kg i.v. over 10 min, maximum total dose 150 mg) is the most appropriate therapy.

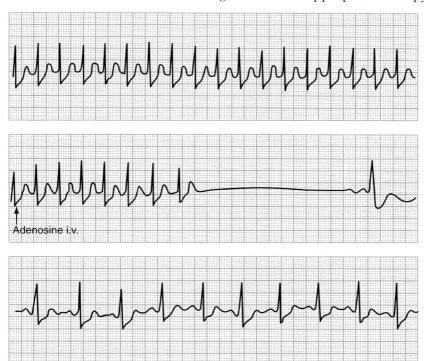

Fig. 22.3   A narrow complex supraventricular tachycardia is terminated by a bolus of intravenous adenosine. There is a 3-second pause on restoration of sinus rhythm. With resumption of sinus rhythm a delta wave is apparent, revealing the underlying diagnosis of Wolff–Parkinson–White syndrome. Continuous rhythm strips.

MANAGEMENT OF PULMONARY OEDEMA

A venous line should be inserted and the patient should be monitored. If there is an underlying cardiac rhythm disturbance, this should be corrected. Specific measures for the treatment of pulmonary oedema include:

Oxygen

Oxygen (40%) should be given to correct hypoxaemia. Most patients are hypocapnic and CO_2 retention is rarely a problem, but in occasional patients with obstructive airways disease and CO_2 retention, it may be necessary to use a lower inspired oxygen concentration.

Diamorphine

The standard dose of diamorphine is 5 mg given intravenously. It may be necessary to reduce this dose in elderly or frail patients. The diamorphine should be accompanied by an anti-emetic, such as cyclizine.

Nitrates

Administration of a sublingual tablet of glyceryl trinitrate has an immediate effect to lower pulmonary pressures and reduce pulmonary oedema.

Frusemide

The patient should be given intravenous frusemide. The usual dose would be 40 mg, but this may be increased in patients already on diuretic therapy. The immediate benefits of frusemide are related to a direct effect to reduce pulmonary pressures – the benefits from diuresis take longer to occur.

In cases of refractory pulmonary oedema inotropic therapy should be considered. Aminophylline 250 mg i.v. over 10 min is frequently effective. Alternatively, patients may be commenced on a dobutamine infusion, commencing at 5 µg/kg/min.

MANAGEMENT OF PULMONARY EMBOLISM

General management and pain relief

Opiates such as diamorphine are appropriate, but care is needed in hypotensive patients. Hypoxaemia is likely and high concentrations of oxygen (at least 40%) should be administered. It is usual to have high right-sided filling pressures following pulmonary embolism. Any decrease in the right-sided filling pressure is likely to lead to a further decrease in cardiac output. For this reason diuretics and vasodilators should be avoided. If right-sided pressure should fall, it may become necessary to give intravenous fluids to maintain cardiac output.

Anticoagulation

The patient should be heparinized to prevent further embolism. Therapy should be initiated with a bolus of 5000–10 000 units, followed by a maintenance infusion of 1000 units/h, adjusted according to the activated partial thromboplastin time (APTT). The APTT should be maintained at approximately twice the control value.

Thrombolysis

In patients with severe haemodynamic compromise, thrombolytic therapy should be given to dissolve the embolus. A loading dose of 600 000 units of streptokinase should be given over 30 min, followed by a maintenance infusion of 100 000 units hourly, with subsequent adjustment in accordance with clotting parameters.

Embolectomy

Pulmonary embolectomy is rarely undertaken. Its use is confined to patients who continue to deteriorate despite thrombolytic therapy or patients in whom there is an absolute contraindication to the use of thrombolytic agents.

MANAGEMENT OF CARDIAC TAMPONADE

General management

The management of cardiac tamponade depends upon clinical circumstances. In many cases, haemodynamic compromise may be relatively mild and no action may be required other than simple observation. As in pulmonary embolism, patients with cardiac tamponade have high right-sided filling pressures. Diuretics and vasodilators should be avoided. Further elevation of right-sided pressures with intravenous fluids may be of value and gain a temporary improvement in cardiac output while awaiting more definitive therapy.

In other cases of more severe haemodynamic compromise, intervention may be necessary. If the patient is not critical and if there is an underlying cause of tamponade which is likely to recur, formal surgical drainage with the formation of a pericardial window to the pleural cavity is most appropriate.

In cases of severe haemodynamic compromise, where urgent action is required, pericardial aspiration is indicated. In all but the most severe emergencies, the pericardial effusion should be defined with an echocardiogram. This facilitates assessment of the best approach for drainage, which in most cases will be subcostal. In a few cases, however, there may be a greater separation of pericardium from myocardium over the apex and in these circumstances an apical approach should be considered.

Pericardial aspiration – subcostal approach

The patient should be sitting at an angle of 45° with the back supported. Local anaesthetic is infiltrated just to the left of the xiphisternum. An 18- or 16-gauge aspiration needle is then inserted, directed towards the left shoulder. Prior echocardiography can demonstrate the correct angulation of the needle. A sterile, insulated wire with a crocodile clip at each end is attached to the needle and to a V lead of an appropriate ECG machine. The needle is advanced slowly applying gentle suction until either pericardial fluid is aspirated or ST elevation becomes apparent on the electrocardiogram recorded from the needle – ST elevation indicates that the needle has contacted the myocardium (Fig. 22.4). A sudden 'give' will usually be felt when the pericardial space is entered. If blood is withdrawn it should be observed for clotting to determine whether the specimen has been obtained from a cardiac chamber – fluid from a haemopericardium will not clot. Once the needle is in the pericardial space a guidewire is passed and the needle replaced by a blunt cannula or a catheter such as a pigtail catheter.

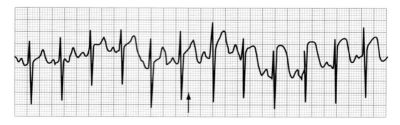

Fig. 22.4   Pericardial aspiration. An ECG has been recorded by attaching the V lead of an ECG machine to the aspiration needle. The development of marked ST elevation indicates that the tip of the needle is in direct contact with myocardium.

TEMPORARY CARDIAC PACING

Temporary cardiac pacing is most frequently undertaken using the Seldinger technique via a subclavian approach. The skin is anaesthetized about 1 cm below the mid-point of the clavicle, a local anaesthetic infiltrated upwards underneath the clavicle and then medially towards the sternal notch. A longer needle attached to a saline-filled syringe is then substituted and passed in the same direction, whilst aspirating. When the subclavian vein is entered a guidewire is passed through the needle and along the vein, under fluoroscopic guidance to the right atrium. The needle is then withdrawn and an introducer passed over the guidewire. The guidewire itself is then withdrawn and a bipolar temporary pacing wire passed through the sheath.

The pacing wire is passed to the right atrium. In general, it is difficult to advance the pacing wire directly across the tricuspid valve and this can only be achieved by forming a loop in the right atrium. The wire should be positioned along the floor of the ventricle with its tip in the apex. The pacing threshold is then determined by attaching the wire to an external pacemaker box. In general the threshold should be less than 1 V, at a pulse duration of 0.5 ms. Occasionally, particularly in patients with a right ventricular infarction, it may be necessary to accept higher thresholds.

Complications of temporary pacing

Pneumothorax. After any subclavian venous puncture, a chest radiograph should be requested to check for a pneumothorax. Angling the exploring needle as close as possible to the undersurface of the clavicle minimizes the risk of pneumothorax. In patients with severe respiratory disease, in whom a pneumothorax might provoke respiratory failure, alternative pacing routes should be considered (see below).

Subclavian artery puncture. Even in the most experienced hands it is possible to puncture the subclavian artery rather than the subclavian vein. If arterial puncture should occur, serious consequences are rare. The exception, however, is in thrombolysed patients, where severe bleeding may result. As the subclavian artery is inaccessible to apply pressure, bleeding may be difficult to control. For this reason, where possible, subclavian access should be avoided, when temporary pacing becomes necessary following thrombolysis in acute myocardial infarction. Venous access for pacing can also be achieved by the antecubital vein, the femoral vein or the jugular vein.

Lead displacement. This results in a loss of capture or variable capture and necessitates reposition of the pacing wire.

Lead perforation.   This may occur acutely during lead positioning or due to gradual erosion over a number of days. It causes a rise in the threshold and may result in loss of pacing. The threshold should be checked every day in a patient with a temporary wire to detect any change in the threshold which might indicate perforation. When perforation occurs it may result in pericardial pain and may, occasionally, cause cardiac tamponade.

HYPERTENSIVE CRISIS

If the diastolic blood pressure exceeds 140 mmHg, there is considerable danger of stroke or hypertensive encephalopathy and urgent treatment is necessary to lower the blood pressure. Urgent treatment is also required in patients with bilateral fundal haemorrhages or exudates.

Although urgent control of blood pressure is desirable, excessively rapid reducton may be equally dangerous. Rapid pressure reduction may result in hypoperfusion of the brain, and cause irreversible cerebral damage.

For patients who are alert and in no immediate danger, oral therapy alone may be satisfactory. Nifedipine, 10 mg orally or sublingually, lowers the blood pressure by about 25% in 30 min. The dose may be repeated in a further 30 min if needed. In occasional patients the fall in blood pressure may be excessive and result in cerebral ischaemia.

If more urgent control of blood pressure is required, this can be achieved by parenteral drug administration. A nitroprusside infusion is frequently chosen and provides a rapid pressure reduction in all patients. The starting dose is 0.25 µg/kg/min, which can be titrated up according to response. Great care is necessary, because a slightly excessive dose may cause severe hypotension and result in cerebral ischaemia. One of the advantages of nitroprusside is that the hypotensive effect disappears in minutes once the drug is stopped. Direct intra-arterial pressure measurements are indicated to guard against excessive pressure reduction.

Labetalol is sometimes chosen as an alternative for its combined alpha- and beta-antagonism. The drug is best given as an infusion with a starting dose of 2 mg/min. The infusion should be continued until a satisfactory blood pressure response is achieved and then stopped. The effective dose is usually in the range 50–200 mg.

Further reading

Handley, A. J. (1997) Basic life support. *British Journal of Anaesthesia* **79**: 151.
Robertson, C. E. (1997) Advanced life support guidelines. *British Journal of Anaesthesia* **79**: 172.
Vincent, R. (1997) Drugs in modern resuscitation. *British Journal of Anaesthesia* **79**: 188.

Clinical Trials and their Influence on Clinical Practice

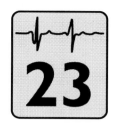

23

It is now widely recognized that practice should be based on sound scientific evidence and that the best guide to treatment is the randomized clinical trial. Fortunately in cardiology and, particularly, in ischaemic heart disease and hypertension, there are now a large number of excellent trials which should provide the basis for rational therapeutics. It is important for clinicians to understand the principles upon which trials can be judged, because there are many that do not achieve an adequate standard. One must also be aware of their limitations.

Essential characteristics of a good clinical trial

Every trial should have a clearly stated hypothesis: the concept that the trial sets out to evaluate. It should define one or, at the most, two primary outcomes or end-points. It should be randomized so that the two or more groups being compared are as similar as possible in their characteristics at the start of the trial. Preferably, it should be double blind so that neither the patients nor those treating them are aware who is in the active treatment group and who is a control. Patients enrolled in the trial should be fully informed of its nature and give informed consent.

Those designing the trial should state what they anticipate as the probable event rate in the control and treated groups, and provide the statistical basis on which the number of patients to be recruited was decided. The trial must be large enough to make it unlikely that an apparently significant result was due to chance. In the past, most trials were too small.

Limitations of trials

Some clinical situations do not lend themselves to randomized clinical trials. Thus, if the mortality rate associated with a condition is predictably extremely high without treatment (such as cardiac arrest), it would be unethical to have a placebo group when clearly effective therapy is available (such as cardiopulmonary resuscitation). In some cases, it is impractical to obtain informed consent, such as in those with mental impairment. It is often possible to recruit only a relatively small proportion of patients with the condition under study for a variety of reasons (such as anticipated non-compliance), and it may then be difficult to extrapolate from the population included to those not included in the study.

Systematic reviews and meta-analyses

There are some trials, such as those cited above, that give a definite answer to a clinical question. However, it is often the case that trials are too small to answer convincingly any or all of the questions that are important to clinicians. By pooling the results of several trials, it may be possible to reach conclusions on the basis of the accumulated data and, furthermore, to do so about specific subgroups that are seldom possible from a single trial. Thus, most individual trials in ischaemic heart disease have had too little information about women·or the elderly; reviews, however, have produced clinically useful information by pooling the results of several trials.

A good example is the 'aspirin papers', in which many trialists collaborated to produce a detailed review of all the aspirin trials in cardiovascular disease. As a consequence, it was possible to show what was not clearly demonstrated in single trials, for example that aspirin was effective in preventing venous thrombosis and in the long-term management of patients after myocardial infarction.

Examples of clinical trials

Listed below are some of the major trials that have changed the practice of cardiology over the past two decades.

THROMBOLYSIS IN ACUTE MYOCARDIAL INFARCTION

GISSI

Over 11 000 patients presenting within 12 h of the onset of chest pain were randomized to receive either streptokinase or conventional treatment. Mortality at 21 days was reduced by streptokinase from 13.0% to 10.7%. Analysis of subgroups within the study suggested that patients who presented early benefited most; for patients treated within the first hour, the reduction in mortality rate was almost 50%.
Lancet 1987; **ii**: 871–4.

ISIS-2

In this study, two agents (aspirin 160 mg and streptokinase 1.5 mega units) were each compared against placebo in a study of over 17 000 patients. As in the GISSI study, streptokinase significantly reduced the mortality rate from 12.0% to 9.2%. What was less expected was that aspirin also significantly reduced the mortality rate from 11.8% to 9.4% and that the effect of the two agents in combination was cumulative. In patients who received both streptokinase and placebo, the mortality rate was 8.0% compared with 13.2% for those who received both placebo preparations.
Lancet 1988; **ii:** 349–60.

GISSI-2

Some 12 000 patients were randomized to receive either streptokinase or tissue plasminogen activator (tPA) with or without heparin. The overall mortality in the study was low (in keeping with the beneficial effects of thrombolysis) but there were no significant differences between the two agents used.
Lancet 1990; **336:** 65–71.

ISIS-3

This trial of over 40 000 patients compared the effects on mortality of three different thrombolytic agents, namely streptokinase, anistreplase and tPA. As in GISSI-2, no major differences in mortality were noted between the three thrombolytic regimes.
Lancet 1992; **339:** 753–70.

GUSTO

This study compared an accelerated tPA regimen with streptokinase and with the combination of streptokinase and tPA. The 30-day mortality rate was lower in the tPA group than in patients treated either with streptokinase alone or with the combination. The differences between the groups, however, were small (death plus non-fatal stroke 6.9% for accelerated tPA, 7.7% for streptokinase with subcutaneous heparin and 7.9% for streptokinase with intravenous heparin).
New England Journal of Medicine 1993; **329:** 673–82.

Comment

All patients with a hisory suggestive of acute myocardial infarction and ST segment elevation on the ECG should be considered for thrombolytic therapy. Patients with new bundle branch block will also benefit from thrombolysis. The benefit is greatest when the thrombolytic agent is given within a few hours of the onset of pain and is small if the time interval between the onset of pain and drug administration exceeds 12 h. There is some evidence that tPA is superior to streptokinase but the differences are small and many physicians in the UK continue to use streptokinase because of its substantially lower cost.

BETA-BLOCKERS IN MYOCARDIAL INFARCTION

The Norwegian TIMOLOL trial

This randomized multi-centre double-blind placebo-controlled study examined the effect of timolol (10 mg twice daily) on reinfarction and death in 1884 patients after myocardial infarction. Treatment was started at a mean of 11.5 days after myocardial infarction and the average duration of follow-up was 17 months. Treatment with timolol lowered the mortality rate from 16.2% to 10.4% and reduced the risk of reinfarction from 14% to 10%.
New England Journal of Medicine 1985; **313**: 1055–8.

Beta-Blocker Heart Attack trial

This study was similar in design to the Norwegian TIMOLOL trial but used propranolol in a variable dose which was adjusted according to serum levels. Some 3738 patients were followed for a mean period of 25 months. The event rate was lower than in the Norwegian study, probably because the patients tended to be younger. As in the TIMOLOL study, however, propranolol significantly reduced both the overall mortality rate (from 9.8% to 7.2%) and the risk of reinfarction.
Journal of the American Medical Association 1982; **247**: 1701–14.

ISIS-1

Unlike the two beta-blocker studies described above, ISIS-1 examined the effects of beta-blockers given acutely in myocardial infarction. A total of 16 027 patients presenting within 12 h of the onset of symptoms were randomized to receive either a single dose of intravenous atenolol followed by oral atenolol for 1 week or standard medical therapy. The trial was not placebo controlled. The mortality rate at 14 days was reduced by 15% in the atenolol group. Although the trial medication was given for only 7 days, the benefit, in terms of mortality reduction, was still present at 1 year.
Lancet 1988; **8591**: 921–23.

Comment

Although beta-blockers have not been 'retested' in the post-thrombolysis era, most physicians accept that they have been shown to reduce mortality and reinfarction when given both acutely during myocardial infarction and as part of secondary prevention. Despite the fact that ISIS-1 included the use of a single dose of intravenous beta-blocker, this is not common practice in the UK. Most physicians, however, do commence treatment with a beta-blocker soon after admission. The choice of beta-blocker is probably not important but there is some evidence that those with intrinsic sympathomimetic activity, which do not slow the resting heart rate, are less effective agents for secondary prevention than beta-blockers without this property.

ANGIOTENSIN-CONVERTING ENZYME (ACE) INHIBITORS FOLLOWING MYOCARDIAL INFARCTION

These studies can be broadly divided into so-called 'non-selective' studies in which all patients with myocardial infarction were randomized to receive either an ACE inhibitor or placebo and 'selective' studies in which only certain subgroups of patients with infarction were selected for randomization, usually in the belief that they were at greater than average risk.

GISSI-3

Just over 20 000 patients with myocardial infarction were randomized to receive either lisinopril or placebo. In those treated with lisinopril, the mortality rate at 6 weeks was reduced by 6%.
Lancet 1994; **343:** 1115–22.

ISIS-4

In this non-selective study of 58 000 patients with myocardial infarction, captopril reduced the 5-week mortality rate from 7.69% to 7.19%.
Lancet 1995; **345:** 669–85.

AIRE

In the AIRE study, only patients with myocardial infarction and clinical evidence of left ventricular failure were randomized to receive either an ACE inhibitor (ramipril) or placebo. The reduction in the mortality rate in the active (treatment) group was greater (approximately 20%) in this study than in any of the other ACE inhibitor studies, probably because the study design selected out those patients at greatest risk of subsequent death.
Lancet 1993; **342:** 821–8.

SAVE

In this study, patients with myocardial infarction were selected for inclusion if they had impaired left ventricular function by radionuclide ventriculography, defined as a left ventricular ejection fraction of less than 40%. Some 1556 patients were randomized; at 42 months, the group treated with the ACE inhibitor (captopril) showed a 14% reduction in mortality rate.

New England Journal of Medicine 1992; **327:** 669–77.

Comment

Should ACE inhibitors be given to all patients following myocardial infarction? Although the two large studies looking at all patients with myocardial infarction were positive (ISIS-4 and GISSI-3), the overall benefit was small and most cardiologists in the UK appear to favour selective use of ACE inhibitors after myocardial infarction. Patients who should be treated with ACE inhibitors include those with clinical radiological evidence of left ventricular failure during their hospital stay and also those with impaired left ventricular function on echocardiography.

ACE INHIBITORS IN CARDIAC FAILURE

CONSENSUS study

This was the first randomized mortality study of ACE inhibitors in patients with congestive cardiac failure. A total of 253 patients with severe cardiac failure (grade IV) were randomized to receive either enalapril or placebo in addition to conventional therapy. After just 6 months of treatment, the total mortality rate was reduced from 52% to 36%. This is equivalent to a relative risk reduction of 40%. The benefit appeared to be due to prevention of the progression of heart failure rather than to the prevention of sudden cardiac death.

New England Journal of Medicine 1987; **316:** 1429–35.

V-HeFT-II

In this study, the addition of enalapril was compared with that of both hydralazine and a nitrate in patients with established heart failure. Some 804 patients were followed for a period of 2.5 years. The relative risk reduction in mortality for enalapril compared with conventional vasodilator therapy at 2 years was 28%.

New England Journal of Medicine 1991; **325:** 303–10.

SOLVD

This study comprised two 'arms', a SOLVD treatment arm which consisted of patients with evidence of heart failure requiring treat-

ment and a SOLVD prevention arm in which patients had no clinical evidence of heart failure and were not already receiving treatment. All patients, however, had impaired left ventricular function as defined by an ejection fraction of less than 35% on echocardiography. As in the other studies, treatment with enalapril in the SOLVD treatment arm significantly reduced the mortality rate over a period of 5 years. In patients without overt congestive cardiac failure at randomization (the SOLVD prevention group), enalapril treatment produced a small but insignificant reduction in mortality but did reduce the number of patients developing clinical heart failure and the number of hospitalizations for treatment of cardiac failure.
New England Journal of Medicine 1981; **325**: 293–302 and 1992; **327**: 685–91.

Comment

The loop diuretics (frusemide, bumetanide) remain the first choice of therapy in patients with congestive cardiac failure and provide better symptom relief than the ACE inhibitors used alone. However, the ACE inhibitors have now been shown to improve the prognosis in patients with moderate and severe heart failure, and to retard the development of overt heart failure in those with asymptomatic left ventricular dysfunction. It seems reasonable, therefore, that all patients who require a loop diuretic should also be considered for concomitant ACE inhibitor therapy.

CHOLESTEROL LOWERING AND CORONARY EVENTS

Scandinavian Simvastatin Survival Study (the 4S study)

This was the definitive secondary prevention trial of cholesterol-lowering medication. A total of 4444 patients with definite coronary artery disease and a cholesterol level in the range of 5.5–8.0 mmol/l were randomized to receive either simvastatin or placebo. The median follow-up period was 5.4 years. The results were striking: simvastatin reduced the mortality rate from coronary disease by 42%. There was no increase in non-cardiovascular deaths (such as cancer or suicide) and the reduction in the rate of all-cause mortality (i.e. all deaths) was 30%. In addition to reducing mortality, treatment also appeared to reduce coronary morbidity, with a significant reduction in the treatment group of patients requiring coronary angioplasty or coronary artery bypass surgery.
New England Journal of Medicine 1994; **331**: 1383–9.

WOSCOPS (West of Scotland Coronary Prevention Study)

Just as the 4S study is regarded as the definitive secondary prevention trial, so WOSCOPS is regarded as the definitive primary prevention trial of cholesterol lowering. This study followed a number of large, but inconclusive, studies that had taken place in the 1960s and 1970s. The main difference between WOSCOPS and older primary prevention trials was that, like the 4S study, the agent being tested was an HMG CoA reductase inhibitor (in this case pravastatin) which effectively and safely lowered plasma cholesterol levels. A fixed dose of 40 mg daily was used in a placebo-controlled study of 6595 men with moderately raised cholesterol levels. After a follow-up period of just under 5 years, the reduction in the combined rate of death and non-fatal myocardial infarction was 30%. As in the 4S study, there was no evidence of increased mortality from other causes. The reduction in the all-cause mortality rate in this study was very close to statistical significance (3.2% for pravastatin, 4.1% for placebo).
New England Journal of Medicine 1995; **333:** 1301–7.

CARE study

In this secondary prevention study, 4159 patients with proven myocardial infarction and with 'normal' cholesterol levels were randomized to receive either pravastatin or placebo and followed for a period of 5 years. The combined rate of fatal and non-fatal myocardial infarction was reduced by 24% (13.2% in the placebo group, 10.2% in the pravastatin group). As in the 4S study, there was also a reduction in the requirement for coronary angioplasty and coronary artery bypass surgery in the treatment group.
New England Journal of Medicine 1996; **335:** 1001–9.

Comment

The appearance of the 'statin' drugs has revolutionized the treatment of hypercholesterolaemia. These drugs reliably and safely lower plasma cholesterol levels and have been shown in angiographic studies to slow the progression of coronary atheroma. They may also stabilize atheromatous plaques to reduce the chance of plaque rupture with subsequent myocardial infarction.

Who, then, should be given these drugs? The evidence is strongest for those with proven coronary artery disease. Thus most patients with angina, or with a history of myocardial infarction, coronary angioplasty or coronary bypass grafting, and a cholesterol level above 5.5 mmol/l, should be considered for treatment, which is likely to be lifelong. At the other end of the spectrum, asymptomatic individuals with a moderate increase of the plasma cholesterol level but no other risk factors should probably not be treated because their absolute risk of a major coronary event is low. In between, there are many patients with moderate hypercholesterolaemia who do not yet have manifest coronary artery disease but who do have other risk factors such as hypertension, diabetes or a strongly positive family history. It seems likely that many of these patients would benefit from cholesterol-lowering therapy, and studies to address this issue are presently being conducted.

ASPIRIN IN THE PREVENTION OF MYOCARDIAL INFARCTION

The American Physicians Health Study

In this placebo-controlled double-blind primary prevention study, 220 171 male doctors were randomized to receive either 325 mg of aspirin daily or matching placebo. Follow-up for an average of 5 years demonstrated a low event rate (suggesting that American doctors are relatively healthy) but did show a 44% reduction in the risk of myocardial infarction among those taking aspirin. This benefit was seen only in those aged 50 years and over.
New England Journal of Medicine 1989; **321:** 129–35.

The Antiplatelet Triallists Collaboration

This is not a single study but a meta-analysis of almost 300 randomized controlled trials of over 100 000 patients. While antiplatelet therapy (most commonly aspirin) was effective in both primary and secondary prevention of cardiovascular events, the benefit was greatest when the event rate was highest. In patients with acute myocardial infarction, the risk of a further major event within the next month was reduced from 14.4% to 10.6%; post-myocardial infarction, chronic treatment reduced the risk of a further event from 17.1% to 13.5%. In primary prevention, where the absolute number of events is much lower, the benefit was smaller and was not statistically significant (4.9% with placebo, 4.5% with aspirin over a period of 62 months).
British Medical Journal 1994; **308:** 81–106.

Comment

Aspirin is cheap, widely available, and relatively free from side-effects. Its efficacy in secondary prevention has been established beyond any reasonable doubt and all patients with a history of angina, myocardial infarction, coronary angioplasty or coronary artery bypass grafting should take aspirin for life. Different trials have used different dosages, ranging from 75 to 1200 mg per day. Most physicians prescribe either 75 or 150 mg daily; there appears to be no additional benefit in exceeding 150 mg once daily.

Aspirin's role in primary prevention is less clearly defined. It seems logical, however, that patients with multiple risk factors for coronary artery disease should be considered for long-term aspirin therapy, particularly if their other risk factors (such as hypertension, diabetes and hypercholesterolaemia) are being treated actively.

ANTICOAGULANTS FOR ATRIAL FIBRILLATION

The Copenhagen AFASAK study

Just over 1000 patients with chronic non-rheumatic atrial fibrillation were randomized to receive warfarin, aspirin or placebo. The follow-up period was 2 years. Thrombo-embolic events were significantly reduced by warfarin but not by aspirin. Bleeding complications were more common in the warfarin group but none of these was fatal.
Lancet 1989; **i:** 175–9.

The Boston Area Anticoagulation Trial for Atrial Fibrillation

Warfarin was compared with placebo in this study of 420 patients with non-rheumatic atrial fibrillation. This differed from other studies in that low-dose warfarin was used, the target prothrombin time ratio being just 1.2–1.5. Although the numbers were small, the effects were striking: there were just two strokes in the warfarin group compared with 13 in the control group. Furthermore, all-cause mortality was also significantly reduced in the warfarin group. With the low doses of warfarin used, bleeding complications appeared to be no more common than in the control group.
New England Journal of Medicine 1990; **323:** 1505–11.

Comment

Atrial fibrillation is common and its frequency in the population rises with age. Until recently, it was considered that elderly people should not be commenced on long-term anticoagulation because the risks of bleeding were high. However, recent studies have shown that it is the elderly who are at highest risk of stroke and who stand to gain most from anticoagulation, provided this can be monitored safely.

Index

Abdominal palpation 49
Acromegaly 363
Actin filaments 1, 2
Action potential 3, 9–13
Adams-Stokes attack 39, 204, 205–6
Adenosine 185, 220, 399, 400, 401
Adrenaline 396
Advanced life support 394–7
Afterload 4
AIDS 224, 226, 235, 358
AIRE 411
Alcohol consumption 104, 323, 333
Alcoholic cardiomyopathy 238, 366
Aldosteronism, primary 326–7
Alpha-blockers 335, 336
Ambulatory blood pressure
    monitoring 331
Ambulatory ECG monitoring 76–7,
    78, 208
Amiloride 165
Amiodarone 140, 219, 222, 242, 396,
    400
Amlodipine 113
Anacrotic pulse 42
Anaemia 56, 59, 154, 371
Anaesthesia 379
Anaphylactic shock 171
Angina pectoris 35–6, 95–6, 106–13,
    276
    coronary artery bypass surgery
        117–20, 122
    drug treatment 111–13, 120–1
    percutaneous transluminal
        coronary angioplasty (PTCA)
        113–16, 121, 122
    risk factor modification 110–11,
        121
    unstable 120–1
Angiotensin receptor antagonists 335

Angiotensin-converting enzyme
    (ACE) inhibitors
    dilated cardiomyopathy 237
    heart failure 166–7, 412–13
    hypertension 334–5, 336
    myocardial infarction 137, 146,
        150, 411–12
Anistreplase 136
Ankylosing spondylitis 366
Antiarrhythmic drugs 217–22, 237–8
Antibiotics 293, 294, 295
Anticoagulant therapy 137, 194, 238,
    265, 294, 403, 416
Anti-hypertensive drugs 334–7
Anti-tachycardia pacing 214, 399,
    400
Anxiety states 377–8
Aortic aneurysm
    dissecting 94, 338–40, 341
    saccular/fusiform 342–3
Aortic intramural haematoma 340–1
Aortic penetrating atherosclerotic
    ulcer 341–2
Aortic regurgitation 42, 58, 281–5
    with aortic stenosis 285
    with mitral stenosis 261–2
Aortic stenosis 85, 274–81, 299
    physical signs 42, 49, 51, 52, 53,
        55, 56, 57, 277
    with aortic regurgitation 285
Aortic trauma 342
Aortic valve calcification 274
Apex beat 47–8
Arrhythmias 177–222
    carotid sinus massage 194–5
    heart failure 159
    investigations 90, 91, 208
    management 208–22
        pacing 208–13

Arrhythmias (*contd*)
  mechanisms 177–9
  post-myocardial infarction 124,
    134, 138–41, 147–8, 149
  postoperative 385
  sinus node abnormalities 179–82
  supraventricular 182–94
  surgical risk 380–1
  ventricular 195–200
Arrhythmogenic right ventricular
  dysplasia 243–4
Arteriovenous fistulae 94
Ascites 37, 162
Aspartate transaminase 129
Aspirin 111, 121, 134–5, 151, 391,
  415–16
Asysole 394, 396
Atheromatous plaque 95, 96, 98
  rupture 96, 123
Atherosclerosis 94, 95–9, 175, 342
Athletes 370
Atrial ectopic beats 182–3
Atrial fibrillation 42, 191–4
  anticoagulant therapy 194, 416
  carotid sinus massage 194
  management 213, 399–400
  mitral stenosis 256
  post-myocardial infarction 139–40
  Wolff-Parkinson-White syndrome
    401
Atrial flutter 185, 186, 189–91
  carotid sinus massage 194–5
  management 400
  post-myocardial infarction 139–40
Atrial natriuretic peptide 157
Atrial septal defect 51, 56, 68, 83,
  299, 300–3
Atrioventricular (heart) block 140,
  202–4, 212–13
  complete heart block 46, 51, 140,
    205–6
  first degree 203
  second degree Mobitz type 1
    (Wenckebach block) 203, 204
  second degree Mobitz type 2 203,
    204
Atrioventricular node 11, 13
Atrioventricular re-entry tachycardia
  185, 186
Atropinine 396
Auscultation 49–50
Austin Flint murmur 58

Automatic implantable cardioverter
  defibrillator 197, 214, 217

Balloon valvuloplasty 265–6
Basic life-support 392, 394
Beriberi 365
Beta-adrenoceptor blocking drugs
  angina pectoris 112, 121
  heart failure 168
  hypertension 334, 336
  myocardial infarction 137, 149–50,
    151–2, 410–11
Bicuspid aortic valve 274
Bile acid sequestrants 102
Bjork-Shiley prosthetic valve 387
Blood pressure 321–2
  measurement 43–4
Bretylium 220, 396
Broad complex tachycardias 399
Bumetanide 165
Bundle branch block 21, 22, 25–9,
  30, 141, 206–8
Bundle branches 11, 13
Bundle of His 11, 13

Calcium antagonists 112–13, 121,
  237, 335
Cannon waves 46–7
Carbon dioxide retention 33, 353,
  354
Carcinoid syndrome 363–4
Cardiac arrest 200, 392–7
Cardiac catheterization 82–5
  aortic regurgitation 283
  aortic stenosis 85, 279–80
  mitral regurgitation 270–1
  mitral stenosis 261
Cardiac catheters 87
Cardiac cycle 6–8, 45
Cardiac enzymes 129–31
Cardiac output 1
  heart failure 156
  measurement 84
Cardiac pain 34–6
Cardiac surgery 382–5
Cardiac transplantation 173–5
Cardiac tumours 368
Cardiogenic shock 124, 141–3, 171
Cardiomyopathy 233, 235–6
  alcoholic 238

Cardiomyopathy (*contd*)
arrhythmogenic right ventricular
dysplasia 243–4
dilated 236–8
hypertrophic 238–42
pregnancy 374
restrictive/infiltrative 242–3
Cardiopulmonary bypass 383–4
CARE 414
Carey Coombs murmur 58, 246
Carotid sinus hypersensitivity 195,
213
Carotid sinus massage 194–5, 401
Carotid sinus syncope 39
Carpentier-Edwards prosthetic valve
387, 388
Chagas' disease (trypanosomiasis)
234, 358–9
Chest compression 393, 394
Chest inspection 47
Chest palpation 47–9
Chest x-ray 61–8
Cheyne-Stokes respiration 34
Cholesterol lowering drugs 102,
413–15
Cholestyramine 102
Chordae tendinae rupture 268
Chorea (St Vitus' dance) 247
Clinical trials 407–16
Clubbing 60, 292
Coarctation of aorta 43, 299, 307–10,
328
Collapsing (waterhammer) pulse 42,
282
Colour flow mapping 74
Complete heart block 46, 51, 140,
205–6
Conduction disorders 202–8
Congenital heart disease 297–319
abnormal left-right
communications 299, 300–7
combined obstructive and shunt
lesions 312–16
displacement lesions 300, 316–19
embryology 297–9
management in newborn 318–19
obstructive lesions 299–300,
307–12
pregnancy 373
CONSENSUS 412
Continuous-wave Doppler 73–4
Contraception 328, 345, 374

Cor pulmonale (pulmonary heart
disease) 353–5
Coronary angiography 85–7, 89
Coronary artery bypass surgery
117–20, 121, 122
Coronary artery disease 93–105
atherosclerosis 95–7
dietary fat intake 102–3
familial factors 103
post-myocardial infarction risk
stratification 148–9
preventive public health measures
104–5
psychological factors 376–7
risk factors 99–104
surgical risk 379–80
Coronary artery spasm 94
Coronary artery stents 114–16, 117,
118
Coronary circulation 92–3
Corticosteroids 174, 249
Creatine phosphokinase 129
Cushing's syndrome 326
Cyanosis 37–8, 60, 319
Cyclosporin 174, 175

D.C. cardioversion 193, 213, 396, 401
Defibrillation 396
Dextrocardia 318
Diabetes mellitus 99, 101, 104, 363
Diamorphine 391, 402
Diet 102–3, 323
Digoxin 24, 140, 168–70, 220, 221,
400
Dilated cardiomyopathy 236–8
Diltiazem 112
Diphtheria 357
Directional atherectomy 116
Diuretics 164–6, 237
Dobutamine 172, 173
Dopamine 172, 173
Doppler echocardiography 72–4
Dyspnoea 32–4

Ebstein's anomaly 317–18
Echocardiography 69–75
aortic regurgitation 283, 284
aortic stenosis 278, 279
colour flow mapping 74
Doppler examination 72–4

Echocardiography (*contd*)
  hypertension 331–2
  hypertrophic cardiomyopathy 240
  infective endocarditis 292
  M-mode 69–70
  mitral regurgitation 270, 271, 272
  mitral stenosis 259–61, 262, 263
  pericardial effusion 227, 228
  pericardial tamponade 229
  transoesophageal 74–5
  two-dimensional 70–2
Eisenmenger syndrome 314–16, 351,
    352
Ejection click 53
Electro-mechanical dissociation 394,
    396–7
Electrocardiogram 9, 11–30
  acute pericarditis 225
  angina pectoris 107–8
  aortic regurgitation 283
  aortic stenosis 277
  athletes 370
  atrial ectopic beats 182–3
  atrial fibrillation 191, 192–3
  atrial flutter 185, 186, 190
  atrial septal defect 30, 302, 303
  atrioventricular (heart) block 203,
    204, 205
  bundle branch block 21, 22, 25–9,
    30, 207
  cardiac pacing 208–9
  digitalis therapy 24
  genesis 11–14
  hypertension 330, 331
  interpretation 30
  junctional (nodal) rhythm 183
  leads/electrodes 14–17
  left heart failure 160
  mean frontal QRS axis 29–30
  mitral regurgitation 270
  mitral stenosis 258
  myocardial infarction 19, 22, 23,
    125–8, 129, 130, 131
  myocardial ischaemia 24
  myxoedema 22
  normal 14, 17–24
  paroxysmal supraventricular
    tachycardia 184
  pericarditis 23
  pulmonary embolism 347–8
  pulmonary hypertension 352
  sick sinus syndrome 181

sinu-atrial block 202
  sinus tachycardia 24, 179, 180
  torsades de pointes 198–9
  tricuspid stenosis 287
  ventricular ectopic beats 21,
    195–6
  ventricular fibrillation 199
  ventricular hypertrophy 21, 22,
    24–5
  ventricular tachycardia 22, 196,
    200, 201
    benign 198
  Wolff-Parkinson-White syndrome
    19, 187, 188
Electrophysiological studies 87,
    90–1, 208
Embryology of heart 297–9
Endocarditis
  infective *see* Infective endocarditis
  prosthetic heart valves 389
  rheumatic 246
Endocrine disease 326–8, 360–4
Endothelium 97–8
Erythema marginatum 247
Essential hypertension 323–4
Excitation-contraction coupling 3
Exercise 104, 333, 370
  angina pectoris provocation 107
  cardiovascular changes 5–6
Exercise testing 75–7, 149

Faint, simple (vasomotor syncope)
    39
Fat intake 102–3, 323
Fibrates 102
Fibrinogen 104
Flecainide 219, 222, 400
Foam cells 95, 98
Frusemide 165, 402
Functional capacity 40
Fundoscopy 330

Gallop rhythm 53
General examination 60
GISSI trials 408, 409, 411
Glyceryl trinitrate 111–12
Glycogen storage disease 364
Gout 364
Graham Steel murmur 58, 289, 351
GUSTO 409

Haemochromatosis 364
Haemoptysis 38
Heart failure 52, 53, 153–75
  arrhythmias 159
  causes 154
  clinical syndromes 159–62
  in newborn 319
  management 162–70, 412–13
  neuroendocrine response 156–7
  pathophysiology 154–9
  pulmonary heart disease (cor
    pulmonale) 353–4
  surgical risk 380
Heart rate 42
Heart sounds 50–3, 54
Heart valve replacement 386–7
Heart-lung transplantation 175
Heparin 348
Hepato-jugular reflux 46
Hepatomegaly 162, 354
High-density lipoprotein 101
HIV myocarditis 235
HMG CoA reductase inhibitors
    (statins) 102, 111, 150–1
Hydralazine 166, 167
Hyperkalaemia 22
Hyperlipidaemia 98, 99–102
  treatment 102, 110–11, 413–15
Hypertension 51, 321–37
  drug treatment 334–7
  endocrine disease 326–8
  ischaemic heart disease association
    99, 103
  postoperative 385
  psychological factors 376–7
  renal disease 324–6
  surgical risk 380
Hypertensive crisis 406
Hyperthyroidism (thyrotoxicosis)
    360–2
Hypertrophic cardiomyopathy 48,
    238–42
Hyperventilation 32
Hypokalaemia 22, 24
Hypoplastic left heart syndrome 310
Hypothermia 24
Hypothyroidism 22, 362–3
Hypovolaemic shock 171

Immunosuppressive treatment 174
Infective endocarditis 256, 268,
    289–95

antibiotic prophylaxis 294–5
antibiotic treatment 293–4
anticoagulant therapy 294
infective agents 289, 290
native valve 289
patients at risk 295
pregnancy 373
prosthetic valve 290
surgery 294
Inotropic agents 172–3
Insulin resistance 99, 104
Intra-aortic balloon pump 143, 173,
    386
Intravenous drug abuse 289–90
Investigations
  invasive 82–91
  non-invasive 61–81
Ischaemic heart disease *see* Coronary
    artery disease
ISIS trials 409, 410, 411
Isosorbide mononitrate 112

Jugular venous pressure 45, 161–2
Jugular venous pulse 44–5
Junctional (nodal) ectopic beats 183
Junctional (nodal) rhythm 183

Korotkoff sounds 44

Lactate dehydrogenase 129–30
Laser angioplasty 116
Left bundle branch block 25–6, 27,
    51, 206–8
Left heart failure 124, 141, 159–61
  pulmonary congestion 158–9, 160
Left ventricular function 85
Lignocaine 218–19, 396
Lipids 98, 330–1
Long QT interval 22
Loop diuretics 165
Low-density lipoprotein 98, 101

Macrophages 98, 99
Magnetic resonance imaging 81
Marfan syndrome 342, 343, 367–8
Mean frontal QRS axis 29–30
Mental stress 104
Micturition syncope 39

Mitral regurgitation 49, 52, 56, 57,
   253, 267–73
  echocardiography 270, 271, 272
  electrocardiogram 270
  medical treatment 273
  surgery 273
Mitral stenosis 254–67
  with aortic regurgitation 261–2
  balloon valvuloplasty 265–6
  cardiac catheterization 85, 261
  echocardiography 259–61, 262,
   263
  electrocardiogram 258
  medical treatment 265
  physical signs 42, 48, 49, 51, 53,
   58, 59, 257–8
  radiological appearances 258
  surgery 265–6
  with tricuspid regurgitation 263,
   287–8
Mitral valve 6, 7, 252–3
Mitral valve prolapse 267, 270, 271,
  272
Mitral valvotomy 389
Mouth to mouth ventilation 393
Murmurs 53, 55–9
  continuous 59
  diastolic 57–8
  presystolic 58–9
  systolic 55–7
Mycotic aneurysm 292
Myocardial contractility 4–5
Myocardial infarction 94, 123–52
  anticoagulant therapy 137
  clinical features 34–6, 123–4
  complications 124, 138–48
  diagnosis 132–3
  drug treatment 134–8, 149–50,
   410–12, 415–16
  electrocardiogram 19, 22, 23,
   125–8, 129, 130, 131
  infarct expansion 97, 144, 146
  management 133–8, 391–2
  pain relief 133, 391
  pathology 96–7
  physical signs 42, 124–5
  prognosis 138
  rehabilitation 151–2
  risk stratification at discharge
   148–9
  secondary prevention 151–2
  serum enzymes 129–31

thrombolysis 135–6, 391–2,
   408–10
  ventricular remodelling 146, 155
Myocardial ischaemia 24, 34–6
Myocardial perfusion studies 79–80
Myocarditis 233–5, 246, 357, 358
Myosin filaments 1
Myxoma 368, 369

New York Heart Association
   classification 40
Nicardipine 113
Nicotinic acid 102
Nifedipine 113, 406
Nitrates 111–12, 121, 166, 167, 402

Obesity 103, 323, 364–5
Oedema 36–7, 162
Opening snap 53, 54
Oral contraceptive pill 328, 345
Orthopnoea 33
Osler's nodes 60, 291

P wave 14, 18
  abnormalities 18–19
Pacemaker codes 211–12
Pacemaker, physiological 11
Pacing 208–13
  anti-tachycardia 214, 399, 400
  dual-chamber 210–11
  modes 211–12
  permanent 209–11
  rate-responsive 211
  temporary 209, 405–6
Pain relief 133, 391
Palpitation 36
Pancreatitis, acute 171
Papillary muscle rupture 144
Paroxysmal dyspnoea 33–4, 160, 161
Paroxysmal supraventricular
   tachycardia 184–7, 194, 401
Pectus excavatum (funnel chest) 47
Percussion 49
Percutaneous transluminal coronary
   angioplasty (PTCA) 113–16,
   121, 122
  coronary artery stents 114–16, 117,
   118
  directional atherectomy 116

Percutaneous transluminal coronary angioplasty (PTCA) (*contd*)
laser angioplasty 116
restenosis 113
rotational atherectomy 116
Pericardial aspiration 404
Pericardial effusion 64, 227, 228
Pericardial friction (rub) 59, 224–5
Pericarditis 23, 36, 145, 358
acute 223–7
constrictive 43, 51, 52, 230–2
rheumatic 247
Pericardium 223
Persistent ductus arteriosus 42, 49, 58, 59, 68, 83, 299, 306–7
Phaeochromocytoma 327–8
Pickwickian syndrome 365
Plain radiography 61–8
Platelets 98
Polyarteritis 367
Polycythaemia 354
Postural syncope 39–40
Potassium-sparing diuretics 165–6
PR interval 14, 19
Pregnancy 56, 59, 372–4
mitral stenosis 265, 267
termination 374
Preload 4
Prinzmetal's angina (vasospastic angina) 95
Propafenone 219
Prosthetic heart valves 387–8
complications 388–9
pregnancy 373
Prosthetic valve endocarditis 290, 389
Pseudoxanthoma elasticum 367
Psychological factors 376–8
Pulmonary artery wedge pressure 82
Pulmonary circulation abnormalities 66–8
Pulmonary embolectomy 349, 403
Pulmonary embolism 145, 256, 345–9
electrocardiogram 347–8
management 348–9, 402–3
prevention 345–6
recurrent 349
Pulmonary heart disease (cor pulmonale) 353–5
Pulmonary hypertension 48, 53, 67–8, 349–52

primary ('unexplained') 352
Pulmonary oedema 34, 402
left heart failure 158–9, 160, 161
Pulmonary regurgitation 288–9
Pulmonary stenosis 84, 288, 299, 310–11
physical signs 48, 49, 51, 52, 53, 55–6, 57
Pulse
arterial 41–3
venous 44–7
Pulsed Doppler echocardiography 72–3
Pulsus alternans 43, 160
Pulsus bigeminus 42
Pulsus bisferiens 42
Pulsus paradoxus 43
Purkinje system 11, 13

Q wave abnormalities 21
QRS complex 14, 20–1
QT interval 22

Radiofrequency ablation 91, 188–9, 214–17
Radionuclide imaging 79
myocardial perfusion studies 79–80
ventriculography 80–1
Re-entry arrhythmias 177–9
Regional anaesthesia 379
Reiter's disease 366
Renal artery stenosis 324
Renal blood flow 157
Renal disease 324–6
Renin-angiotensin-aldosterone system 156, 325
Restenosis 113
Restrictive cardiomyopathy 242–3
Rheumatic fever, acute 245–50
Rheumatic valve disease 58, 250–1, 254, 267, 274, 281, 286, 287
infective endocarditis 289, 290
pregnancy 372–3
Rheumatoid arthritis 366
Right bundle branch block 51, 206, 207
electrocardiogram 26, 28, 29
Right heart failure 143, 161–2
Right-sided aorta 318

Rotational atherectomy 116

St Jude prosthetic valve 387
Salicylates 249, 250
Salt retention 157–8, 164–6
Sarcoidosis 367
Sarcomere 1–3
SAVE 411–12
Scandinavian Simvastatin Survival
    Study 413
Scleroderma 367
Septicaemic shock 171
Serum glutamic-oxalo-acetic
    transaminase (aspartate
    transaminase) 129
Shock (acute circulatory failure) 42,
    170–3
Sick sinus syndrome 181
Silent ischaemia 94
Sinu-atrial block 202
Sinus arrest 202
Sinus arrhythmia 181–2, 212
Sinus bradycardia 180–1
Sinus node 11, 13
Sinus tachycardia 24, 179–80, 194
Sinus of Valsalva aneurysm 343–4
Smoking 99, 103, 110
Sodium bicarbonate 396
SOLVD 412–13
Sotalol 220
Spironolactone 165
Splenomegaly 60, 292
Splinter haemorrhage 60, 291
ST segment 22–4
    abnormalities 23
Starling's law 3
Starr-Edwards prosthetic valve 387
Statins 102, 111, 150–1
Streptokinase 136, 349, 391
Sudden death 22, 96, 110, 134, 148,
    187, 199, 240, 242, 277, 280
Supraventricular tachycardia 182–94
    ventricular tachycardia
        differentiation 200–2
Surgery 379–90
Surgical risk 379–81
    estimation 381, 382
Swan-Ganz catheterization 82, 84,
    142
Sympathetic nervous system 156
Syncope 38–40

Syphilis 94, 274, 281, 342, 343,
    359–60
Systemic embolism 145, 256, 292
Systemic lupus erythematosus 366
Systemic manifestations 60
Systolic venous pulsation 47

T wave 14, 21–2
    abnormalities 22, 23
Tachyarrhythmias 396, 397
Tamponade 43, 229, 403–4
Tendon xanthomata 60
Tetralogy of Fallot 300, 312–14
Thallium scan 79–80, 380
Thiazide diuretics 165, 334, 336
Thrills 48–9
Thrombolytic agents 136
Thrombolytic therapy 136
    myocardial infarction 135–6,
        391–2, 408–10
    pulmonary embolism 349, 403
Thyrotoxicosis (hyperthyroidism) 56,
    154, 192, 360–2
Tissue plasminogen activator 136
Torsades de pointes 22, 198–9, 399
Toxoplasmosis 359
Transoesophageal echocardiography
    74
Transposition of great arteries
    316–17
Trauma 368, 370
Triamterene 165
Tricuspid atresia 312
Tricuspid regurgitation 47, 56, 162,
    287–8
    with mitral disease 263, 287–8
Tricuspid stenosis 58, 59, 84, 286–7
Tricuspid valve 7, 286
Troponin subunit markers 130
Trypanosomiasis (Chagas' disease)
    358–9
Tuberculous pericarditis 225, 358

U wave 24
Unipolar leads 15–17
Unstable angina 120–1

v-HeFT-II 412
Valve calcification 65–6

Valve repair 389–90
Vasodilator therapy 166–8, 335–6
Vasospastic angina (Prinzmetal's angina) 95
Venous hum 59
Venous pressure 46
Ventricular aneurysm 146–7
Ventricular arrhythmias 195–200
Ventricular ectopic beats 21, 139, 195–6
Ventricular fibrillation 139, 199–200, 394, 396
Ventricular septal defect 49, 56, 58, 68, 83, 143–4, 299, 304–5
Ventricular tachycardia 22, 46, 139, 196–7, 200, 201

benign 197–8
management 213, 397
supraventricular tachycardia differentiation 200–2
Ventriculography 80–1, 85
Verapamil 112, 220, 221
Viral myocarditis/pericarditis 224, 225, 234, 235, 358

Wolff-Parkinson-White syndrome 19, 87, 90, 187–9, 208, 222, 401
WOSCOPS 414

Xanthelasma 60

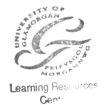